Studies in Computational Intelligence

Volume 1133

The series “Studies in Computational Intelligence” (SCI) publishes new developments and advances in the various areas of computational intelligence—quickly and with a high quality. The intent is to cover the theory, applications, and design methods of computational intelligence, as embedded in the fields of engineering, computer science, physics and life sciences, as well as the methodologies behind them. The series contains monographs, lecture notes and edited volumes in computational intelligence spanning the areas of neural networks, connectionist systems, genetic algorithms, evolutionary computation, artificial intelligence, cellular automata, self-organizing systems, soft computing, fuzzy systems, and hybrid intelligent systems. Of particular value to both the contributors and the readership are the short publication timeframe and the world-wide distribution, which enable both wide and rapid dissemination of research output.

Indexed by SCOPUS, DBLP, WTI Frankfurt eG, zbMATH, SCImago.

All books published in the series are submitted for consideration in Web of Science.

Khalid Raza · Surender Singh
Editors

Artificial Intelligence and Autoimmune Diseases

Applications in the Diagnosis, Prognosis, and Therapeutics

Springer

Editors
Khalid Raza
Department of Computer Science
Jamia Millia Islamia
New Delhi, Delhi, India

Surender Singh
Department of Pharmacology
All India Institute of Medical Sciences
New Delhi, Delhi, India

ISSN 1860-949X ISSN 1860-9503 (electronic)
Studies in Computational Intelligence
ISBN 978-981-99-9028-3 ISBN 978-981-99-9029-0 (eBook)
https://doi.org/10.1007/978-981-99-9029-0

This Springer imprint is published by the registered company Springer Nature Singapore Pte Ltd.
The registered company address is: 152 Beach Road, #21-01/04 Gateway East, Singapore 189721, Singapore

Paper in this product is recyclable.

To our family,

For their unwavering love, encouragement, and understanding during the countless hours we spent researching, writing, and pondering the complexities of both artificial intelligence and autoimmune diseases.

To mentors and colleagues,

Thank you for your guidance, expertise, and relentless pursuit of knowledge. Your insights and collaborations have enriched the content of this book and inspired to push the boundaries of our understanding.

To the patients,

Whose courage in the face of autoimmune diseases serves as a constant reminder of the real-world impact of our work. Your stories drive our passion for finding innovative solutions.

To the AI community,

For pioneering technologies that hold the promise of transforming the diagnosis and treatment of autoimmune diseases.

This book is dedicated to all those who believe in the power of knowledge, innovation, and compassion to improve the lives of those affected by autoimmune diseases. May our collective efforts bring us closer to a future of better understanding and more effective treatments.

With heartfelt gratitude,

Khalid Raza and Surender Singh

Preface

Autoimmune diseases represent a complex condition for a variety of painful syndromes. Autoimmunity is defined as the development of the immune system's response against an unknown trigger, in the form of auto-antibodies and T-cell responses toward self-structures, and the immune system may begin to attack the body's own tissues instead of fighting infections. In autoimmune diseases, the inflammation becomes chronic, causing pain and severe damage to the tissues. Nearly 4% of the worldwide population is affected by more than 80 different types of autoimmune diseases. Some common autoimmune disorders are *Multiple Sclerosis, Rheumatoid Arthritis, Sjögren Syndrome, Myasthenia Gravis, Pernicious Anemia, Reactive Arthritis, Systemic Lupus Erythematosus, Type I Diabetes, Autoimmune Hepatitis, Insulin-dependent Diabetes Mellitus, Thyroiditis, Crohn's Disease, Psoriasis, Scleroderma,* and *Graves Disease.* These diseases are difficult to diagnose because the specific disorders have numerous possible symptoms and individual symptoms vary. Treatment for autoimmune diseases generally focuses on reducing the immune system's activity.

Artificial Intelligence (AI) and machine learning are handy tools today for improved and early diagnosis of diseases, understanding their progression, and better disease treatment planning and drug discovery. These technologies can target autoimmunity and digital health technologies to improve patient diagnosis, prognosis, and treatment. However, AI efficacy, cost, and scalability evaluations are needed. Data scientists use healthcare analytics to help doctors make accurate diagnoses and choose the best treatments. Predictive and prescriptive analytics can forecast and monitor illness, and AI and machine learning pipelines can examine and learn from various data sources.

The purpose of this book is to provide an overview of various autoimmune disorders and how AI and machine learning might be utilized for the diagnosis, prognosis, and treatment of these disorders. AI algorithms are used to create synthetic patient populations with the properties of actual patient cohorts, build personalized predictive models of drug combinations, and unravel complex relationships between diet, microbiome, and genetic line-up to determine the comparative treatment response.

The main aim of this book is to encapsulate and occupy recent advances and state-of-the-art applications of AI and machine learning techniques in the diagnosis, prognosis, and therapeutics of various autoimmune diseases, including Rheumatoid Arthritis, Multiple Sclerosis, Type I Diabetes, Systemic Lupus Erythematosus, Sjogren Disease, Addison's Disease, Inflammatory Bowel Disease, and so on.

New Delhi, India

Khalid Raza
Surender Singh

Acknowledgments

Editing a book is a journey that requires the collective efforts and support of numerous individuals and institutions. We express our heartfelt gratitude to all those who have contributed to the creation of "Artificial Intelligence and Autoimmune Diseases—Applications in the Diagnosis, Prognosis, and Therapeutics."

Contributing Authors

First and foremost, we extend our sincere thanks to the contributing authors of this volume. Your dedication, expertise, and commitment to advancing the field of autoimmune diseases through the lens of artificial intelligence are truly commendable. Your insightful contributions have enriched this book and will undoubtedly inspire future generations of researchers and practitioners.

Reviewers and Peer Contributors

We are grateful to the reviewers and peer contributors who meticulously examined the content, providing invaluable feedback and ensuring the highest quality of scholarship in this volume. Your expertise and rigorous evaluation have been instrumental in shaping the final product.

Supportive Institutions

Our sincere appreciation goes to the institutions and organizations that have supported our research endeavors. Your infrastructure, resources, and encouragement have been instrumental in facilitating the research and collaboration necessary for this book's success.

Family and Friends

To our families and friends, we owe a debt of gratitude for your unwavering support and understanding during the often demanding process of writing and editing. Your encouragement and patience have been a source of strength throughout this journey.

Readers and the Healthcare Community

We extend our thanks to the readers of this book, including healthcare professionals, researchers, students, and anyone interested in the intersection of artificial intelligence and autoimmune diseases. Your curiosity and commitment to improving healthcare through AI are what drive our passion for this field.

The Publishing Team

A special acknowledgment goes to our publisher Springer, editors, and production team for their dedication to bringing this book to fruition. Your expertise, guidance, and commitment to excellence have been invaluable.

Last but not least, we extend our heartfelt appreciation to each and everyone who contributed to this project. This book would not have been possible without the collective effort and support of a vast network of individuals and institutions. Together, we are advancing the frontiers of knowledge and healthcare through the power of AI.

Khalid Raza
Surender Singh

About This Book

Advancements in medical science and technology have revolutionized healthcare, and one of the most promising frontiers in this domain is the intersection of Artificial Intelligence (AI) and autoimmune diseases. "**Artificial Intelligence and Autoimmune Diseases—Applications in the Diagnosis, Prognosis, and Therapeutics**" is a groundbreaking edited volume that delves deep into the transformative potential of AI in the realm of autoimmune diseases. This volume encapsulates fundamental concepts related to autoimmune diseases, basics of artificial intelligence (AI), and machine learning, recent applications of AI and machine learning techniques in the diagnosis, prognosis, and therapeutics of various autoimmune diseases, along with a few case studies. Some of the autoimmune diseases covered in this volume are Rheumatoid Arthritis (RA), Multiple Sclerosis (MS), Type 1 Diabetes (T1D), Systemic Lupus Erythematosus (SLE), Sjogren Disease (SD), Addison's Disease (AD), Inflammatory Bowel Disease (IBD), etc. This edited volume contains 15 chapters, divided into four parts.

The book begins with the first part which covers a comprehensive overview of autoimmune disorders, including their types, symptoms, and risk factors. Authored by experts in the field, Chapter "Autoimmune Disorders: Types, Symptoms, and Risk Factors" sets the stage by elucidating the fundamental aspects of these diseases. Chapter "Autoimmune Diseases: Recent Insights on Epidemiology, Pathogenesis, and Prevalence Rate" complements this foundation by offering recent insights into the epidemiology, pathogenesis, and prevalence rates of autoimmune diseases, providing readers with a current and holistic perspective.

The heart of this volume lies in the second part, where the role of AI in diagnosing and prognosticating autoimmune disorders is explored. Chapters "The Role of Artificial Intelligence and Machine Learning in Autoimmune Disorders" and "Autoimmune Autonomic Disorder: AI-Based Diagnosis and Prognosis" present the transformative potential of AI in the diagnosis and prognosis of these diseases. From AI-based diagnosis of autoimmune autonomic disorders to the use of Convolutional Neural Networks (CNN) for detecting Rheumatoid Arthritis, these chapters showcase the innovative approaches that AI brings to the table. Chapters "The Emerging Applications of Machine Learning in the Diagnosis of Multiple Sclerosis"–"Exploring Challenges and Opportunities for the Early Detection of Multiple Sclerosis Using Deep Learning" extend this exploration to the diagnosis of Multiple Sclerosis, elucidating the emerging applications, challenges, and opportunities in using machine learning and deep learning for early detection. Chapter "AI-Assisted Model for Risk Detection of Autoimmune Diseases" introduces a model for AI-assisted detection of risk for autoimmune diseases, emphasizing the proactive aspect of AI in healthcare, which can lead to early intervention and improved patient outcomes.

The third part shifts the focus to treatment planning and management, with chapters dedicated to the application of AI in the diagnosis and treatment of Rheumatoid Arthritis. These chapters present a detailed examination of the current status and future prospects of AI-enhanced treatment strategies, illustrating how AI is poised to revolutionize the management of autoimmune diseases.

The fourth part presents a collection of case studies, showcasing the real-world impact of AI in the diagnosis of autoimmune diseases. Chapter "Artificial Intelligence and Machine Learning Techniques in the Diagnosis of Type I Diabetes: Case Studies" discusses the application of AI and machine learning techniques in the diagnosis of Type I Diabetes, offering concrete examples of how AI is already making a difference in patient care. Chapter "Computational Intelligence Methods for Biomarkers Discovery in Autoimmune Diseases: Case Studies" explores computational intelligence methods for biomarker discovery in autoimmune diseases, highlighting the potential for AI to uncover novel insights that can aid treatment strategies.

The contributing authors of this volume are experts in their fields and they are from various reputed universities and institutions across the globe. The "Artificial Intelligence and Autoimmune Diseases—Applications in the Diagnosis, Prognosis, and Therapeutics" is a comprehensive and forward-thinking volume that explores the exciting fusion of AI and autoimmune diseases. It is an essential resource for healthcare professionals, researchers, and students seeking to understand and harness the potential of AI in transforming the landscape of autoimmune disease diagnosis, prognosis, and treatment. With its diverse array of chapters authored by experts in the field, this book serves as a valuable reference for those on the cutting edge of healthcare innovation and AI integration.

Contents

Editors and Contributors

About the Editors

Dr. Khalid Raza is an Associate Professor at the Department of Computer Science, Jamia Millia Islamia (Central University), New Delhi, India. He has also served as the ICCR Chair Visiting Professor at the Faculty of Computer & Information Sciences, Ain Shams University, Cairo, Egypt. Dr. Raza has over 13 years of teaching and research experience. He has contributed over 110 peer-reviewed research articles in refereed international journals, conference proceedings, and book chapters. Dr. Raza has authored/edited 7 Books published by reputed publishers like Springer-Nature, Elsevier, and CRC Press. Dr. Raza is an Academic Editor of PeerJ Computer Science, and Guest Editor of the Journal Natural Product Communications. He has active collaborations with scientists from leading institutions in India and abroad. He has received grants for two Govt. funded research projects and worked as Principal Investigator. Dr. Raza has delivered several keynote addresses, invited talks, public lectures, and seminars at National and International conferences and workshops, and chaired technical sessions at various National and International conferences. Dr. Raza has been featured in the list of the World's Top 2% Scientists released by Stanford University (USA) in collaboration with Elsevier for two consecutive years 2021 and 2022. He is a Life Member of the Computer Society of India (CSI) and Soft Computing Research Society, and a Regular Member of Machine Intelligence Research (MIR) Lab, USA.

Dr. Surender Singh is Professor at the Department of Pharmacology, All India Institute of Medical Sciences (AIIMS), New Delhi, India. Dr. Singh has teaching and research experience of more than 30 years. He is Fellow of National Academy of Medical Sciences (FAMS), India, Fellow of Royal Society of Chemistry (FRSC), UK, Fellow of International Medical Science Academy (FIMSA), India, Fellow of Institution of Chemists (FIC), India, Fellow of International Council of Ayurveda (FICA), India, Member of New York Academy of Sciences, USA, and D.Sc. (Honoris Causa), Colombo, Sri Lanka. Dr. Singh has published over 150 Research Papers, authored/edited over 10 Books and Scientific Series, guided over 65 theses (MD, MDS, M Pharm, MSc, PhD, PDF), and completed over 35 research projects funded by various finding agencies including ICMR, DBT, AIIMS, AYUSH, Govt. of India. His research interest lies in autoimmune diseases, and AI applications in autoimmune diseases.

Contributors

Muhammad Kalamuddin Ahamad Department of Computer Application, Integral University, Lucknow, U.P, India

Ahmad A. L. Ahmad Advanced Structures and Composites Center, University of Maine, Orono, ME, USA

Faiz Akram Faculty of Engineering and Technology, Department of Computer Engineering, Jamia Millia Islamia, A Central University, New Delhi, India

Usama Akram Central Council for Research in Unani Medicine, Ministry of Ayush, Government of India, New Delhi, India

Afroj Alam Department of Computer Application, Integral University, Lucknow, U.P, India;
Department of Computer Science Engineering, School of Engineering Presidency University, Bangalore, India

Mohammad Amjad Faculty of Engineering and Technology, Department of Computer Engineering, Jamia Millia Islamia, A Central University, New Delhi, India

Taushif Anwar Department of Computer Science and Engineering, Koneru Lakshmaiah Education Foundation, Vaddeswaram, India

Akshita Arora Department of Pharmaceutics, ISF College of Pharmacy, Ghal Kalan, Moga, Punjab, India

Mohammad Asim Department of Clinical and Experimental Medicine, University of Surrey, Guildford, UK

Danish Aslam Department of Computer Science, Jamia Millia Islamia, New Delhi, India

Shafaque Aziz Faculty of Engineering and Technology, Department of Computer Engineering, Jamia Millia Islamia, A Central University, New Delhi, India

Nagmi Bano Department of Computer Science, Jamia Millia Islamia, New Delhi, India;
International Centre for Genetic Engineering and Biotechnology (ICGEB), New Delhi, India

Debmalya Barh Federal University of Minas Gerais, Belo Horizonte, Brazil

K. R. Dasegowda School of Applied Sciences, REVA University, Bangalore, Karnataka, India

Syed Akramah Ahmad Faizi Delhi Technological University, New Delhi, India

Mohammed Abdul Kareem Department of Biochemistry, Indira Gandhi National Open University, New Delhi, India

Ritu Karwasra Central Council for Research in Unani Medicine, Ministry of Ayush, Government of India, New Delhi, India

Dhirender Kaushik Department of Pharmaceutical Sciences, Gurugram University, Gurugram, India

M. Y. Kavyasree Department of Biotechnology, Ramaiah Institute of Technology, Bangalore, KA, India

Fatima Nazish Khan Department of Biotechnology, New Delhi, India

Saurav Kumar Department of Pharmaceutical Sciences, Gurugram University, Gurugram, India

R. S. M. Lakshmi Patibandla Koneru Lakshmaiah Education Foundation (Deemed to be University), Guntur, Andhra Pradesh, India

Ahmed A. Mohamed Department of Chemistry, University of Sharjah, Sharjah, UAE

K. O. Mohammed Aarif Department of Electronics & Communication Engineering, School of Engineering, Presidency University, Bangalore, India

Awelani Mutshembele South African Medical Research Council (SAMRC), Pretoria, South Africa

Gunjan Nautiyal Department of Pharmaceutical Sciences, Gurugram University, Gurugram, India

Pakruddin Department of Computer Science Engineering, Presidency University, Bangalore, India

Richa Pal Department of Pharmaceutics, ISF College of Pharmacy, Ghal Kalan, Moga, Punjab, India

Parijat Pandey Department of Pharmaceutical Sciences, Gurugram University, Gurugram, India

Azra Parveen Postdoctoral Research Fellow, IIIS Delhi, New Delhi, India

H. Prabhavathi Department of Cytogenomics, Bangalore, KA, India

Mohammad Irfan Qureshi Department of Biotechnology, New Delhi, India

M. Ramakrishna Murthy Anil Neerukonda Institute of Technology and Sciences, Visakhapatnam, Andhra Pradesh, India

Majji Rambabu School of Applied Sciences, REVA University, Bangalore, Karnataka, India

Mritunjay Kr. Ranjan School of Computer Science &, Engineering Sandip University, Nashik, MH, India

Khalid Raza Department of Computer Science, Jamia Millia Islamia, New Delhi, India

J. Riyazulla Rahman Department of Computer Science Engineering, Presidency University, Bangalore, India

Iqra Sajid Department of Computer Science, Jamia Millia Islamia, New Delhi, India

Neha Sami Department of Biosciences, A Central University, New Delhi, India

Arif Md. Sattar Department of Computer Science, Anugrah Memorial College, Gaya, India

Anshul Sharma Department of Pharmaceutics, ISF College of Pharmacy, Ghal Kalan, Moga, Punjab, India;
Department of Pharmacy, Birla Institute of Technology And Science, Pilani (BITS Pilani), Pilani, Rajasthan, India

Isha Sharma Department of Pharmaceutical Sciences, Gurugram University, Gurugram, India

Nitin Sharma Department of Pharmaceutics, ISF College of Pharmacy, Ghal Kalan, Moga, Punjab, India;
Department of Pharmaceutics, Amity Institute of Pharmacy, Amity University, Uttar Pradesh, Noida, India

Shiv Kant Sharma Department of Pharmaceutical Sciences, Gurugram University, Gurugram, India

Sneha Sharma Department of Pharmaceutical Sciences, Gurugram University, Gurugram, India

Faizan Siddiqui International Medical Faculty, Osh State University, Osh City, Kyrgyzstan

Surender Singh Department of Pharmacology, All India Institute of Medical Sciences, New Delhi, India

Mohamed Soudy Bioinformatics Program, Faculty of Computer Science and Information, Ain Shams University, Cairo, Egypt

Kapil Suchal Department of Internal Medicine, School of Medicine, Texas Tech University Health Sciences Centre, Lubbock, TX, USA

Khushnuma Tanveer Department of Computer Science, Jamia Millia Islamia, New Delhi, India

B. Tarakeswara Rao Kallam Haranadhareddy Institute of Technology, Guntur, Andhra Pradesh, India

Sanjay Kr. Tiwari P.G. Department of Mathematics, Magadh University, Bodh-Gaya, India

Karthick Vasudevan School of Applied Sciences, REVA University, Bangalore, Karnataka, India

Preliminaries

Autoimmune Disorders: Types, Symptoms, and Risk Factors

Saurav Kumar, Dhirender Kaushik, and Shiv Kant Sharma

Abstract The immunity generally safeguards against bacteria, viruses, toxins, or any other foreign body. Upon detection of foreign invaders, the organism deploys a legion of combatant cells to initiate an assault against the intruders. Immune systems usually have the ability to discriminate between alien and self-cells. When the immune system doesn't resist the foreign bodies and starts killing of own healthy cells it gives rise to autoimmune disorders. Autoimmune disorders have the potential to impact multiple organs and tissues, such as blood vessels, connective tissue, endocrine glands (e.g., thyroid and pancreas), muscles, joints, skin, and red blood cells. Over 80 autoimmune diseases have been reported from these affected areas, and many more are yet to be identified. Genetics, diet, infections, and chemical exposure can all play a role. Autoimmune disorders are difficult to diagnose because the specific disorders have numerous possible symptoms and individual symptoms vary. Symptoms of autoimmune diseases vary depending on the affected body part. Many types of autoimmune diseases cause fatigue, redness, swelling, heat and pain. This chapter reviews some autoimmune risk factors, indications and different types of autoimmune disorders.

Keywords Autoimmune disorders · Autoimmune disease · Immunity · Prevalence · Autoimmune types

1 Introduction

A category of illnesses known as "autoimmune disorders" develops when the individual's immune system unintentionally targets its own tissues and organs. The immune system is obliged to safeguard the body against detrimental pathogens like viruses and bacteria. However, it can become dysregulated and mistakenly target healthy cells, tissues and organs, resulting in a diverse array of incapacitating and potentially fatal disorders that impact several bodily regions, including the joints,

S. Kumar · D. Kaushik · S. K. Sharma (✉)
Department of Pharmaceutical Sciences, Gurugram University, Gurugram 122003, India
e-mail: shivkantvats@gmail.com

K. Raza and S. Singh (eds.), *Artificial Intelligence and Autoimmune Diseases*, Studies in Computational Intelligence 1133, https://doi.org/10.1007/978-981-99-9029-0_1

skin, thyroid and nervous system. Autoimmune disorders are difficult to diagnose, as their symptoms can be non-specific and overlap with those of other conditions. They can also be challenging to treat, as the immune system is complex and can respond differently to various therapies. Nevertheless, medical researchers and clinicians have made significant progress in understanding autoimmune disorders and developing treatments that can help alleviate symptoms, decline disease development, and improve health. Living with an autoimmune disorder can be challenging, both physically and emotionally. People with these conditions may experience pain, fatigue, and disability, and they may need to make significant lifestyle changes to manage their symptoms. Support from family, friends, and healthcare professionals can be crucial in helping people with autoimmune disorders manage their conditions and improve their health. The pathophysiology of autoimmune disorders varies depending on the specific disorder. In general, autoimmune disorders are depicted by the abidance of autoantibodies, which are antibodies that target the body's own cells, tissues, and organs. These autoantibodies can cause damage to the targeted cells and tissues, leading to inflammation and tissue destruction [1].

This book chapter provides an overview of autoimmune disorders, their causes and risk factors, common symptoms and diagnostic methods, and current treatment options. It also highlights some of the latest research and innovations in the field, as well as the ongoing challenges in managing these complex diseases. By providing a comprehensive and up-to-date perspective on autoimmune disorders, this chapter aims to increase awareness and understanding of these conditions and help patients and their families make informed decisions about their care.

This chapter's bibliographic research involved examining scholarly articles and peer-reviewed textbooks, as well as consulting internationally renowned scientific search engines from the past six decades. In order to compile peer-reviewed publications, bibliographic databases such as Google Scholar, Scopus, SCIELO, and PubMed were searched. We only looked at pertinent papers that were published in English.

Autoimmune disorders can be classified in different ways, based on the criteria used. One possible way to categorize the several autoimmune disorders is based on the type of tissue or organ that is affected. Here's an attempt to group them into categories based on the organs affected.

2 Classification of Autoimmune Disorder

Autoimmune disorders refer to a collection of illnesses that emerge as a result of the immune system's erroneous assault on the body's healthy cells and tissues. There are over 100 different autoimmune disorders that have been identified. Here's an attempt to classify them into different categories based on their primary targeted organ (Fig. 1 and Table 1).

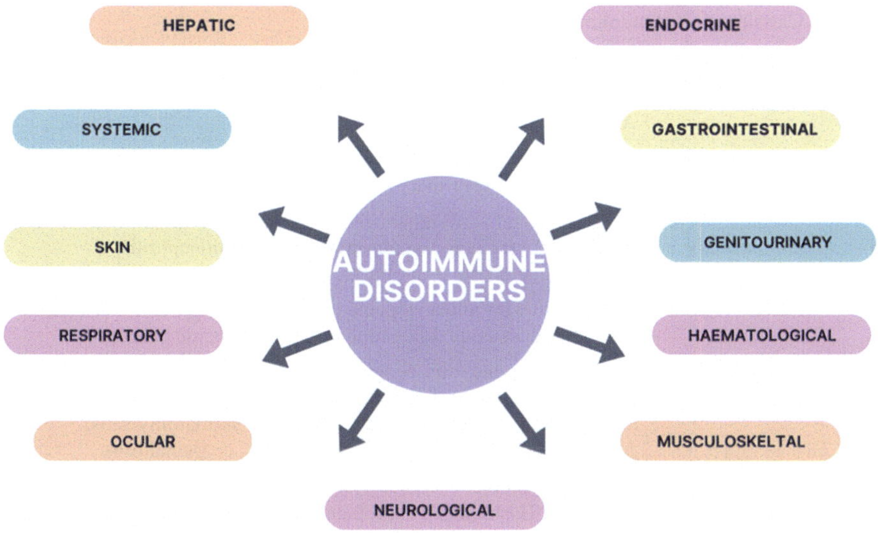

Fig. 1 Classification of autoimmune disease

2.1 *Endocrine Autoimmune Disorders*

Endocrine autoimmune disorders pertain to a cluster of autoimmune ailments that impact the endocrine system, the physiological system responsible for manufacturing and regulating hormones. These disorders materialize as a result of the immune system's misidentification of the body's endocrine glands, subsequently resulting in their impairment and malformation.

2.1.1 Addison's Disease

Addison's disease, also recognized as primary hypoadrenalism, is an infrequent autoimmune disorder characterized by immune-mediated damage to the adrenal glands. This condition affects both sexes and all age groups, with a higher incidence in people aged 30–50 years. The global prevalence of Addison's disease is estimated to range from 1–5 in 100,000 individuals, although this could be an underestimation as some cases may remain undiagnosed due to the non-specific nature of its symptoms. Addison's disease can be challenging to diagnose, as its symptoms can be ambiguous and non-specific. General indications include fatigue, faintness, loss in weight, bradycardia, hyperpigmentation, and cravings for salty food, with additional symptoms such as abdominal pain, muscle and joint pain, vomiting, and nausea occurring less commonly. Autoimmune disorders such as early onset diabetes, thyroiditis, and vitiligo, and certain medications and infections can increase the risk of developing Addison's disease. The main approach to managing Addison's disease

Table 1 Classification of autoimmune disorders

S.no	Organ	Disease
1	Endocrine	Addison's disease, Hashimoto's thyroiditis, IDDM, Graves' disease, Autoimmune polyendocrine syndrome
2	Gastrointestinal	Celiac disease, Inflammatory bowel disease, Crohn's disease, Ulcerative colitis, Primary sclerosing cholangitis, Primary biliary cirrhosis
3	Genitourinary	Interstitial cystitis, IgA nephropathy, Glomerulonephritis, Autoimmune orchitis, Autoimmune oophoritis
4	Haematological	Autoimmune thrombocytopenic purpura, Cold agglutinin disease, Haemolytic anaemia, Idiopathic thrombocytopenic purpura
5	Musculoskeletal	Ankylosing spondylitis, Sjogren's syndrome, Polymyositis, Rheumatoid arthritis, Scleroderma, Psoriatic arthritis, Reactive arthritis, Polymyalgia rheumatica, Juvenile dermatomyositis, Juvenile idiopathic arthritis, Systemic lupus erythematosus
6	Neurological	Autoimmune inner ear disease, Multiple sclerosis, Guillain–Barre syndrome, Hashimoto's encephalopathy, Lambert-Eaton myasthenic syndrome, Myositis, Narcolepsy, Neuromyelitis optica, Neuropathy, Optic neuritis, Stiff-person syndrome, Sydenham chorea, Sydenham chorea, Myasthenia gravis
7	Ocular	Ocular cicatricial pemphigoid, Scleritis
8	Respiratory	Goodpasture's syndrome
9	Skin	Alopecia areata, Bullous pemphigoid, Dermatitis herpetiformis, Herpes gestations, Lichen planus
10	Systemic	Amyloidosis, Antiphospholipid syndrome, Behcet's disease, Cardiomyopathy, Castleman disease, Chagas disease, Chronic inflammatory demyelinating polyneuropathy, Chronic recurrent multifocal osteomyelitis, Sarcoidosis
11	Hepatic	Autoimmune hepatitis, Primary biliary cholangitis, Primary sclerosing cholangitis

is hormone replacement therapy, and typically involves corticosteroids like hydrocortisone or prednisone, and mineralocorticoids like fludrocortisone to replace the deficient hormones. Hormone levels should be managed carefully as both under- and over-replacement of hormones can result in severe health consequences. Moreover, managing concomitant conditions such as thyroid disorders or diabetes may require additional medication. However, with the complete regimen, patients with Addison's disease can live a normal life [2].

2.1.2 Hashimoto's Syndrome

Hashimoto's syndrome, or Hashimoto's thyroiditis, is a persistent self-reactive disease that adversely alters the thyroid gland, triggered by immune-mediated destruction of the thyroid tissue, leading to a variety of symptoms. In the United

States, Hashimoto's syndrome is the most prevalent cause of hypothyroidism, and it is estimated to impact approximately 5% of the population. The infirmity is more general in women, and it usually affects middle-aged women. The symptoms of Hashimoto's syndrome can be vague and non-specific, making it a challenging condition to diagnose. Common symptoms are fatigue, gain in weight, sensitivity to cold, constipation, flaky skin, hair loss and depression. Additionally, some people may experience a swelling in the front of their neck, known as a goitre. The exact causes of Hashimoto's syndrome are not fully intuited, but genetic factors are thought to play a role. Additionally, women are more targeted to develop the condition than men, and the risk increases with age. The treatment for Hashimoto's syndrome typically involves a thyroid hormone replacement regimen, which enacts taking medication to exchange the hormones that the damaged thyroid gland is not able to produce. This typically includes levothyroxine, a synthetic form of the thyroid hormone. It is important to carefully manage hormone levels, as both over- and under-replacement can have serious health consequences. Additionally, people with Hashimoto's syndrome may need to make dietary changes, such as avoiding goitrogenic foods, which can interfere with thyroid hormone production. With complete intervention, preeminent people with Hashimoto's syndrome can lead healthy lives [3].

2.1.3 Graves' Disease (GD)

Graves' disease (GD) is an autoimmune disorder that leads to an increase in thyroid due to the overproduction of thyroid hormones, caused by the immune system attacking the thyroid gland. It is the prevailing cause of hyperthyreosis, impacting around 1–2% of the population, more commonly women aged between 30 and 50. Symptoms include anxiety, irritability, insomnia, weight loss, increased appetite, tremors, muscle weakness, fatigue, heat intolerance and increased heart rate. Eye problems such as bulging eyes or double vision can also occur. The exact causes of GD are not fully understood, but genetic factors and environmental factors such as stress, smoking, pregnancy and certain viral infections may play a role. Treatment may include medication, surgery or supportive therapies, such as eye drops, to manage the symptoms and reduce thyroid hormone production. With proper regimens, patients with GD can lead normal lives [4]. Some of the important characteristics of Grave's Disease are shown in Fig. 2.

2.2 Gastrointestinal Autoimmune Disorders

Gastrointestinal autoimmune diseases (GI-AID) are a cluster of autoimmune disorders that affect the digestive system. These problems occur when the immune mechanism mistakenly impacts the body's own digestive tissues, causing inflammation and damage. GI-AID can affect various parts of the digestive system, including the oesophagus, stomach, small and large intestines, liver, and pancreas.

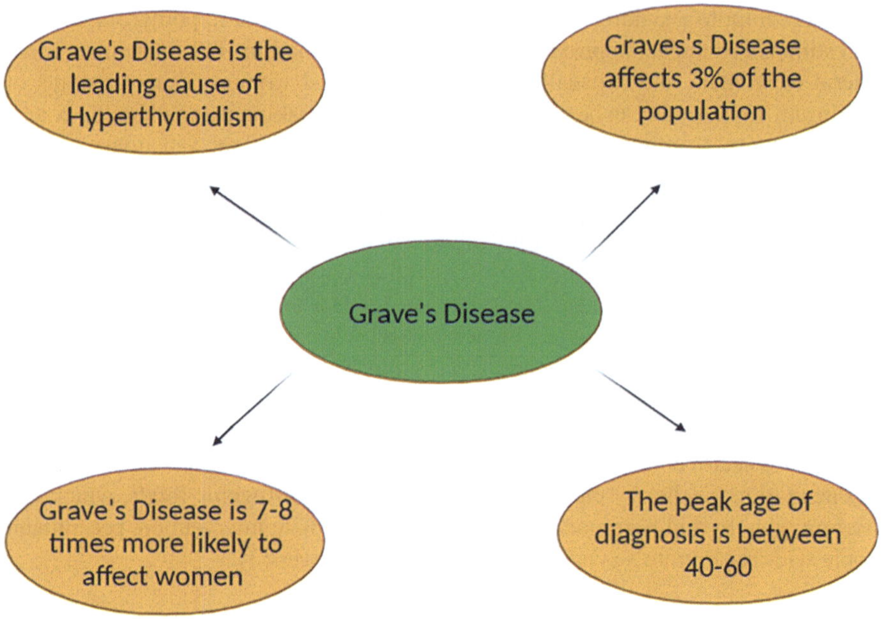

Fig. 2 Characteristics of Grave's disease

2.2.1 Inflammatory Bowel Disease (IBD)

Inflammatory bowel disease (IBD) is a collection of gastrointestinal-related perpetual inflammatory diseases. IBD is divided into two categories: Crohn's disease and ulcerative colitis, both of which involve soreness and injure the gastric lining. IBD is a relatively usual malady, impacting lakhs of people globally. The exact prevalence of IBD varies by region, but it is estimated that approximately 1 in 250 people in North America and Europe are affected by the condition. The manifestations of IBD can vary reliant on the severity and type of the condition, but common symptoms include abdominal distress, diarrhoea, bloody stools, fatigue, and loss in weight. Additionally, some people with IBD may experience fever, joint pain, and skin rashes. The unambiguous cause of IBD is presumed to involve a melding of environmental and genetic factors. Individuals with a genetic history of IBD may be at increased risk of blooming the condition, as are individuals who smoke or use non-steroidal anti-inflammatory drugs, or have an aggravated fat diet and processed foods. IBD treatment commonly incorporates a blend of medication, lifestyle adjustments, and, in some cases, surgical interventions. Medications used to treat IBD may include immunosuppressants, anti-inflammatory drugs, and biological therapies. Living changes may encompass dietary adjustments, stress reduction, and regular exercise. In certain instances, surgery might be required to remove affected parts of the gastric tract. With appropriate treatment and continuous management, numerous individuals with IBD can effectively handle their symptoms and maintain regular, healthy lives [5].

2.2.2 Crohn's Disease

Crohn's disease is a prolonged IBD that results in soreness and damage to the lining of the digestive tract. The condition is relatively common and affects about 1 in 1,000 people. It can occur at any age but is usually diagnosed in individuals aged 15–35. Crohn's disease symptoms differ based on which part of the digestive tract is involved. Symptoms often include bloody stools, abdominal pain, loss in weight, diarrhoea, and fatigue. Some people may also experience fever, joint pain, and skin rashes. While the cause of Crohn's disease is not completely understood, it is presumed to be a melding of environmental factors and genetics. People with a family past of IBD, as well as those who smoke or have used non-steroidal anti-inflammatory drugs (NSAIDs), may be at higher risk for blooming Crohn's disease. The regimen for Crohn's disease is multifaceted and includes medication, lifestyle modifications, and sometimes surgery. Medications utilized for managing Crohn's disease encompass anti-inflammatory drugs, immunosuppressants, and biological therapies. Lifestyle adjustments might entail dietary modifications, stress reduction techniques, and physical activity. If necessary, surgery could be needed to eliminate affected segments of the digestive tract. Proper treatment and management can help individuals with Crohn's disease control their symptoms and live healthy, normal lives [6].

2.2.3 Ulcerative Colitis

Ulcerative colitis is classified as a type of IBD that induces long-term soreness and ulcers in the lining of the colon and rectum. The disease commences in the rectum and may extend throughout the colon. This ailment affects around 1 in 1,000 individuals and can happen at any phase of life, but it is frequently treated in individuals between the ages of 15 and 30. The symptoms of ulcerative colitis can vary in severity, but general symptoms include abdominal distress, diarrhoea, rectal bleeding, an urgent and frequent need for bowel movements, fatigue, and weight loss. Additionally, some individuals with ulcerative colitis may experience fever, joint pain, and skin rashes. The unerring cause of ulcerative colitis is not completely understood, but it is presumed to arise from a melding of environmental and genetic factors. Individuals with an ancestry of IBD, smokers, or those with a diet high in fat and processed foods have an increased risk of developing ulcerative colitis. Treating ulcerative colitis typically involves medication, lifestyle shifting, and sometimes surgery. Regimens used may include biological therapies, anti-inflammatory drugs, and immunosuppressants. Lifestyle changes may involve dietary modifications, stress reduction, and regular exercise. In certain cases, surgery might be required to remove the colon and rectum.

With appropriate treatment and ongoing management, many individuals with ulcerative colitis can effectively handle their symptoms and lead normal, healthy lives [7].

2.3 Genitourinary Autoimmune Disorders

Genitourinary autoimmune disorders are a cluster of autoimmune conditions that affect the organs and tissues of the urinary and reproductive systems. These conditions arise from the immune system erroneously targeting and damaging healthy tissues in these regions, causing inflammation.

2.3.1 Autoimmune Orchitis

Autoimmune orchitis is a rare situation in which the body defence attacks the testicles, causing inflammation and damage to the tissues. It is classified as a type of autoimmune disorder, in which the immune system erroneously targets healthy tissues and organs in the body. Autoimmune orchitis is a relatively rare condition and its exact prevalence is not known. It is commonly treated in men over the age of 40. The symptoms of autoimmune orchitis can include pain and swelling in the testicles, as well as fever, fatigue, and general malaise. In some cases, the condition may lead to infertility or other complications. Men who have had other autoimmune disorders, such as rheumatoid arthritis or lupus, may have a greater chance of developing autoimmune orchitis. The usual approach to treating autoimmune orchitis involves medications such as non-steroidal anti-inflammatory drugs or corticosteroids to alleviate soreness and pain. In some instances, immunosuppressants may be used to limit the immune system's activity and deter additional harm to the testicles. Surgery to eliminate damaged tissue or repair the testicles may be necessary in severe instances. Treatment is aimed at reducing symptoms, preserving fertility, and preventing further damage to the testicles [8].

2.3.2 Autoimmune Oophoritis

Autoimmune Oophoritis is a situation that transpires when the immune mechanism attacks ovarian tissue due to an autoimmune disorder. Autoimmune disorders can stimulate the immune mechanism to mistakenly impact healthy tissues and organs. The exact prevalence of autoimmune oophoritis is unknown, but it can affect women of all ages, with the ubiquitous age of diagnosis being between 17 and 48 years old. Symptoms of oophoritis can include hot flashes, night sweats, and vaginal dryness. Women with family history of autoimmune disorders may be at an aggravated in developing autoimmune oophoritis compared to those without such a history. Treatment for oophoritis usually involves medication to subdue the immune system and decrease inflammation. It can be used to manage symptoms of menopause through hormone replacement therapy. In severe cases, ovarian tissue may have to be removed. Reducing symptoms preserving fertility and preventing further damage to the ovaries are some of the objectives of the treatment program [9].

2.4 Haematological Autoimmune Disorders

Haematological autoimmune disorders are a cluster of circumstances in which the defence system storms blood cells and/or components of the blood. These disorders can affect different elements of the blood, such as white blood cells, red blood cells, plasma proteins, and platelets.

2.4.1 Cold Agglutinin Disease (CAD)

Cold agglutinin disease (CAD) is a rare autoimmune disorder that attacks the blood cells. When red blood cells are exposed to cold temperatures, the immune system in CAD creates antibodies that attach to them and cause them to aggregate (agglutinate). The estimated prevalence rate is 5–10 cases per million persons, CAD is a rare illness. Haemolytic anaemia, which happens when red blood cells clump together and begin to break down (haemolyze) and release haemoglobin into the bloodstream, is the most prevalent sign of CAD. Shortness of breath, pallor, weariness, weakness, and jaundice are just a few symptoms that might result from this. Organ damage, such as renal failure, can occur as a result of CAD in extreme circumstances. As the precise cause of CAD is unknown, and certain factors such as age and pre existing conditions like lymphoma, leukaemia, or viral infections may increase the liklihood of developing CAD. The severity of the anaemia and the underlying cause of the illness will determine how to treat CAD. Treatment may not be required in moderate cases, but in more severe ones, drugs like rituximab, corticosteroids, or immunosuppressants may be used to stifle the immune system and stop the destruction of RBCs. To replenish red blood cells and eliminate antibodies from the bloodstream, plasmapheresis or blood transfusions may occasionally be required. The purpose of treatment is to reduce symptoms and guard against haemolytic anaemia consequences [10].

2.4.2 Haemolytic Anaemia

Haemolytic anaemia develops when the body invades red blood cells at a faster rate than it can produce them, arising in a shortage of oxygen-carrying red blood cells in the body. This can cause symptoms such as fatigue, weakness, and pallor. Various factors can cause haemolytic anaemia, including genetic disorders, infections, medications, and autoimmune diseases. In autoimmune haemolytic anaemia (AIHA), the immune system erroneously attacks its own red blood cells, leading to their destruction. Warm antibody haemolytic anaemia is a general type of AIHA, depicted by the incursion of antibodies that react with RBCs at body temperature, while cold agglutinin disease (CAD) is described by the markers of antibodies that react with RBCs at cold temperatures. The treatment for haemolytic anaemia varies based on the chief cause and the degree of the condition. To curb the immune mechanism and prevent the destruction of red blood cells in AIHA, corticosteroids, immunosuppressants, or rituximab may be utilized. In severe cases, blood transfusions or plasmapheresis may be necessary to replace red blood cells and remove antibodies from the bloodstream. The target of cure is to improve symptoms and restore normal red blood cell counts [11].

2.4.3 Idiopathic Thrombocytopenic Purpura (ITP)

Idiopathic thrombocytopenic purpura (ITP) is a disorder in which the individual's immune mechanism faultily invades platelets, causing destruction and a decrease in the number of platelets in the blood. Platelets facilitate blood clotting, and a shortage of platelets can result in bruising, bleeding, and prolonged bleeding after injury. The occurrence of Idiopathic thrombocytopenic purpura is quantified to be around 3.3 per 100,000 persons per year in adults and 50–100 cases per 1,000,000 children per year. It is common in women and perpetually occurs in young adults or children. The incidence of ITP varies widely in different populations and geographical areas. The reason for ITP is not fully understood, and it is considered an autoimmune disorder. It can occur in children as well as in adults and is more common in women. In some cases, ITP may be activated by viral pathogens, medications, or pregnancy. Symptoms of ITP include easy bruising, petechiae (small purple or red spots), delayed bleeding from cuts, nosebleeds, and bleeding gums. In severe cases, internal bleeding may occur, which can be life-threatening. Diagnosis for ITP depends on the seriousness of the condition and the presence of bleeding symptoms. Normal cases may not require treatment, while more severe cases may require medications to suppress the immune system and prevent platelet destruction. Corticosteroids, immunoglobulins, and thrombopoietin receptor agonists are some of the medications used to treat ITP. In some cases, splenectomy may be necessary to improve platelet counts [12].

2.5 Musculoskeletal Autoimmune Disorders

Musculoskeletal autoimmune disorders are a cluster of circumstances that affect the muscles, bones, and joints. These disorders develop when the body's defence mistakenly injures the body's own tissues, causing inflammation and damage.

2.5.1 Ankylosing Spondylitis (AS)

Ankylosing spondylitis (AS) is characterized as a form of chronic inflammatory arthritis that firstly targets the spine and sacroiliac joints—the joints linking the lower back to the pelvis. It is a type of musculoskeletal autoimmune disorder that promotes pain and stiffness in the affected areas, and in severe cases, can result in the fusion of the spine, leading to a loss of mobility. Ankylosing spondylitis (AS) is a relatively rare condition, with a ubiquity of approximately 0.1–0.5% in most populations worldwide. However, the prevalence can be higher in certain populations, such as in people of North European descent, where it can be as high as 1–2%. AS typically develops in early adulthood, with symptoms usually appearing before the age of 30. It occurs in men than women, with a male ratio female to approximately 3:1. The manifestations of AS include stiffness in the lower back and buttocks and chronic pain which may worsen with rest and improve with exercise. Fatigue, loss of appetite, and difficulty breathing are the other symptoms of AS. Treatment for AS focuses on reducing pain and stiffness, improving mobility, and preventing or slowing down the development of the disease. This could apply to pharmaceuticals like biologics that target particular immune system proteins, disease-modifying antirheumatic therapies, and NSAIDs. Regular exercise and physical treatment can also assist to increase mobility and lessen discomfort. Surgery may be required in extreme circumstances to repair broken joints or to address spinal abnormalities [13].

2.5.2 Sjögren's Syndrome

Sjögren's syndrome is an autoimmune disorder that mainly impacts the glands responsible for producing tears and saliva, resulting in dryness of the eyes and mouth. It can also attack anatomically, such as the skin, joints, lungs, kidneys, and nervous system. The prevalence of Sjögren's syndrome is low, ranging from 0.05% to 1% in most populations globally, but it can be higher among specific groups, such as women over 50, where it can be as high as 10%. Approximately 1–4 million people in the US are affected by Sjögren's syndrome, with a higher incidence in women than men, at a ratio of approximately 9:1. The disease is more common to people between the ages of 40–60. Common symptoms include joint pain, fatigue, dry eyes, skin rashes dry mouth, and vaginal dryness. Diagnosis involves physical examination, medical history, and laboratory tests such as blood tests and a biopsy of the salivary gland. Although there is no proper regimen for Sjögren's syndrome, treatment can help alleviate symptoms and prevent complications. This may include the use of artificial tears and saliva substitutes, medications to reduce inflammation, and immune system suppressants. In severe cases, surgery may be necessary to alleviate complications such as corneal damage [14]. The characteristics of Sjogren's Syndrome are presented in Fig. 3.

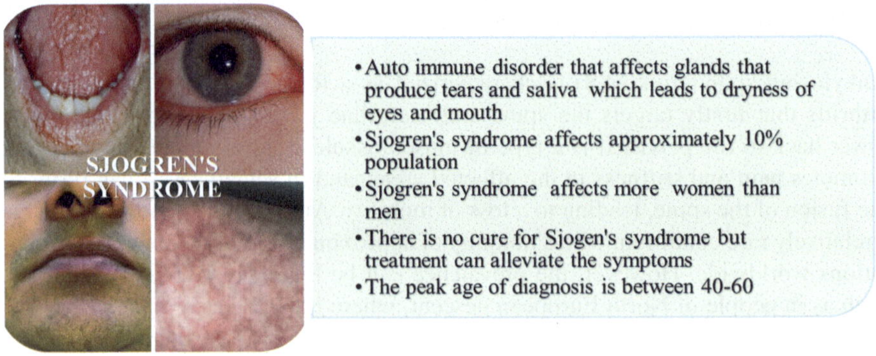

Fig. 3 Characteristics of Sjogren's syndrome

2.5.3 Scleroderma

Scleroderma, also recognized as systemic sclerosis, is an infrequent autoimmune disease that impacts connective tissues in the body. Scleroderma is a situation where the skin and internal organs become hardened and stiff, which can result in impairment and malfunction. The precise reason for scleroderma is unknown, but it is thought to be caused by genetic factors. In Canada and the United States, scleroderma affects roughly 47 individuals per million [15] with a higher incidence in women and African Americans. It can harm at any age but is frequent in adults of the ages of 30–50. The manifestations of scleroderma can vary widely reliant on the extent and urgency of the disease. The ubiquitous symptom is thickening and hardening of the skin, especially on the hands and face. Other symptoms may include Raynaud's phenomenon, joint pain and stiffness, muscle weakness, fatigue, gastrointestinal problems, and lung or heart problems. The root cause of scleroderma is investigated, but a few aspects may aggravate a person's risk of nurturing the disease, including genetics, exposure to toxins, and certain viral infections. Scleroderma is primarily classified into two main types: limited cutaneous scleroderma and diffuse cutaneous scleroderma. Skin that is thickened and hardened on the hands, face, and feet is a sign of restricted cutaneous scleroderma. Skin thickening and hardening that affects significant portions of the body, as well as internal organs like the lungs, heart, and kidneys, are symptoms of diffuse cutaneous scleroderma. Scleroderma has no known treatment, but medications can aid with symptom management and reduce the disease's progression. Medications to reduce immune system activity and inflammation, physical therapy to increase muscular strength and range of motion, and surgery to remove injured tissue or increase blood flow to the affected areas are all possible forms of treatment. Additionally, modifying one's lifestyle by giving up smoking, eating a healthy diet, and avoiding stress or exposure to cold temperatures may help in recovery [16].

2.5.4 Reactive Arthritis

Reactive arthritis, also recognized as Reiter's syndrome, is an inflammatory arthritis that occurs as a result of an infection in another anatomy. The condition typically affects the joints, eyes, urethra, and skin. Reactive arthritis is relatively uncommon, with a prevalence of approximately 5 in 1000 people. The condition typically affects young adults, with a peak incidence in the 20 s and 30 s. Mostly men are more affected than women. The symptoms of reactive arthritis can vary but typically include joint pain, stiffness, and swelling, particularly in the knees, ankles, and feet. The condition can also cause ocular inflammation, urethra, and skin. Other symptoms may include fatigue, fever, and weight loss. The root cause of reactive arthritis is not completely known, but it is thought to be activated by an infection in the body, typically in the gut or urinary tract. The condition is more common in people who have a genetic predisposition to developing it, and it is also an augmented predisposition in those who have had a recent bacterial infection. Treatment for reactive arthritis typically involves addressing the underlying infection, if present, and managing the symptoms of the condition. Non-steroidal & anti-inflammatory drugs may be used to reduce pain and inflammation, and corticosteroids may be used in more severe cases. In some cases, disease-modifying antirheumatic drugs may be prescribed to help prevent joint damage. Reactive arthritis typically resolves within a few months, although in some cases it can become a chronic condition. Long-term follow-up may be required in some cases to monitor for potential complications, such as joint damage or eye problems [17].

2.5.5 Systemic Lupus Erythematosus (SLE)

Systemic lupus erythematosus (SLE) is a systemic autoimmune disorder that can cause soreness and injure the various parts of the body, such as internal organs, skin, and joints. This condition is associated with the production of autoantibodies that mistakenly attack healthy tissues and organs. SLE has a prevalence of about 20 to 150 cases per 100,000 people, with women being affected about 10 times more frequently than men. The disease often appears in people of age 15 and 45. The signs of SLE can exhibit significant variation among individuals and may encompass skin rashes, fatigue, fever, hair loss, and joint pain. Other possible symptoms include chest pain, difficulty breathing, and kidney problems. The right cause of SLE is unknown. Risk factors for SLE include family history of the disease, exposure to certain medications, and certain infections. There are various types of SLE, including drug-induced lupus, which is caused by certain medications; cutaneous lupus, which affects only the skin; and neuropsychiatric lupus, which affects the nervous system. Treatment for SLE often involves the melding of regimens and lifestyle shifts. Typically used regimens include corticosteroids, antimalarials, and immunosuppressants. Lifestyle changes may include getting regular exercise, avoiding sun exposure, and eating a healthy diet. While SLE is incurable, many individuals with the condition can manage their manifestations and lead relatively normal lives with proper regimens and management [18].

2.5.6 Rheumatoid Arthritis (RA)

Rheumatoid arthritis (RA) is an impersistent autoimmune disorder that induces inflammation, pain, and stiffness in the joints. It is the most common form of inflammatory arthritis and can also affect other organs such as the lungs and heart. RA is more prevalent in women than men and typically develops in people between 30 and 50 years of age. Around 1% of the global population has RA, with a higher incidence in developed countries and among certain ethnic groups such as Native Americans and those of Scandinavian descent. The risk of developing RA increases with age, and women are three times more likely than men to develop the condition. Although symptoms vary from person to person, stiffness, swelling, and pain in the hands, wrists, and feet are common. Fever, weight loss, and exhaustion may also occur. The cause of RA is unknown, but genetics, smoking, and obesity are risk factors. Seropositive RA, seronegative RA, juvenile idiopathic arthritis (JIA), and Felty's syndrome are some types of RA. Treatment aims to reduce inflammation, relieve pain, and improve joint function and includes non-steroidal anti-inflammatory medicines, disease-modifying antirheumatic drugs, biological agents, and corticosteroids. Additionally helpful in controlling RA symptoms and enhancing joint function are physical therapy and occupational therapy [19] (Table 2).

2.6 Neurological Autoimmune Disorders

Neurological autoimmune disorders are a cluster of autoimmune diseases in which the immune mechanism mistakenly impacts the nervous system, leading to damage or dysfunction of the nerves. These disorders can impact other parts of the nervous system, comprising the brain, spinal cord, and peripheral nerves.

2.6.1 Multiple Sclerosis (MS)

Multiple sclerosis (MS) is a complex and more frequent disabling neurological autoimmune disorder where the immune system of the body erroneously impacts the myelin sheath, which covers nerve fibres in the brain and spinal cord, causing damage to the nervous system. This damage to the myelin sheath results in the formation of scar tissue (sclerosis), which can interfere with nerve signals between all the body parts and the brain. The prevalence of MS varies widely between populations, with an estimated 25 lakh people affected globally. Multiple Sclerosis (MS) is more prevalent in women and typically appears between the people of 20 and 40 years. The signs of MS can differ significantly based on the extent and location of myelin sheath

Table 2 Current Treatment of Rheumatoid Arthritis

S.no	Category	Examples
1	Non-steroidal anti-inflammatory medicines	Aspirin, Ibuprofen, Indomethacin, Diclofenac, Nabumetone [20]
2	Glucocorticoids	Prednisone, methylprednisolone [21]
3	Disease-modifying antirheumatic drugs (DMARDs)	Methotrexate, Hydroxychloroquine, Sulfasalazine, Leflunomide [22]
4	Other antirheumatic drugs	Gold sodium thiomalate, cyclosporine, and tetracyclines [23]
5	Biological agents • Anti-TNF-α • IL-1 inhibitors • Stimulation blockers • β-cell targeted therapies	Infliximab, etanercept, Anakinra Abatacept Rituximab [23]
6	Lifestyle	Regular exercise and running [24]
7	Surgery	Synovectomy, joint replacement surgery
8	Physiotherapy	Physiotherapy, heat application, electronic stimulation, hydrotherapy, cryotherapy [25]
9	Compression gloves	Compression gloves are specialized handwear designed to help prevent medical conditions associated with blood circulation issues in the hands and wrists. Although they can provide relief for arthritis symptoms, their medical effectiveness may be limited [26]
10	Dietary supplements	Fatty acids, Vitamins, Diets, Minerals, Herbal [27]
11	Vaccination	It is recommended to receive the inactivated influenza vaccine every year. For people under the age of 65, the pneumococcal vaccine should be given twice, while for those over 65, it should be given once [28]

damage. Common symptoms of MS encompass muscle weakness, limb numbness or tingling sensations, coordination and balance issues, vision problems, fatigue, and cognitive impairment (Fig. 4). The symptoms of MS may also come and go, with periods of remission and relapse. Individuals with a family history of the disease, of Northern European ancestry, or exposed to certain environmental factors like viral infections or low levels of vitamin D, may be at higher risk. Currently, there is no specific regimen for MS, but regimens are available to manage its manifestations and attenuate its progress. These treatments may involve the use of medications to reduce inflammation, immunosuppressants to suppress the immune system's response, and physical therapy to enhance coordination and strength [29].

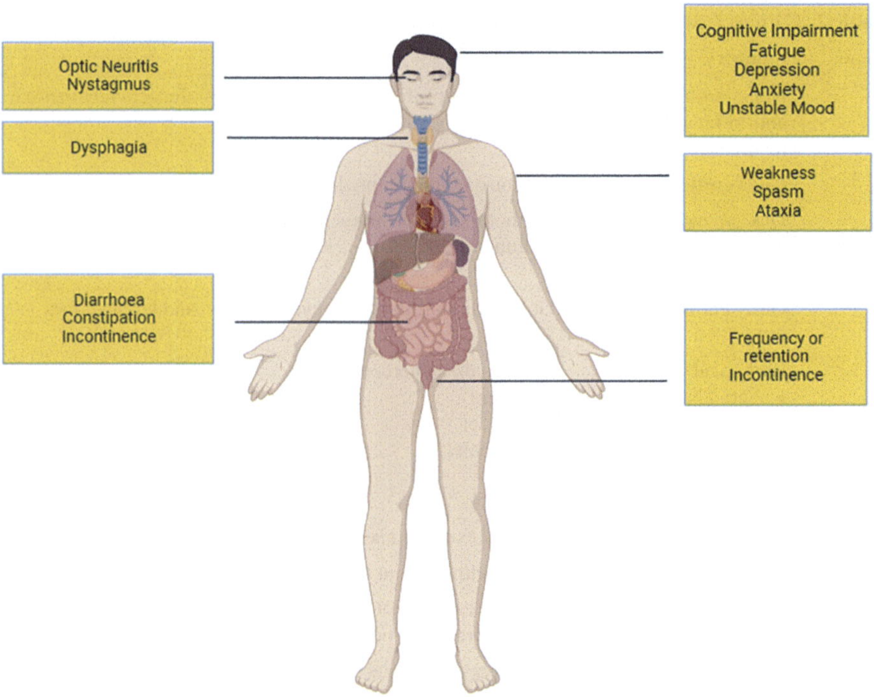

Fig. 4 Symptoms of multiple sclerosis

2.6.2 Guillain–Barre Syndrome (GBS)

Guillain–Barre syndrome (GBS), is a peculiar yet Critical autoimmune illness that impacts the PNS. Its symptoms include sudden muscle weakness, tingling sensations, and numbness, which can quickly progress to paralysis of the respiratory and limb muscles. GBS is typically triggered by a preceding bacterial or viral infection, such as respiratory or gastrointestinal infections, and it affects about 1 in 100,000 people per year. Although GBS can be acquired at any phase, it is more general in adults than children, and men are more likely to develop it than women. The symptoms usually develop over several days to a few weeks, and they can be severe enough to require hospitalization. The potential risks for GBS include ancestry of infections, autoimmune disorders, and recent vaccinations. In some cases, GBS can also be associated with certain types of cancer. There are 3 different types of GBS: Acute Inflammatory Demyelinating Polyradiculoneuropathy (AIDP), Miller-Fisher Syndrome (MFS), and Chronic Inflammatory Demyelinating Polyradiculoneuropathy (CIDP). With 90% of cases being AIDP, it is the most prevalent type. Hospitalization, supportive care, and treatment to address the disorder's underlying cause are frequently used in the treatment of GBS. Patients with serious conditions could need mechanical ventilation to help them breathe. Treatments include plasma exchange therapy and intravenous immunoglobulin (IVIG) can assist in lessening the severity of symptoms and minimize the length of the condition. While most patients with GBS eventually recover from their symptoms, the recovery process can be slow and can take several months to a year. Some patients may experience residual weakness or other long-term complications as a result of the disorder [30].

2.6.3 Hashimoto's Encephalopathy (HE)

Hashimoto's encephalopathy (HE), also recognized as steroid-responsive encephalopathy associated with autoimmune thyroiditis (SREAT), is a relatively uncommon autoimmune disorder that affects the brain. The condition is often linked to Hashimoto's thyroiditis, an autoimmune disease that primarily complicates the thyroid gland. Hashimoto's encephalopathy is not well understood, and its precise causes and mechanisms are still being studied. However, the exact relationship between the two conditions is unclear. The prevalence of HE is not known, as it is often underdiagnosed or misdiagnosed. It is more common among women in comparison to men and usually occurs in middle-aged or older adults. Clinical manifestations of Hashimoto's encephalopathy can vary widely but may include confusion, memory loss, seizures, hallucinations, headaches, and stroke-like symptoms such as weakness or numbness on one side of the body. The symptoms may develop gradually or suddenly and can be mild or severe. The root cause of this is still investigative, but research suggests that HE is a complex and multifactorial autoimmune disorder. This implies that the body's immune mechanism erroneously attacks healthy brain tissue, causing soreness and damage. Some risk factors for developing Hashimoto's encephalopathy may include having Hashimoto's thyroiditis, other autoimmune disorders, or a family history of autoimmune disease. Treatment for Hashimoto's encephalopathy usually involves the use of corticosteroids, which can help to attenuate soreness and relieve symptoms. Other immunosuppressive medications may also be used in some cases. In addition to medication, supportive care such as physical therapy and speech therapy may be effective for those with neurological symptoms. Overall, HE is a rare and complex autoimmune disorder that can be less predictable to diagnose and treat. To ascertain the underlying cause of the condition and receive adequate treatment, it is crucial to seek medical attention promptly when experiencing neurological symptoms such as confusion, memory loss, or seizures [31].

2.6.4 Myasthenia Gravis

Myasthenia gravis is a condition of autoimmunity that affects the interaction between the nerves and muscular tissues. This disorder causes weakening of the skeletal muscles, which are responsible for movements like chewing, walking, and talking. Myasthenia gravis is caused by antibodies that target the acetylcholine receptors in the muscles. The antibodies block or destroy these receptors, which reduces the ability of nerves to activate muscles. The incidence of myasthenia gravis is reported to be around 20 cases/100,000 people. It acquires all genders, and it can be visible in any age group, although it is more visible in women <40 years and men >60 years. The clinical manifestations of myasthenia gravis include muscle weakening and fatigue, which complexes with more actively working and gets better with rest. The manifestations can vary in severity and may affect different muscle groups, such as the eyes, face, limbs, and respiratory muscles. Some people may experience double vision, drooping eyelids, slurred speech, and difficulty swallowing. There are several risk factors that may enhance the likelihood of occurrence of myasthenia gravis, including having a family history of the disorder, being female, and having Comparable autoimmune illnesses like lupus/rheumatoid arthritis. Certain medications such as beta blockers and quinidine may also aggravate the risk of myasthenia gravis. The treatment for myasthenia gravis aims to improve muscle strength and reduce symptoms. The medications used include anticholinesterase drugs, which increase the availability of acetylcholine, and immunosuppressants, which reduce the production of the antibodies that attack the muscles. In some suffers, thymectomy, the surgical removal of the thymus gland, might be recommended. Overall, while myasthenia gravis can be a challenging disorder to manage, with proper therapy, most people are able to live casual and fulfilling lives [32]. Symptoms and characteristics of Myasthenia Gravis are presented in Fig. 5.

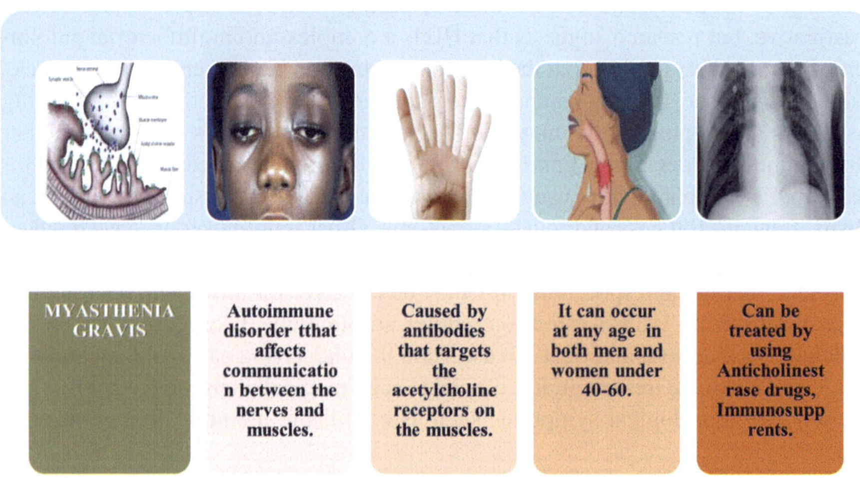

Fig. 5 Symptoms and characteristics of Myasthenia Gravis

2.7 *Ocular Autoimmune Diseases*

Ocular autoimmune disorders are a category of medical ailments in which the immune system of the body mistakenly impacts healthy cells in the eyes and the surrounding tissues. This results in inflammation, tissue damage, and in severe cases, vision loss.

2.7.1 Ocular Cicatricial Pemphigoid (OCP)

Ocular cicatricial pemphigoid (OCP), OCP, or mucous membrane pemphigoid, is an autoimmune disorder that affects the mucous membranes such as the conjunctiva and oral mucosa. The condition causes inflammation, scarring, and deterioration in the affected tissues, particularly in the eyes and surrounding tissues. Although it can affect individuals of all ages, it is more prevalent in women aged 60 and above. Symptoms of OCP may include redness, itching, burning, tearing, and sensitivity to light. As the disease progresses, it can cause scarring of the conjunctiva, which can lead to eyelid deformities, dry eyes, and vision loss. OCP can also affect the mouth and throat, causing difficulty with swallowing and speaking. The specific aetiology of OCP remains uncertain, but it is hypothesized to be an autoimmune disease. The immune mechanism erroneously assaults the body's own tissues, including those of the eyes and mouth. Risk factors for developing OCP include older age, female gender, and a history of other autoimmune disorders. The regimen for OCP focuses on managing manifestations and preventing complications. This may involve the use of lubricating eye drops, topical steroids, and other medications to reduce inflammation and scarring. In severe cases, surgical intervention may be necessary to correct eyelid deformities and restore vision. Ongoing monitoring and management by an ophthalmologist and other healthcare providers is important to prevent further damage and complications [33].

2.7.2 Scleritis

Scleritis is a category of autoimmune disorder prominently affecting the sclera, which is the white outer layer of the eye. It is characterized by inflammation of the sclera, which can lead to severe eye pain, redness, and swelling. Scleritis is a relatively rare condition and can affect people of varying ages although it is more commonly occurring in women and those over the age of 50. Scleritis comes in two primary varieties: anterior and posterior. The front of the eye is affected by anterior scleritis, whereas the back is affected by posterior scleritis. The more prevalent variety, anterior scleritis, frequently coexists with autoimmune diseases including lupus and rheumatoid arthritis. Scleritis symptoms may include redness, discomfort, and swelling in the affected eye, depending on the kind and degree of the disorder. Some people may also experience blurred vision, sensitivity to light, and tearing. In severe cases, scleritis can lead to vision loss. Risk factors for scleritis include a history of autoimmune disorders, such as autoimmune arthritis and lupus, as well as blood infections and certain medications. NSAIDs, corticosteroids, immunosuppressive medications, and surgery are all possible treatments for scleritis. If you have signs of scleritis or any other eye issue, you should contact a doctor to help maintain your eyesight and prevent further complications [34].

2.8 *Respiratory Autoimmune Disorders*

A category of diseases known as respiratory autoimmune disorders affects the airways, lungs, and other respiratory system organs. When the body's defence system impacts healthy cells and tissues in the respiratory system unintentionally it leads to damage to associated tissues and results in severe inflammation.

2.8.1 Goodpasture's Syndrome

Goodpasture's syndrome is an uncommon autoimmune disease affecting both the lungs as well as kidneys. It is associated with the association of autoantibodies targeted against the basement membrane inside the listed organs. The antibodies can result in damage to the covering of the lungs and the filtering units of the kidneys, leading to respiratory failure and kidney failure. The incidence of Goodpasture's syndrome is reported to be around 1 in 1 million people. The condition is most commonly present in young adults and is more common in males than females. The symptoms of Goodpasture's syndrome may include cough, shortness of breath, chest pain, fatigue, urine with blood, and inflammation in the legs and feet. The symptoms may appear suddenly and can rapidly worsen if left untreated. Smoking has been identified as a major cause of the condition. The treatment for Goodpasture's syndrome is associated with suppression of the immune system with drugs such as corticosteroids, plasmapheresis, and immunosuppressants. Plasmapheresis is a procedure that removes the autoantibodies from the blood. If the kidneys are severely damaged, dialysis or kidney transplantation may be necessary. Early diagnosis and treatment are essential for a good outcome in Goodpasture's syndrome. Without treatment, the condition can quickly lead to respiratory failure and kidney failure, which can be life-threatening [35].

2.9 *Skin Autoimmune Disorders*

Skin autoimmune disorders are medical conditions in which the anatomical immune system mistakenly impacts its own skin cells. These disorders can affect people of any age and may present with a wide range of symptoms, including rash, blisters, itching, and skin thickening.

2.9.1 Alopecia Areata

Alopecia areata is a form of autoimmune disease that can result in hair loss on the scalp as well as other body parts. This medical condition arises when the immune mechanism attacks hair follicles by mistake, resulting in hair loss. The condition can occur abruptly and progress quickly, or it may take a long time to develop. While alopecia areata can affect anyone, it is most prevalent in individuals under the age of 30, with up to 2% of the general population being affected. Some researchers have linked the condition to stress, infections, and particular drugs. It is also most common in people with other autoimmune malfunctioning such as vitiligo, lupus, and thyroid disease. The symptoms of alopecia areata include hair loss on the scalp or different body areas, as well as alteration in hair thickness or texture. Some individuals may experience hair regrowth, while others may suffer permanent hair loss. Therapy for alopecia areata relies upon the extent of hair loss and the individual's response to treatment. Some people may choose to simply wait and see if hair regrows on its own, while others may opt for treatment with corticosteroids, topical immunotherapy, or other medications. In some cases, hair transplantation may be an option. While there is currently no permanent cure for alopecia areata, ongoing research is being conducted to better understand the condition and develop new treatment options [36].

2.9.2 Dermatitis Herpetiformis

Dermatitis herpetiformis is a chronic autoimmune skin disorder characterized by a blistering rash that generally occurs on the elbows, buttocks, knees, and scalp. In the entire world, 10 in 10,000 people have this rare disease. The autoimmune disorder celiac disease, which affects the small intestine, is strongly related to the syndrome. Symptoms of dermatitis herpetiformis usually include small, itchy, fluid-filled blisters that appear on the skin. These blisters may be grouped together in clusters and can be painful or cause a burning sensation. In some cases, the skin may become red and inflamed. The rash can come and go and may be triggered by certain foods or medications. Dermatitis herpetiformis is thought to be caused by an atypical immune interaction with gluten, which is a protein commonly present in wheat, barley, and rye, although the exact cause of the condition remains unknown. The antibodies produced in response to gluten can deposit in the skin and cause inflammation and blistering. Diagnosis of dermatitis herpetiformis typically involves a skin autopsy, in which a minor skin is used for histology. Blood tests may also be used to detect the existence of antibodies associated with celiac disease. Treatment for dermatitis herpetiformis typically involves a gluten-free diet and medication to relieve symptoms. Topical corticosteroids or oral medications, such as dapsone, can help to reduce inflammation and itching. In a few cases, immunosuppressive medications may be helpful to help control the immune response. With proper treatment, the symptoms of dermatitis herpetiformis can be controlled [37].

2.9.3 Herpes Gestations

Herpes gestations, also known as gestational pemphigoid or pemphigoid gestations, is a rare autoimmune disorder that occurs during pregnancy. It is described by the formation of itchy, blistering skin abrasions that typically start in the abdomen and can transmit to other body parts. The accurate cause of herpes gestations is still investigated, but it is assumed to be an autoimmune disorder in which the mother's immune mechanism faultily harms the skin cells of the developing foetus. The disorder is associated with the presence of autoantibodies to bullous pemphigoid antigen 180 (BPAG1), a protein found in the skin and placenta. Herpes gestation affects approximately 1 in 50,000–60,000 pregnancies and is most commonly diagnosed during the second or third trimester. The indications usually resolve after delivery but may recur with subsequent pregnancies. Treatment for herpes gestations typically involves topical or oral corticosteroids to attenuate inflammation and itching. In harsh cases, immunosuppressive regimens may be needed. It is important for pregnant women with herpes gestations to be closely monitored by their healthcare providers to ensure the health of the mother as well as of the developing foetus [38].

2.10 Systemic Autoimmune Disorder

A set of illnesses known as systemic autoimmune disorders affect many body organs and tissues. These conditions develop when the immune system unintentionally damages and inflames healthy cells, tissues, and organs. Chronic and frequently relapsing–remitting conditions are associated with systemic autoimmune diseases.

2.10.1 Amyloidosis

Amyloidosis is an unusual and complex disease that occurs when atypical proteins called amyloids build up in organs and tissues. These amyloid proteins originate in the bone marrow and can accumulate in various organs such as the heart, kidneys, liver, spleen, or nervous system, causing organ damage and dysfunction. There are several types of amyloidosis, classified based on the type of protein involved. Some types of amyloidosis are acquired, meaning they develop as a result of another disease or condition, such as multiple myeloma, while others are hereditary, meaning they are passed down from parent to child. The symptoms of amyloidosis can vary depending on which organs are affected. Some common symptoms include fatigue, shortness of breath, weight loss, swollen ankles or legs, numbness in hands or feet, and an enlarged tongue. The diagnosis of amyloidosis often involves different tests, including blood tests, imaging studies, and biopsies of affected organs or tissues. Treatment options depend on the type and seriousness of amyloidosis but may include stem cell transplantation, chemotherapy, or medications to control signs and attenuate the growth of the disease. Overall, amyloidosis is a rare and complex disease that can affect multiple organs and tissues in the body. Early treatment is important for improving outcomes and managing symptoms [39].

2.10.2 Behcet's Disease

Behcet's disease, also called Behcet's syndrome, is a prolonged autoimmune disorder that impacts multiple organs in the body and is rare. The first description of this condition was made by the Turkish dermatologist, Hulusi Behcet, in 1937. While the disease can affect people of any age, it most commonly occurs in 20–40 years of age and is more prevalent in the Middle East and Asia. The disease is characterized by episodes of inflammation in the blood vessels of the body, which can cause a wide range of manifestations. Common manifestations include recurrent oral and genital ulcers, skin lesions, joint pain, eye inflammation, and gastrointestinal problems. In severe cases, the disease can also affect the brain, spinal cord, and other organs. The procuring of Behcet's disease is often based on clinical manifestations and exclusion of other diseases. Although there is no specific test to confirm the diagnosis, imaging studies and blood tests can be used to help rule out alternative diagnoses. Medication to stifle the immune mechanism and lessen inflammation is typically used to treat Behcet's disease. The intensity of the symptoms and the organs that are affected determine the medication to be taken. Corticosteroids, immunosuppressive medications, and biologic pharmaceuticals are among the often-prescribed drugs. Behcet's disease must be continuously managed and observed because it is a chronic disorder. Although the condition cannot be cured, early detection and treatment can help control symptoms and avoid complications [40].

2.10.3 Cardiomyopathy

Cardiomyopathy is a medical condition that impairs the function of the heart muscle, leading to difficulty in pumping blood to other parts of the body. Cardiomyopathy can be dilated, hypertrophic, restricted, or arrhythmogenic in the right ventricular region. The most prevalent type is dilated cardiomyopathy, when the heart weakens and enlarges, making it less effective at pumping blood. Thickening of the heart muscle caused by hypertrophic cardiomyopathy makes it challenging for the heart to promote blood to the body's other organs. The heart's muscles harden as a result of restrictive cardiomyopathy, making it challenging for the heart to fill with blood. Rarely occurring arrhythmogenic right ventricular cardiomyopathy causes aberrant cardiac rhythms by replacing the heart muscle with scar tissue. Shortness of breath, exhaustion, swelling in the legs, feet, or abdomen, irregular heartbeats, chest pain, and fainting are some of the indications of cardiomyopathy. Some people might not exhibit any symptoms, especially in the beginning. A family history of cardiomyopathy, high blood pressure, diabetes, obesity, alcoholism, drug misuse, and specific infections including viral myocarditis are risk factors for the illness. Medication to enhance heart function, regulate heart rhythm, and prevent blood clots may be part of the treatment for cardiomyopathy. Surgery or a heart transplant may be required in extreme circumstances. A healthy weight, quitting smoking, consuming less alcohol and caffeine, and engaging in regular exercise can all help manage the illness [41].

2.10.4 Sarcoidosis

Sarcoidosis is a systemic autoimmune disease expressed by the development of protuberances (inflammatory cells) notably in the lungs, lymph nodes, and skin. Additionally, they can impact the eyes, liver, heart, spleen, nervous system, and other organs. The accurate cause of sarcoidosis is an abnormal immune response to an unknown trigger, such as an infection or environmental factor. Sarcoidosis can affect people of any age room, gender, or ethnicity, but it is general in people of African or Scandinavian descent and in women. The ubiquity of sarcoidosis varies widely reliant on the population studied, with an aggravated incidence in northern European and African American populations. Indications of sarcoidosis can depend on the organs affected but may include fatigue, shortness of breath, cough, skin rash, joint pain, and fever. In some cases, sarcoidosis can be asymptomatic and is identified incidentally on imaging studies done for other reasons. The appraisal of sarcoidosis can be strenuous, as there is no particular test to appraise the disease. It is usually based on a combination of clinical manifestations, imaging studies, and biopsy findings. Blood tests, pulmonary function tests, and imaging studies like chest X-ray, CT scan, and MRI can help in the diagnosis. Biopsy of affected organs, such as the lungs or skin, is often necessary to confirm the diagnosis. Treatment of sarcoidosis is reliant on the extent and harshness of the disease and the organs involved. In some cases, no treatment is necessary, as the disease may go into remission on its own. In other cases, treatment may include corticosteroids, immunosuppressive agents, and other medications to decrease inflammation and prevent organ damage. In rare cases, surgery is necessary to remove granulomas. The prognosis for sarcoidosis varies widely, with some people experiencing mild symptoms that do not require treatment, while others may have chronic disease that requires lifelong monitoring and treatment. In severe cases, sarcoidosis can lead to significant organ damage and even death [42].

2.10.5 Hepatic Autoimmune Disorders

Hepatic autoimmune disorders are a cluster of diseases that affect the liver and are caused by an abnormal immune response. The body's defence which normally protects the body from outsiders, mistakes healthy liver cells for outsider substances and attacks them. This causes inflammation and injury to the liver tissue, leading to various symptoms and complications. Symptoms of Autoimmune Disorders are mentioned in Fig. 6.

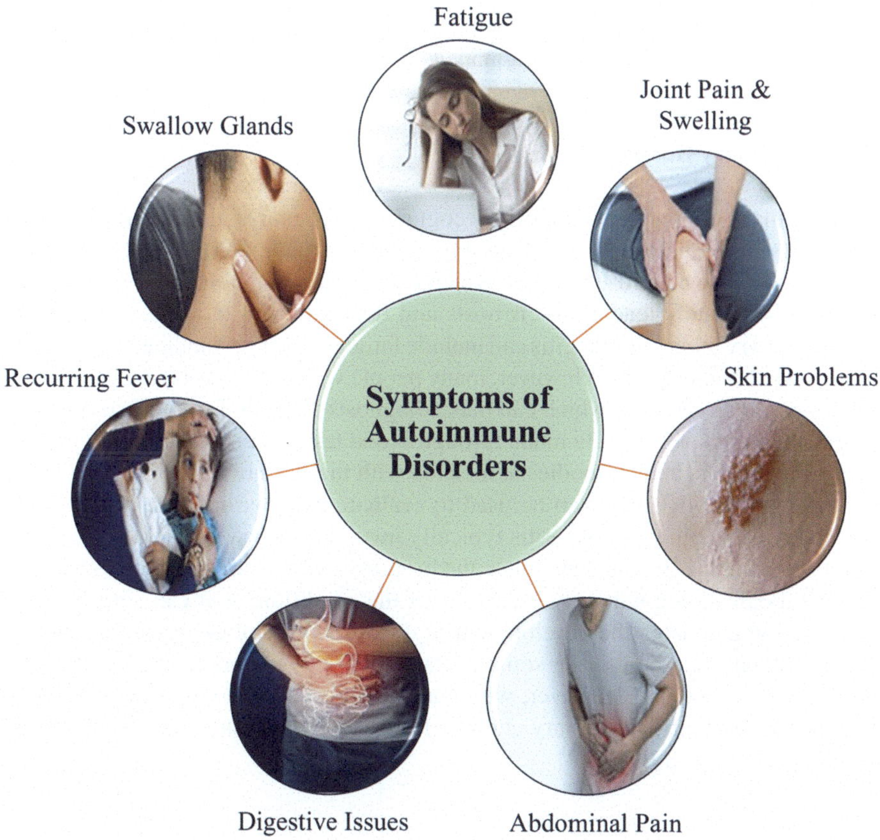

Fig. 6 Symptoms of autoimmune disorders

2.10.6 Autoimmune Hepatitis

Autoimmune hepatitis is a persistent liver disease that arises when the body's immune mechanism impacts liver cells, leading to soreness and damage. According to estimates, there are 1 to 2 cases of autoimmune hepatitis for every 100,000 individuals globally. Women are more influenced than males to have the condition. The condition can affect anyone at any age, more likely to 15–40 age group. Autoimmune hepatitis symptoms might range; however, they may include fatigue, nausea, joint pain, itching, and jaundice. If the illness is not treated, it may result in liver cirrhosis, liver failure, and even death. Blood testing, imaging tests, and liver biopsies are all used to diagnose autoimmune hepatitis. Immunosuppressive medications, like corticosteroids and azathioprine, are frequently used in treatment to suppress the immune system and lessen liver inflammation. A liver transplant might be required in specific circumstances. People with autoimmune hepatitis should seek ongoing medical attention, refrain from drinking alcohol, and take certain medications because they can worsen liver damage. Many patients with autoimmune hepatitis are able to live normal, healthy lives with the right care and management [43].

2.10.7 Primary Biliary Cholangitis

Primary biliary cholangitis, formerly recognized as primary biliary cirrhosis, is an autoimmune liver disease that leads to injury and destruction of the bile ducts in the liver. This leads to a build-up of bile, which causes inflammation and damage to the liver cells, ultimately leading to cirrhosis and liver failure if left untreated. Symptoms of primary biliary cholangitis can include fatigue, itching, jaundice, dry eyes and mouth, and abdominal pain. However, many people with the condition may not experience symptoms early on, which can make diagnosis difficult. Diagnosis of primary biliary cholangitis is typically made through blood tests that measure levels of liver enzymes, bilirubin, and antibodies associated with the condition. Imaging tests such as ultrasound or MRI may also be used to evaluate the liver and bile ducts. Treatment for primary biliary cholangitis typically involves medications that help reduce inflammation in the liver and attenuate the progress of the disease. Ursodeoxycholic acid is a medication commonly used to treat the condition, as it can help improve liver function and delay the development of cirrhosis. Immunosuppressants such as prednisone may also be used in some cases. In more advanced cases, a liver transplant may be necessary. However, with early diagnosis and appropriate treatment, many people with primary biliary cholangitis are able to manage the condition and live relatively normal lives [44].

2.10.8 Primary Sclerosing Cholangitis (PSC)

Primary sclerosing cholangitis (PSC) is a chronic liver disease that is rare and distinguished by inflammation, fibrosis, and strictures in the bile ducts. This results in hindered bile flow, causing damage to liver cells and leading to cirrhosis and liver failure in advanced cases. Both men and women can be affected by PSC, which typically manifests in individuals aged 30–50, although it can develop at any age, PSC is an autoimmune disease in which the body's immune mechanism erroneously targets the bile ducts, resulting in inflammation and scarring. PSC is frequently entwined with other autoimmune disorders, such as inflammatory bowel disease (IBD). Symptoms of PSC can vary, but typically include fatigue, itching, jaundice, and abdominal pain. As the disease progresses, complications such as cirrhosis, portal hypertension, and liver failure may develop. Diagnosis of PSC is often made through blood tests to assess liver function and imaging studies such as magnetic resonance cholangiopancreatography (MRCP) to evaluate the bile ducts. Liver biopsy may also be enacted to assure the diagnosis. There is currently no cure for Primary Sclerosing Cholangitis (PSC), and treatment is fixated on controlling symptoms and attenuating the progression of the disease. Medications such as ursodeoxycholic acid may be used to improve liver function and delay the need for liver transplantation. In advanced cases, liver transplantation may be necessary to prolong survival. Overall, the prognosis for PSC varies depending on the harmfulness of the disease during diagnosis and the effectiveness of treatment. Early detection and treatment are important in improving outcomes and preventing complications [45].

3 Discussion and Conclusion

Autoimmune disorders encompass a diverse array of diseases, each with unique characteristics. They arise from an overactive immune system that mistakenly attacks the body's own tissues. Common autoimmune disorders include rheumatoid arthritis, lupus, multiple sclerosis, and Type 1 diabetes. Symptoms vary widely depending on the disease but often include fatigue, joint pain, inflammation, and, in severe cases, organ damage. These disorders result from a complex interplay of genetic, environmental, and immunological factors. Genetic predisposition plays a significant role, but environmental factors like infections, toxins, and diet also contribute. Hormonal changes, stress, and gender influence risk. Lifestyle modifications, such as a balanced diet and stress management, can help reduce the risk of autoimmune disorders in individuals with genetic susceptibility.

In conclusion, autoimmune disorders are a diverse group of diseases with complex origins. Early diagnosis and personalized treatment strategies are becoming more feasible due to advancements in genetic research. Increased awareness among healthcare professionals and the public is vital for timely intervention. Collaboration between researchers, healthcare providers, and patients is essential for advancing our understanding of autoimmune disorders. Expectations for the future include targeted therapies and improved management. Continued research will lead to better outcomes and improved quality of life for those affected by autoimmune disorders.

References

1. Vernino S (2020) Autoimmune autonomic disorders. CONTINUUM: Lifelong Learn Neurol 26(1):44–57.
2. Barthel A, Benker G, Berens K, Diederich S, Manfras B, Gruber M, Kanczkowski W, Kline G, Kamvissi-Lorenz V, Hahner S, Beuschlein F, Brennand A, Boehm BO, Torpy DJ, Bornstein SR (2019) An update on addison's disease. Exp Clin Endocrinol Diabetes 127(2–03):165–175. https://doi.org/10.1055/a-0804-2715. Epub 2018 Dec 18 PMID: 30562824
3. Weetman AP (2021) An update on the pathogenesis of Hashimoto's thyroiditis. J Endocrinol Invest 44:883–890
4. Lui DTW, Lee KK, Lee CH, Lee ACH, Hung IFN, Tan KCB (2021) Development of Graves' disease after SARS-CoV-2 mRNA vaccination: a case report and literature review. Front Public Health 23(9):778964. https://doi.org/10.3389/fpubh.2021.778964.PMID:34888290;PMCID: PMC8650637
5. Chang JT (2020) Pathophysiology of inflammatory bowel diseases. N Engl J Med 383(27):2652–2664. https://doi.org/10.1056/NEJMra2002697. PMID: 33382932

6. Roda G, Chien Ng S, Kotze PG, Argollo M, Panaccione R, Spinelli A, Kaser A, Peyrin-Biroulet L, Danese S (2020) Crohn's disease. Nat Rev Dis Primers 6(1):22. https://doi.org/10.1038/s41572-020-0156-2. (Erratum in: Nat Rev Dis Primers. 2020 Apr 6;6(1):26. Erratum in: Nat Rev Dis Primers. 2020 May 20;6(1):42. Erratum in: Nat Rev Dis Primers. 2020 Jun 19;6(1):51. PMID: 32242028)
7. Raine T, Bonovas S, Burisch J, Kucharzik T, Adamina M, Annese V, Bachmann O, Bettenworth D, Chaparro M, Czuber-Dochan W, Eder P (2022) ECCO guidelines on therapeutics in ulcerative colitis: medical treatment. J Crohns Colitis 16(1):2–17
8. Jacobo P (2018) The role of regulatory T Cells in autoimmune orchitis. Andrologia 50(11):e13092
9. Jacob S, Koc M (2015) Autoimmune oophoritis: a rarely encountered ovarian lesion. Indian J Pathol Microbiol 58(2):249
10. Berentsen S (2021) How I treat cold agglutinin disease. Blood J Am Soc Hematol 137(10):1295–1303
11. Gabelli M, Ademokun C, Cooper N, Amrolia PI (2022) Pathogenesis, risk factors and therapeutic options for autoimmune haemolytic anaemia in the post-transplant setting. Br J Haematol 196(1):45–62
12. Vaillant AJ, Gupta N (2023) ITP-immune thrombocytopenic purpura. StatPearls. (6 May 2023)
13. Hwang MC, Ridley L, Reveille JD (2021) Ankylosing spondylitis risk factors: a systematic literature review. Clin Rheumatol 40:3079–3093
14. Aguinaga MDLAG, Martinez FL, Ramos MADLG, Arana HLM, Zuniga LMV, Cepeda SEN, Alcala AED, Soto JMS (2022) Sjogren's syndrome, an update. Int J Appl Dental Sci 2022:1–5
15. Calderon LM, Pope JE (2021) Scleroderma epidemiology update. Curr Opin Rheumatol 33(2):122–127
16. Zhao M, Wu J, Wu H, Sawalha AH, Lu Q (2022) Clinical treatment options in scleroderma: recommendations and comprehensive review. Clin Rev Allergy Immunol 1:1–9
17. Bentaleb I, Abdelghani KB, Rostom S, Amine B, Laatar A, Bahiri R (2020) Reactive arthritis: update. Curr Clin Microbiol Rep 7:124–132
18. Basta F, Fasola F, Triantafyllias K, Schwarting A (2020) Systemic lupus erythematosus (SLE) therapy: the old and the new. Rheumatol Therapy. 7(3):433–446
19. Huang S, Kronzer VL, Dellaripa PF, Deane KD, Bolster MB, Nagaraja V, Khanna D, Doyle TJ, Sparks JA (2020) Rheumatoid arthritis–associated interstitial lung disease: current update on prevalence, risk factors, and pharmacologic treatment. Curr Treat Options Rheumatol 6:337–353
20. Thakur S, Riyaz B, Patil A, Kaur A, Kapoor B, Mishra V (2018) Novel drug delivery systems for NSAIDs in management of rheumatoid arthritis: an overview. Biomed Pharmacother 1(106):1011–1023
21. Ferreira JF, Mohamed AA, Emery P (2016) Glucocorticoids and rheumatoid arthritis. Rheum Dis Clin 42(1):33–46
22. Köhler BM, Günther J, Kaudewitz D, Lorenz HM (2019) Current therapeutic options in the treatment of rheumatoid arthritis. J Clin Med 8(7):938
23. Gaffo A, Saag KG, Curtis JR (2006) Treatment of rheumatoid arthritis. Am J Health Syst Pharm 63(24):2451–2465
24. Chehade L, Jaafar ZA, El Masri D, Zmerly H, Kreidieh D, Tannir H, Itani L, El Ghoch M (2019) Lifestyle modification in rheumatoid arthritis: dietary and physical activity recommendations based on evidence. Curr Rheumatol Rev 15(3):209–214
25. Küçükdeveci AA (2019) Nonpharmacological treatment in established rheumatoid arthritis. Best Pract Res Clin Rheumatol 33(5):101482
26. Hammond A, Jones V, Prior Y (2016) The effects of compression gloves on hand symptoms and hand function in rheumatoid arthritis and hand osteoarthritis: a systematic review. Clin Rehabil 30(3):213–224
27. Philippou E, Petersson SD, Rodomar C, Nikiphorou E (2021) Rheumatoid arthritis and dietary interventions: systematic review of clinical trials. Nutr Rev 79(4):410–428

28. Friedman MA, Winthrop K (2016) Vaccinations for rheumatoid arthritis. Curr Opin Rheumatol 28(3):330–336
29. Hauser SL, Cree BA (2020) Treatment of multiple sclerosis: a review. Am J Med 133(12):1380–1390
30. Shahrizaila N, Lehmann HC, Kuwabara S (2021) Guillain-Barré syndrome. The Lancet 397(10280):1214–1228
31. Pinedo-Torres I, Paz-Ibarra JL (2018) Current knowledge on Hashimoto's encephalopathy: a literature review. Medwave 18(06)
32. Bubuioc AM, Kudebayeva A, Turuspekova S, Lisnic V, Leone MA (2021) The epidemiology of myasthenia gravis. J Med Life 14(1):7
33. Schonberg S, Stokkermans TJ (2023) Ocular pemphigoid. In: StatPearls. StatPearls Publishing
34. van Laar J (2020) Current insights in the pathogenesis of scleritis. Experimental Eye Res
35. Hellmark T, Segelmark M (2014) Diagnosis and classification of Goodpasture's disease (anti-GBM). J Autoimmun 1(48):108–112
36. Zhou C, Li X, Wang C, Zhang J (2021) Alopecia areata: an update on etiopathogenesis, diagnosis, and management. Clin Rev Allergy Immunol 61(3):403–423
37. Salmi TT (2019) Dermatitis herpetiformis. Clin Exp Dermatol 44(7):728–731
38. Lipatov IS, Tezikov YV, Ovchinnikova MA (2020) Efficiency of gestational and perinatal pathology prevention with a cytokine-like peptide in frequently recurring herpes at the pregravid stage. Obstet Gynecol 15(1):94–102
39. Schwotzer R, Flammer AJ, Gerull S, Pabst T, Arosio P, Averaimo M, Bacher VU, Bode P, Cavalli A, Concoluci A, Dirnhofer S (2020) Expert recommendation from the Swiss Amyloidosis Network (SAN) for systemic AL-amyloidosis. Swiss Med Wkly 150:w20364
40. Davatchi F (2018) Behçet's disease. Int J Rheum Dis 21(12):2057–2058. https://doi.org/10.1111/1756-185X.13465. PMID: 30681276
41. Brieler JA, Breeden MA, Tucker J (2017) Cardiomyopathy: an overview. Am Fam Physician 96(10):640–646
42. Tabukashvili R, Kapetivadze V, Kuparadze M, Avaliani I, Maglapheridze Z, Lazashvili T, Kapetivadze I (2023) Sarcoidosis with prolonged remission–a clinical case report. Exp Clin Med Georg (1)
43. Komori A (2021) Recent updates on the management of autoimmune hepatitis. Clin Mol Hepatol 27(1):58
44. Lleo A, Wang GQ, Gershwin ME, Hirschfield GM (2020) Primary biliary cholangitis. The Lancet 396(10266):1915–1926
45. Dyson JK, Beuers U, Jones DEJ, Lohse AW, Hudson M (2018) Primary sclerosing cholangitis. Lancet 391(10139):2547–2559. https://doi.org/10.1016/S0140-6736(18)30300-3. Epub 2018 Feb 13 PMID: 29452711

Autoimmune Diseases: Recent Insights on Epidemiology, Pathogenesis, and Prevalence Rate

Gunjan Nautiyal, Isha Sharma, Parijat Pandey, and Shiv Kant Sharma

Abstract Autoimmune diseases (ADs) represent a complex condition for a variety of painful syndromes including malfunction of the body's immune system. It is characterized as the emergence of a body's defense system response against an unknown trigger, manifested as autoantibodies and T cell responses toward its own structures. In ADs, the inflammation becomes chronic, causing pain and severe damage to the tissues involved. Many autoimmune disorders have been strongly associated with genetic predisposition and/or environmental factors. Nearly 4% of the worldwide population is affected by more than 80 different types of ADs, which encompass both systemic and tissue-specific ailments including, systemic lupus erythematosus, insulin-dependent diabetes mellitus, autoimmune hepatitis, rheumatoid arthritis, thyroiditis, Crohn's disease, psoriasis, multiple sclerosis, etc.; with a higher prevalence rate in women in comparison to men. Till now, there is no specific cause associated with ADs reported; they only show patterns of remission and recurrence. They are difficult to diagnose because the specific disorders have numerous possible symptoms and individual symptoms vary. Treatment for autoimmune diseases generally focuses on reducing the immune system's activity. This chapter explores numerous autoimmune disease, their epidemiology, and prevalence rate, concluding with a brief overview of pathogenesis as well as new treatment approaches.

Keywords Autoimmune disorders · Immune system · Prevalence · Rheumatoid arthritis · Pathogenesis

1 Introduction

The network of cells and tissues that protects humans from viruses, germs, and illness is known as a person's immune system. It makes an attempt to track down, neutralize, and eliminate any stimulus that may cause injuries to people [1]. The

G. Nautiyal · I. Sharma · P. Pandey · S. K. Sharma (✉)
Department of Pharmaceutical Sciences, Gurugram University, Gurugram 122003, India
e-mail: shivkantvats@gmail.com

K. Raza and S. Singh (eds.), *Artificial Intelligence and Autoimmune Diseases*, Studies in Computational Intelligence 1133, https://doi.org/10.1007/978-981-99-9029-0_2

body's immune system protects it against illness and infection. Autoimmune disorders (ADs) refer to a group of medical conditions in which the immune system is not able to distinguish between foreign antigens and healthy cells in the body, mistaking them for these potential infectious antigens. Any region of the body might be affected by these attacks, which can degrade physical function or even become life-threatening. This mechanism of self-attack of the immune system to the host body might be determined via the theoretical framework of molecular mimicry. In the context of a healthy individual, the person's immune system fights against foreign invaders, alongside developing a reaction in accordance with them. While, in the situation of people suffering from autoimmunity ailments, the immune system is incapable of recognizing its own body's cells and mistakes them by mimicking them as foreign antigens. Molecular mimicry represents a phenomenon wherein an external antigen shares structural similarities with self-antigens (Fig. 1). Though the relationship between molecular mimicry and autoimmune disorders is still being studied, it is considered a key mechanism involved in triggering autoimmunity [2]. ADs can cause a range of symptoms, self-destructing attacks, and autoimmune reactions that range from mild to life-threatening and can present differently depending on the type of disorder and the age of onset. It is estimated that there are nearly 100 different types of immune-mediated illnesses present in a small minority, affecting approximately 20% of the global population. Around 80% of AD predominantly affects the female population [3, 4]. This chapter contains updated information on their epidemiology, pathogenesis, and prevalence rates. The chapter discusses the most recent research and findings, providing a comprehensive overview of the field's current state of knowledge. It sheds light on the factors that influence the development of autoimmune diseases and highlights the prevalence rates of various conditions, providing researchers, clinicians, and patients with valuable information.

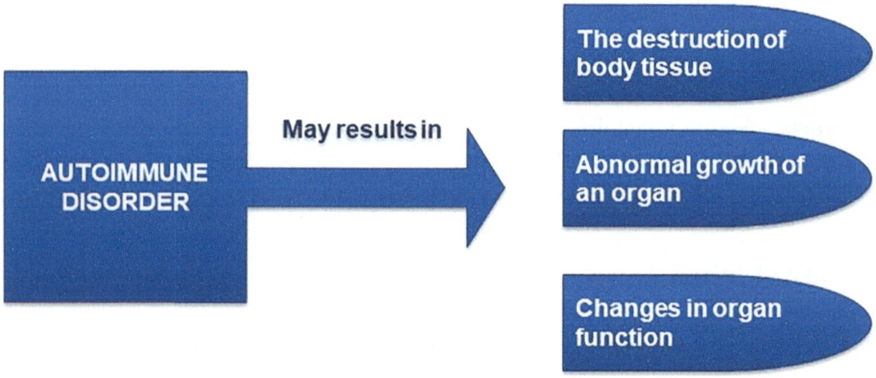

Fig. 1 Key mechanisms in the progression of autoimmune disorders

1.1 Common Symptoms for Various Autoimmune Disorders

Autoimmune medical conditions are a category of disorders in which the immune system assaults the body's self-tissues or organs. It is important to note that the symptoms of autoimmune diseases can vary greatly from person to person, and some people may experience only mild symptoms while others may have more severe symptoms. One of the hallmark symptoms is chronic inflammation, which often leads to pain, swelling, and redness in the affected tissues. Fatigue is another prevalent symptom, as the immune system's constant activity can be draining. Many autoimmune disorders also share symptoms like fever, joint pain, and muscle weakness, which can result from the immune system's attack on joints and muscles. Additionally, skin problems such as rashes, ulcers, and changes in pigmentation can be common, as can gastrointestinal symptoms like abdominal pain, diarrhea, and malabsorption of nutrients. Furthermore, ADs may affect the endocrine system, leading to hormone imbalances and resulting in symptoms like weight changes, mood swings, and changes in blood pressure. Neurological symptoms, including cognitive impairment, headaches, and numbness or tingling in extremities, can also occur due to autoimmune attacks on the nervous system.

If people are experiencing any of these symptoms, it is important to talk to the doctor for an accurate diagnosis and appropriate treatment [4]. The clinical manifestations of autoimmune diseases differ based on the type of disease, but a few common indications have been represented in Fig. 2.

Even while autoimmune diseases come in many different forms, many of them have comparable symptoms. The above-shown symptoms are typical signs of autoimmune disease. Numerous autoimmune diseases impact several bodily parts. The signs and indications vary depending on which region(s) of the body get impacted, such as:

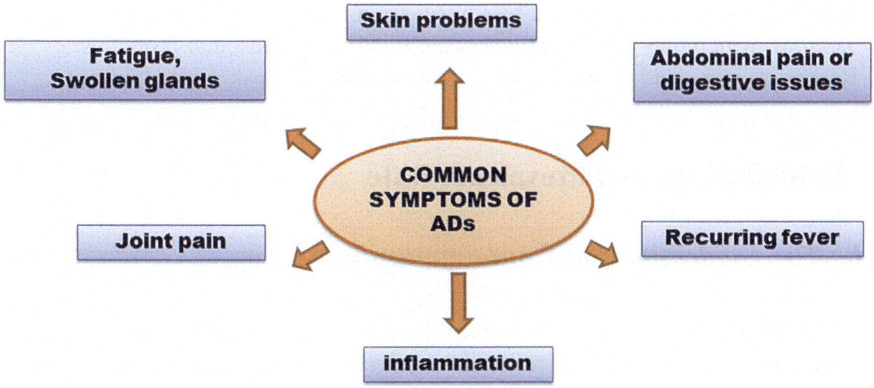

Fig. 2 Common symptoms of Autoimmune Disorders (ADs)

Table 1 Symptoms in relevance to particular Autoimmune Disorder

S.no	Autoimmune disorders	Symptoms
1.	Rheumatoid arthritis	Joint symptoms such as swelling, warmth, discomfort, and stiffness. While RA most typically affects people as they become older, it can begin as early as your 30 s
2.	Psoriasis	Skin cells to develop and then shed when no longer needed. Excessive multiplication of skin cells. Extra cells accumulate and develop inflammatory areas. It may look purple or dark brown with grey scales on darker skin tones
3.	Multiple sclerosis	Numbness, weakness, balance issues, and difficulty walking
4.	Intestinal bowel syndrome	Joint pain, kidney pain, brain pain, heart pain, joint pain, exhaustion, rashes, diarrhea, stomach discomfort, and ulcer bleeding
5.	Addison's disease	Weakness, exhaustion, weight loss, and low blood sugar
6.	Graves' illness	High heart rate (tachycardia), heat intolerance, accidental weight loss, and enlargement of the thyroid gland (goitre). Rarely include skin (Graves' dermopathy) or eye (Graves' ophthalmopathy) symptoms
7.	Hashimoto's thyroiditis	Weight gain, sensitivity to cold, weariness, hair loss, and thyroid swelling (goitre)
8.	Myasthenia gravis	Eye motions, opening and shutting eyelids, swallowing, and facial movements can all be affected by muscle weakness
9.	Celiac disease	Stomach difficulties after ingesting gluten. May cause nausea, vomiting, diarrhea, constipation, and abdominal bleeding
10.	Pernicious anemia	Lack of blood cell formation results in weariness, weakness, and headaches

- Joint discomfort, stiffness, and loss of function are possible outcomes.
- Thyroid, which may trigger fatigue, weight gain, and muscular problems.
- Rashes, blisters, and color changes on the surface of the skin [5] (Table 1).

2 Epidemiology and Prevalence Rate

2.1 The Epidemiology of Autoimmunity

Historically, autoimmune disorders were thought to be rare or less prevalent, but comprehensive epidemiological research revealed that their impact on mortality and morbidity is considerable. Autoimmunity has now been found to affect roughly 3–5% of the global population. Despite huge progress through the detection as well as management of autoimmune illnesses, evidence on the etiological processes that ultimately result in pathological findings remains limited. Epidemiological studies have indicated ADs to be the 10th most common cause of mortality in developing countries [6, 7].

2.2 Prevalence Rate

Nearly 4% of the global population is afflicted with one of over eighty distinct autoimmune diseases, among which the most common are type 1 diabetes, rheumatoid arthritis, multiple sclerosis, lupus, Crohn's syndrome, psoriasis, and sclerosis [7]. The incidence and frequency of ADs varied. Whenever differences in ages, sexes, ethnic backgrounds, and numerous other social variables are examined, geoepidemiology becomes more complicated. ADs can develop at any age, although each disease has a distinct age of start. In almost all cases, the frequency is higher in immediate family members and significantly greater in twins with monozygotic DNA. Women have a higher prevalence of ADs, with a proportion of women to men that varies between 10:1 and 1:1, except Crohn's disease having a gender ratio of 1: 1.2. The sex prejudice of ADs has received a great deal of research, yet it remains unsolved [8].

Multiple sclerosis (MS), for example, is distributed inconsistently around the globe, with incidence ranging from 5 cases/100,000 people in tropical areas and Asia to greater than 200 cases/ 100,000 people in temperate regions. MS is estimated to affect 0.8–8.7 people/100,000 in Europe, 2.7–7.5 people throughout North America, and 0.7–3.6 people in Asia and the Middle East [9]. The average prevalence of T1D in European, American, and Chinese populations is 5–10, 10–20, and 1/100 000 individuals yearly, respectively. The prevalence of coeliac disease (CeD) in the UK increased from 5.2 to 19.1/100,000 person-years between 1990 and 2011 (10). However, between 1999 and 2012, there was a 1.8% yearly drop in the incidence of SLE in the UK, whereas the prevalence climbed from 64.99 to 97.04 per 100,000 people each year. The global prevalence of rheumatoid arthritis (RA) was estimated to be 0.24% in 2010, substantially unchanged from the incidence rate of 0.25% in year 1990 [10]. Conventional geo-epidemiological investigations revealed that gene level vulnerability and surrounding variables are the primary associated risk traits for declined tolerance [11] (Table 2).

The prevalence of ADs varies depending on the specific condition and geographic location, as follows. ADs are more common in women than in men. This gender difference is seen across many ADs, including lupus, rheumatoid arthritis, multiple sclerosis, and Sjogren's syndrome. The reason for this gender difference is not fully understood, but it is thought to be related to hormonal and genetic factors. ADs can occur at any age, but some conditions are more common in certain age groups. For example, juvenile idiopathic arthritis is the most common type of arthritis in children, while rheumatoid arthritis is more common in adults over the age of 40. Multiple sclerosis typically affects people between the ages of 20 and 40. The prevalence of these diseases also greatly varies by ethnicity. For example, lupus is more familiar in African American, Hispanic, and Asian women which are among white women.

Table 2 Worldwide prevalence of various Autoimmune Disorders [12, 13]

S.no	Target organ	Autoimmune diseases	Worldwide prevalence rate (Approximate ratio)
1	Joints	Rheumatoid arthritis	0.5–1%
		Axial spondyloarthritis	0.3%
		Psoriatic arthritis	0.06–0.25%
2	Muscles	Myasthenia gravis	0.02%
		Polymyositis	0.007%
3	Skin	Systemic lupus erythematosus	0.2–3%
		Psoriasis	2–3%
		Vitiligo	0.5–1%
		Pemphigus vulgaris	0.01%
4	Hairs	Alopecia areata	0.1%
5	Gastrointestinal tract	Celiac disease	0.7%
		Inflammatory bowel syndrome	6.8 Million
		Ulcerative colitis	0.2–0.4%
		Crohn's disease	0.2–0.3%
		Autoimmune gastritis	Uncertain
6	Liver	Autoimmune hepatitis	17.7%
		Primary biliary cholangitis	0.03%
7	Central nervous system	Multiple sclerosis	<0.1%
		Narcolepsy	0.03%
		Neuromyelitis optica	0.004%
		Guillian-barre syndrome	0.16–3%
		Chronic inflammatory demyelinating polyneuropathy	1.5–3. 6 Million
8	Endocrine + Exocrine Glands	Type 1 diabetes mellitus	0.4%
		Hashimoto's disease/ hypothyroidism	0.1–2%
		Graves' disease	0.5%
		Sjogren's syndrome	0.2–1%
9	Kidney	Lupus nephritis	0.008–0.2%
		Goodpasture syndrome	0.0001–0.001%
10	Reproductive Organs	Autoimmune orchitis	Uncertain
		Autoimmune oophoritis	Uncertain

Type 1 diabetes is more common in white people and Hispanic populations rather than African Americans and Asian Americans. Several environmental factors such as infections, medications, and exposure to toxins may play a role in the development of ADs. For example, infections with certain viruses such as the Epstein–Barr virus have been linked to an increased risk of developing lupus. Exposure to certain medications such as procainamide and hydralazine has been linked to the development of drug-induced lupus [14, 15].

3 Pathogenesis of Autoimmune Diseases

Researchers are unaware of the precise origins of autoimmune illness, although numerous ideas point to an overactive immune system attacking the body following an infection or damage. The exact cause of ADs is not fully understood, but several factors may contribute to their development, including genetic predisposition, environmental triggers, and dysregulation of the immune system Fig. 3 [16].

Autoimmune illness is caused by a combination of an individual's genetic makeup and the effects of environmental factors such as warm temperatures, infections, drugs, and environmental toxins. The vague nature of this set of conditions, however, indicates our lack of understanding of the etiology of many disorders. Except for a few rare disorders, the onset event(s) of most ADs has not been well characterized.

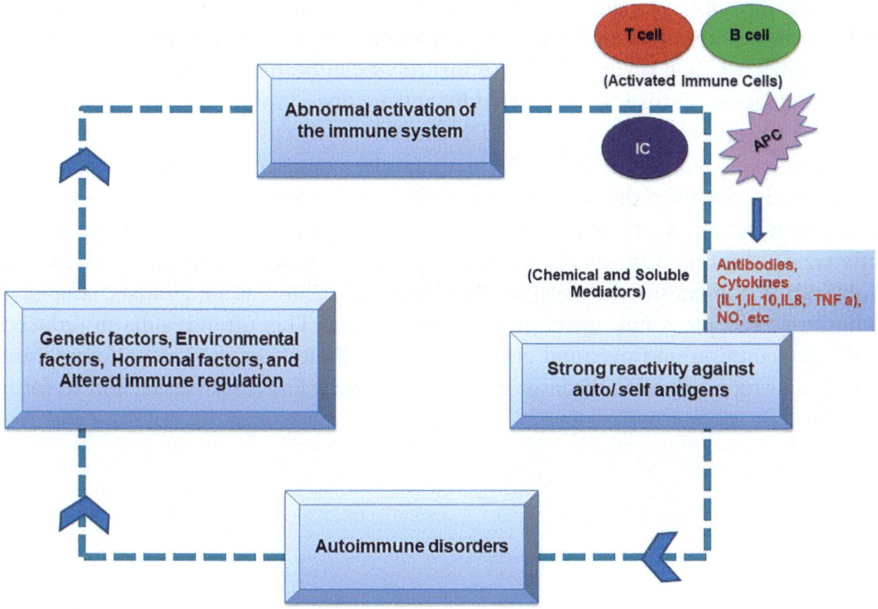

Fig. 3 Pathogenesis of autoimmune disease

There are various plausible explanations for the emergence of autoimmune illnesses, and autoimmunity is most likely caused by a combination of variables. Evidence currently shows that regulatory T and B cells are critical in maintaining tolerance and preventing autoimmune reactions. The regulatory T cells are especially crucial for suppressing autoreactive T cells which enter the thymus after not being destroyed during thymic selection (see T Lymphocytes and Cellular Immunity). Furthermore, antigen mimicry between pathogen antigens and self-antigens can result in cross-reactivity and autoimmunity. Trauma, pharmacological combinations, or disease states can all expose hidden self-antigens, triggering an autoimmune reaction. All of these variables may have a role in autoimmunity. Finally, tissue and organ damage in the autoimmune disease state is caused by inappropriate inflammatory responses that must be treated (Table 3).

4 Target Organs Affected by Several Autoimmune Disorders

There are two types of autoimmune diseases: organ-specific and systemic. An organ-specific disease is one in which the immune system responds to antigens in a particular organ. These are diseases in which autoantibodies are created that target just the tissue of a specific organ, hence harming only that organ. Addison's disease, autoimmune hemolytic anemia, Goodpasture syndrome, Graves' disease, Hashimoto's thyroiditis, idiopathic thrombocytopenic purpura, insulin-dependent diabetes mellitus, myasthenia gravis, pernicious anemia, post-streptococcal glomerulonephritis, and others are examples of such disorders. These disorders can be further classified based on tissue damage as (a) diseases mediated by cell-mediated immunity and (b) diseases mediated by autoantibodies. MS, HTS, Addison's disease, and other conditions are examples. Similarly, diseases are mediated by autoantibody activity. Similarly, autoantibody-mediated diseases include antibodies that behave as agonists, attaching to hormone receptors in place of the usual ligand and promoting inappropriate activity. This frequently results in an excess of mediators or an increase in cell proliferation. Autoantibodies, on the other hand, can behave as antagonists, attaching to hormone receptors but preventing receptor action. This often results in reduced mediator secretion and eventual atrophy of the afflicted organ. The following are some major representative diseases in this group: MG, Graves' disease, and so forth (Fig. 4).

Table 3 Some common mechanisms that can contribute to the development of autoimmune disorders [3, 17–19]

S.no	Factors associated	Key Mechanism
1	Genetic factors	Certain genes may be associated with a higher likelihood of developing autoimmune disorders. These genes could be interfering with the immune system's ability to distinguish between self and non-self, resulting in the production of autoantibodies that can attack healthy tissues
2	Dysregulation of the immune system	The immune system is complex and involves multiple cells and molecules that work together to fight off infections and maintain tissue homeostasis. Dysregulation of the immune system, such as an imbalance between different types of immune cells or defects in immune signaling pathways, can lead to the development of autoimmune disorders
3	Environmental triggers	Environmental factors such as infections, toxins, and stress can trigger autoimmune disorders. For example, viral infections such as Epstein–Barr virus and cytomegalovirus have been linked to the development of multiple sclerosis and lupus
4	Epigenetic modifications	Epigenetic modifications such as DNA methylation, histone modification, and microRNA expression can affect the expression of genes involved in immune regulation and contribute to the development of autoimmune disorders
5	Molecular mimicry	In some cases, the immune system may mistakenly recognize a self-antigen as foreign due to its similarity to a pathogen. This can occur when a pathogen shares a similar amino acid sequence with a self-antigen, leading to the production of autoantibodies that attack both the pathogen and healthy tissues

5 Prevalence of the Most Common Autoimmune Diseases

5.1 Rheumatoid Arthritis

Rheumatoid arthritis (RA) is the most prevalent kind of chronic inflammatory arthritis, affecting around 1% of the population. RA etiology is complicated, with various genetic, environmental, immunologic, and other variables all contributing to disease development and manifestation. It is triggered by intricate connections among genes and the external environment, resulting in a symmetric breakdown of

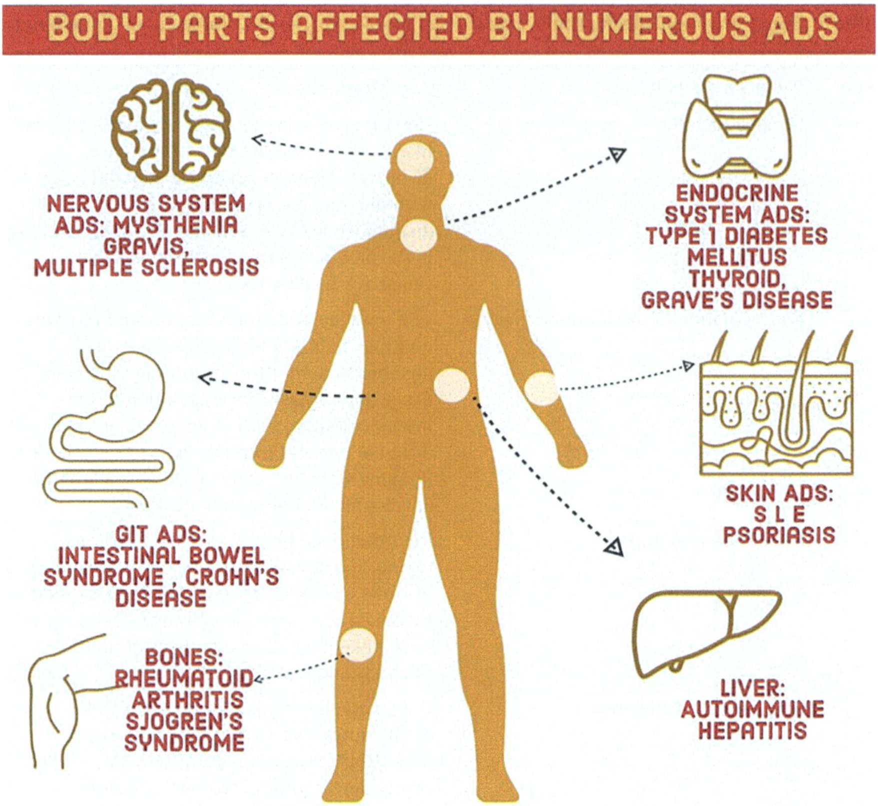

Fig. 4 Body parts affected by numerous Autoimmune Disorders (ADs)

immune tolerance and synovial inflammatory conditions. Inflammation and matrix breakdown, accompanied by cartilage and bone loss, are accelerated and monitored via different mechanisms. Given the variable response to medication, it is obvious that RA is not a single illness; rather, various routes can lead to auto-reactivity and synovial inflammation, resulting in clinical presentations that are comparable [20–23].

Early RA is characterized by prompt reactions to a restricted amount of self-antigenic substances along with minimal generalized inflammation, which is accompanied by a development of growing natural and adaptive reactions and injury to tissues over time as long as a certain level is crossed and medically visible RA occurs. The immune system produces antibodies, which stick to the interior linings of joints. Inflammatory pain, swelling, and discomfort result from immune system cells assaulting the joints. If untreated, rheumatoid arthritis causes irreversible joint degeneration. Rheumatoid arthritis treatments may include a variety of either oral or injection-based drugs that suppress the body's immune system's overactivity [24].

Table 3 shows the prevalence rate of RA, it was found to be higher in North America, Western Europe, and the Caribbean, and relatively lower in Southeast Asia, Oceania, and Western Sub-Saharan Africa [25].

5.2 *Systemic Lupus Erythematosus (Lupus)*

Systemic lupus erythematosus (SLE) is an autoimmune disease that can affect the layers of skin, joints, central nervous system, and the renal system. Women of reproductive maturity and certain racial groups have a greater likelihood of being infected. SLE is closely related to extremely uncommon, inherited, single-gene complement deficiencies, despite the fact that the illness is polygenic in nature in most people. The condition may develop due to genetic connections with socio-environmental variables, particularly exposure to UV radiation, and Epstein–Barr virus exposure, along with hormonal aspects, resulting in immunological dysregulation at the cytokine, T cell, B cell, and macrophage levels. Because of the broad spectrum of SLE, screening is essentially medical, therefore it remains challenging. Despite the fact that classification criteria have improved clinical trials, only one medication (belimumab) was officially approved for SLE therapy in the sixty years since its discovery. A decade rate of mortality has declined, as well as the toxic side effects of earlier treatments such as cyclophosphamide and glucocorticoids were mitigated in part via novel therapies such as mycophenolate mofetil and glucocorticoid-sparing therapies. Patients with lupus develop autoimmune antibodies which may adhere to tissues located throughout the body. Lupus frequently triggers damage to the joints, lung function, and cells in the bloodstream, nerve endings, and kidneys. Prednisone, a steroid that inhibits immune system exertion, is often prescribed as a form of medication [26–29].

5.3 *Inflammatory Bowel Disease*

Diarrhea, hemorrhaging from the rectal area, frequent stool movements, discomfort in the abdomen, a high fever, and diminished appetite are all symptoms of the immune system attacking the gastrointestinal lining. Inflammatory Bowel Disease (IBD) is a persistent inflammatory gastroenteritis that is divided into Crohn's disease and ulcerative colitis. It happens to genetically susceptible individuals as a result of overly aggressive immune reactions to common stimuli such as food or gut bacteria. This exercise discusses the examination and management of inflammatory bowel disease, as well as the role of the interprofessional team in providing better care to individuals with this illness. IBD is characterized by frequent bouts of inflammation in the gastrointestinal tract induced by an inappropriate immune reaction to certain gut bacteria. The concept of "inflammatory bowel disease" refers to two distinct kinds of idiopathic gastrointestinal conditions that differ in their place of origin and degree of colon wall engagement. Ulcerative colitis and Crohn's disease are the two most prevalent kinds of IBD. Ulcerative colitis (UC) has been characterized by widespread intestinal mucosal inflammatory conditions. Proctitis (rectum) is the most common complication of UC, however, it may additionally have an impact on the sigmoid (proctosigmoiditis), beyond the sigmoid (distal ulcerative colitis), or the entire colon (pancolitis). Crohn's disease (CD), generates transmural ulceration of any region of the gastrointestinal tract (GI), more frequently of the terminal ileum along with the colon. These two disorders are categorized based on level of severity (mild, moderate, or severe) as well as location. The CD is further characterized by its phenotypic features that may include inflammatory, structuring, or penetrating. Extraintestinal signs and indications develop in both CD and UC. Even though the medical conditions are capable of being recognized by the vast majority of individuals, in no fewer than 10% of cases, the symptoms are sufficiently similar that the two disorders cannot be separated at first. Immunosuppressive medications, both oral and injectable, can be used to treat IBD [30–32].

5.4 Multiple Sclerosis

Multiple sclerosis (MS) is an autoimmune, inflamed neurological disorder that affects the central nervous system (CNS). MS wreaks havoc on the CNS's myelinated axons, causing varying degrees of damage to both the myelin as well as the axons. MS progression is unpredictable and extremely variable. The majority of patients experience transient psychological issues that are frequently accompanied by steady neurological deterioration. The immune system destroys nerve cells, resulting in pain, blindness, paralysis, poor coordination, and muscular spasms. Greater than 30% of people suffering from MS face modest-to-grievous spastic movements, primarily in their legs. The most prevalent sensory abnormalities in MS patients include paresthesias (numbness and tingling), dysesthesias (burning and "pins and needles"), diplopia, ataxia, vertigo, and bladder (urinary sphincter) difficulties. A common symptom of MS is unilateral numbness affecting one leg that spreads to engulf the second leg and climbs to the pelvis, abdomen, or chest. Sensory abnormalities normally resolve on their own, although they can sometimes progress to persistent neuropathic pain. Trigeminal neuralgia is also a possibility. Optic neuritis is another typical presenting indication of MS, characterized by full or partial visual loss. Over ninety percent of people with MS suffer from bladder dysfunction, which results in incontinence on a weekly or more frequent basis. Constipation affects at least 30% of patients. Fatigue is the most frequent work-related impairment associated with MS, affecting 90% of patients. Sexual issues are rather prevalent. In persons with MS, disease-modifying treatment aims to reduce the length and frequency of acute exacerbations while also providing symptomatic relief. There are presently no FDA-approved medicines for MS that are curative [33–35].

5.5 *Type 1 Diabetes Mellitus*

Type 1 diabetes mellitus (T1DM) is an autoimmune disease in which immune system antibodies attack and damage pancreatic insulin-producing beta cells. When people with type 1 diabetes (T1D) are initially diagnosed, they need insulin injections to survive. T1D involves metabolic, genetic, and immunogenetic diversity, as well as age-related variations, necessitating a tailored treatment plan for each patient. Insulin secretion can cease abruptly or gradually. Adult-onset T1D has greater levels of residual insulin production (detectable/higher c-peptide), but youth-onset T1D has higher levels of diabetic ketoacidosis. A higher level of detectable c-peptide is linked to improved glycemic management. Other autoimmune illnesses, obesity, comorbidities, and the emergence of diabetes-related complications are also prevalent. Individuals with T1D need insulin replacement for the remainder of their lives, which can be accomplished by many daily insulin injections, insulin pump therapy, or the use of an automated insulin delivery system. Diabetic ketoacidosis (DKA) is a potentially lethal condition that arises in the absence of insulin. In addition to insulin therapy, glucose monitoring using (preferably) a continuous glucose monitor (CGM) and a blood glucose monitor if a CGM is not available is recommended. Monitoring, insulin administration, ketone testing, when necessary, food, including carbohydrate estimates, physical activity, ways to avoid and treat hypoglycemia, and sick day restrictions should all be included in self-management instruction and support. Psychosocial concerns must also be identified and treated. Finland and Italy have the highest occurrence rates, while South America has the lowest [36–42].

5.6 *Guillain–Barré Syndrome*

Guillain–Barré syndrome (GBS) is an uncommon but deadly immune-mediated neuropathy caused by an infection that has a 0.4–2 per 100,000 incidences and has a significant impact on the healthcare system. GBS is a potentially fatal post-infectious condition characterized by quickly progressing, symmetrical extremity weakening. It is triggered by autoimmune nerve damage in the peripheral nervous system, including muscles in the legs, arms, and upper torso, resulting in symptoms such as numbness, tingling, and weakness, which can lead to paralysis. GBS cause involves structural imitation, antiganglioside antibodies, and, probably, supplement activation; a genetic predisposition may play a role, but further research is needed. Approximately 25% of individuals develop respiratory insufficiency, and many have autonomic dysfunction. Investigating the immune-mediated pathogenesis of the illness, recognizing the diversity of manifestations, expanding diagnostic modalities and prognostic models, and conducting randomized trials of therapies to enhance outcomes are all examples of advances made in the last century. More diagnostic procedures (such as CSF fluid testing and nerve conduction investigations) may assist in verifying the clinical diagnosis of GBS, which is especially helpful in people who have unique symptoms or are unclear about the cause of their condition. Electromyography and nerve conduction investigations may assist in differentiating GBS from its imitators. The major treatment for Guillain–Barré syndrome is plasmapheresis, which involves filtering the blood [43–45].

5.7 *Chronic Inflammatory Demyelinating Polyneuropathy*

In Guillain–Barré syndrome, the immune system destroys the nerves in CIDP, but the symptoms are significantly more severe. Chronic inflammatory demyelinating polyradiculoneuropathy (CIDP) is an immune-mediated neuropathy that affects peripheral nerves and nerve roots and has a relapsing–remitting or progressive history of symmetric weakening of proximal and distal muscles. The prevalence of CIDP has been observed to range between 0.7 and 10.3 cases per 100,000 persons. Males outweigh girls by a sex ratio ranging between 1.5 and 4. Adults are most commonly affected by CIDP, and the frequency rises with age. The average age of onset has yet to be identified. There are no particular risk factors for CIDP that have been identified [46, 47].

Pathogenesis of CIPD on two major basis:-Although the cause of CIDP and its variants is unknown, there is evidence to suggest that the disorder(s) is immunologically mediated and can be caused by a variety of causes. The cellular and humoral components of the adaptive immune system appear to be involved in the pathogenesis of CIDP and its variants. Neuropathologic symptoms of CIDP include segmental demyelination and remyelination of peripheral nerves, which can result in the formation of onion bulbs. The term "onion bulb formation" refers to the appearance of damaged axons under the microscope in the transverse slice. As a result of recurring episodes of demyelination and remyelination, affected nerve fibers grow as a result of whorls of overlapping and proliferating Schwann cell processes surrounding bare axons. Electrodiagnostic and/or pathologic signs of demyelination, as well as response to immunomodulatory therapies, are used to diagnose CIDP. If not recognized and treated early, over 30% of individuals may be restricted to a wheelchair. CIDP and GBS treatment are generally comparable [48, 49].

5.8 *Psoriasis*

Psoriasis is an immune-mediated illness (a disease of unclear origin marked by inflammation caused by immune system dysfunction) that causes inflammation in the body. Raised plaques (plaques can vary in appearance depending on skin type) and scales on the skin can be visible signs of inflammation. This occurs when an overactive immune system causes skin cell growth to accelerate. Normal skin cells form and shed (fall off) in about a month. Psoriasis skin cells complete this in three to four days. Skin cells amass on the skin's surface rather than shedding. Certain people claim that psoriasis plaques itch, burn, and sting. Plaques and scales can develop everywhere on the body, although they are most common on the elbows, knees, and scalp. Psoriasis-related inflammation can affect different organs and tissues in the body. People who have psoriasis may also have additional health problems. Psoriatic arthritis affects one out of every three people who have psoriasis. Edoema, stiffness, and soreness in the joints and surrounding areas are all indications of PsA. PsA is commonly misdiagnosed, particularly in its milder forms. However, in order to avoid irreparable joint damage, PsA must be treated as soon as feasible. Symptoms are more common between the ages of 15 and 25, however, they can appear at any age. Psoriasis can affect men, women, and children of various skin colors. The immune system causes skin cells to multiply fast, resulting in silvery, scaly plaques on the skin [50–52].

5.9 Graves' Disease

Graves' disease is an autoimmune disorder that causes overactivity of the thyroid gland, leading to hyperthyroidism, and it affects about 1–2% of the general population. It is more common in women than in men, and the onset of the disease usually occurs between the ages of 20 and 40. The precise etiology of Graves' illness is unknown; however, it is likely to be caused by a mix of hereditary and environmental factors. Graves' illness is characterized by an aberrant immunological response in which the immune system creates antibodies that encourage the thyroid gland to release an abnormally large amount of thyroid hormone. Thyroid-stimulating immunoglobulins (TSIs) are antibodies that stimulate the thyroid gland, bind to the receptors on the thyroid gland, and activate them leading to an increase in thyroid hormone production. The overproduction of thyroid hormone leads to hyperthyroidism and a range of symptoms, including weight loss, tremors, and anxiety. Graves' illness is often treated with a combination of medicine, radioactive iodine therapy, and surgery. Medications such as beta-blockers and antithyroid medications can be used to treat hyperthyroidism symptoms, while radioactive iodine therapy can be used to destroy the thyroid gland and limit thyroid hormone production. In certain situations, surgery to remove the thyroid gland may be required, especially if the patient is pregnant or has a significant goiter [53, 54].

5.10 Hashimoto's Thyroiditis

Hashimoto's thyroiditis is an autoimmune disorder that affects the thyroid gland, leading to hypothyroidism. It is the most common cause of hypothyroidism in areas of the world where iodine intake is sufficient. The prevalence of Hashimoto's thyroiditis varies depending on the population studied, but it is estimated to affect around 1–2% of the general population. Hashimoto's thyroiditis is caused by a response in which the immune system produces antibodies that attack the thyroid gland, leading to inflammation and damage. The antibodies involved in Hashimoto's thyroiditis are primarily directed against the thyroglobulin and thyroid peroxidase enzymes, which are essential for the production of thyroid hormones. Over time, the damage to the thyroid gland can lead to decreased production of thyroid hormones and hypothyroidism. Thyroid hormone replacement therapy (levothyroxine) is commonly used to treat Hashimoto's thyroiditis. This entails taking synthetic thyroid hormone (levothyroxine) to replace the hormone that the thyroid gland no longer produces. The goal of treatment is to restore normal thyroid hormone levels and alleviate the symptoms of hypothyroidism [55–57].

5.11 Myasthenia Gravis

Myasthenia gravis (MG) is a relatively rare disorder, affecting approximately 14 to 20 individuals per 100,000 population worldwide. The prevalence of MG is higher in women than in men, with a female-to-male ratio of approximately 2:1.The illness can strike at any age, although it is more frequent in women under 40 and men over 60. In some cases, MG may be associated with other autoimmune disorders such as rheumatoid arthritis, lupus, or thyroid disease. The underlying pathogenesis of myasthenia gravis involves the production of autoantibodies against the acetylcholine receptors (AChR) at the neuromuscular junction. The antibodies disrupt nerve impulse transmission to the muscle, resulting in muscular weakness and tiredness. AChR antibody production is hypothesized to be initiated by an aberrant immune response directed against the body's own tissues. In addition to the AChR antibodies, other autoantibodies such as those against muscle-specific kinase (MuSK) and low-density lipoprotein receptor-related protein 4 (LRP4) have also been identified in a subset of patients with myasthenia gravis. The presence of these antibodies may be associated with a distinct clinical presentation and treatment response. There is additional evidence that thymus dysfunction may contribute to the etiology of myasthenia gravis. Approximately 70% of patients with MG have abnormalities of the thymus gland, ranging from thymic hyperplasia to thymoma (a type of tumor) [58–64].

5.12 Autoimmune Hepatitis

Autoimmune hepatitis (AIH) is a chronic inflammatory liver disease marked by an increase in aminotransferases, the presence of an anti-nuclear antibody or anti-smooth muscle antibody, elevated immunoglobulin G (IgG), and interface hepatitis/plasma-lymphocytic inflammation. The interplay of genetic predisposition, an environmental trigger, and failure of the native immune system leads to continuous inflammation of hepatocytes and subsequent liver fibrosis, according to the proposed mechanism for the development of autoimmune hepatitis. There have been two types of autoimmune hepatitis recognized. Type 1 is distinguished by the presence of anti-smooth muscle antibodies (ASMA) with or without anti-nuclear antibodies (ANA). Type 2 autoimmune hepatitis is distinguished by the presence of anti-liver/anti-kidney microsome (anti-LMK) type 1 antibodies or anti-liver cytosol (anti-LC) type 1 antibodies. Recent epidemiological studies have shown an increasing trend in the prevalence of AIH globally, particularly in male patients; this trend may imply that the environmental triggers of illness onset are changing over time. Because no disease-specific biomarker or histological finding is currently available, AIH requires a clinical diagnosis, and a validated diagnostic scoring system with acceptable specificity and sensitivity has been proposed. In terms of treatment, corticosteroids, and azathioprine are recommended, although second-line medication, such as mycophenolate mofetil, is being investigated in some patients. Overall, patients with full biochemical responses have a great long-term prognosis, albeit life-long maintenance medication may be necessary since stopping immunosuppressive drugs commonly results in disease return [65–68] (Table 4).

6 Diagnosis and Treatment of Various Autoimmune Disorders

6.1 Diagnostic Tests

The introduction of novel molecular immunology technologies and sophisticated evidence-based clinical laboratory testing has resulted in significant advances in diagnosis, disease classification, and prognosis during the last decade. A physical diagnostic test will be performed by the healthcare professional. The symptoms vary according to the type of sickness [70]. Common tests which may be used to detect an autoimmune disorder are described in Fig. 5.

6.2 Therapies

Some common treatment strategies for the cure of ADs:

- Overcome the process of autoimmune disease
- Maintain the body's ability to fight illness by minimizing symptoms (Treatments will vary depending on your condition and symptoms)

Types of therapies include:

- Medications that replenish a material that the body lacks owing to the autoimmune illness, such as thyroid hormone, vitamin B12, or insulin;
- Blood transfusions if the blood is harmed;

Table 4 Prevalence of several ADs/100,000 people in different countries [25, 32, 35, 42, 45, 64, 69]

S.no	Disease	India	US	France	Japan	Germany	Australia	UK	China
1.	Rheumatoid arthritis	100–200	500–1000	300–800	70–130	500–1000	300–400	400–700	100–200
2.	Systemic Lupus Erythematosus	10–60	20–150	20–80	30–150	40–160	20–60	20–150	15–20
3.	Inflammatory Bowel Disease	50–200	60–100	100–200	30–80	60–150	60–120	100–200	1–4
4.	Type 1 diabetes mellitus	5–10	20–25	8–10	4–6	15–20	11–12	15–20	1–2
5.	Guillain–Barré Syndrome	0.4–2	1–2	0.8–1.1	0.5–2	1.1–1.9	0.6–2.4	1.1–1.9	0.4–1.3
6.	Chronic inflammatory demyelinating polyneuropathy	0.5–1.6	1.6–8.9	1.0–2.5	0.8–1.3	0.6–1.9	0.8–2.0	1.9–8.8	0.1–0.7
7.	Graves' disease	20–50	20–30	10–30	20–40	10–30	10–40	20–45	5–15
8.	Hashimoto's thyroiditis	100–300	200–500	100–200	100–200	100–150	150–200	300–500	0.3–1.5
9.	Myasthenia gravis	1–2	14–20	7–10	4–16	7–15	7–12	15–20	3–10
10.	Autoimmune Hepatitis	2–6	10–30	4–20	9–20	8–25	10–20	15–20	1–20
11.	Multiple Sclerosis	0.5–2.3	100–200	80–100	5–10	120–180	80–100	110–140	0.7–1.6
12.	Psoriasis	60–120	100–150	100–200	40–80	100–150	70–130	150–200	20–60

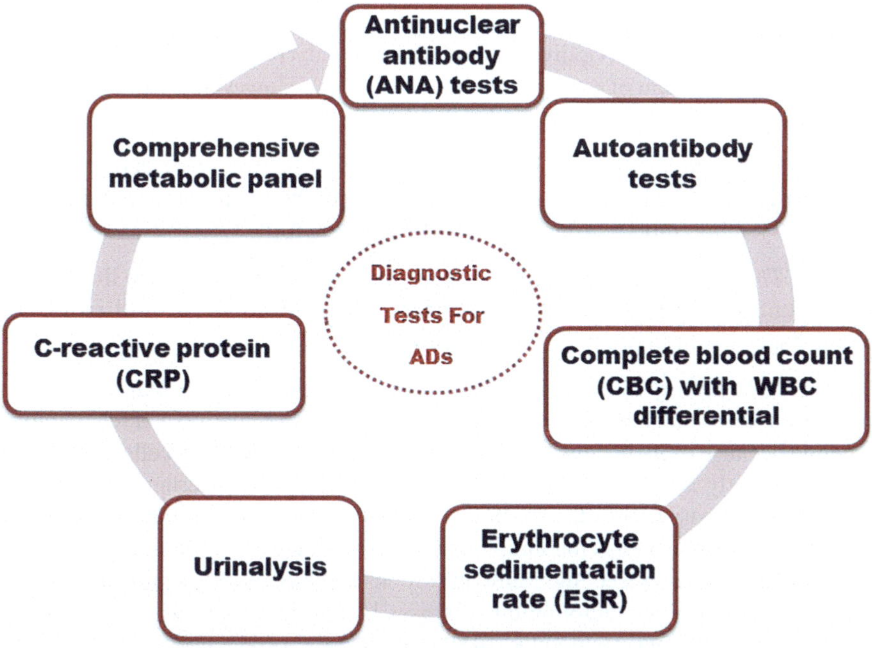

Fig. 5 Diagnostic tests for numerous Autoimmune Diseases (ADs)

- Physical therapy to aid mobility if the bones, joints, or muscles are harmed [71, 72].

6.3 Recent Therapies

Recent therapies for autoimmune disorders have focused on modulating the immune response, reducing inflammation, and promoting tolerance. Here are some recent and emerging therapies, including stem cell therapy:

(a) Biologics and Targeted Therapies: Monoclonal antibodies are a type of biologic that has been designed to target and neutralize immune proteins involved in autoimmune responses. Examples include medications like rituximab (Rituxan) and adalimumab (Humira).

(b) Janus Kinase (JAK) Inhibitors: JAK inhibitors are oral drugs that target the Janus kinase pathway involved in immunological signaling. Examples include tofacitinib (Xeljanz) and baricitinib (Olumiant). They have demonstrated promise in treating conditions like psoriasis and rheumatoid arthritis.

(c) Checkpoint Inhibitors: By altering immune responses, immune checkpoint inhibitors like nivolumab (Opdivo) and pembrolizumab (Keytruda) have been investigated for the treatment of some autoimmune disorders. However, using them carries the chance of escalating autoimmunity.

(d) B cell Depletion Therapy: Drugs like ocrelizumab (Ocrevus) and rituximab (Rituxan) target B cells, which are involved in a number of autoimmune illnesses including systemic lupus erythematosus (SLE) and multiple sclerosis.

(e) Gene Therapy: Emerging gene therapies aim to modify or correct the genetic factors contributing to autoimmune disorders. These therapies are still in experimental stages but hold promise for the future.

(f) Stem Cell Therapy: Stem cell therapy is an area of active research for autoimmune diseases. Stem cells play a crucial role in immunomodulation and regenerative medicine because of their capacity to develop into different types of cells. It has been shown to greatly accelerate the healing process in animals suffering from various autoimmune diseases. Besides healing damaged tissues, Hematopoietic stem cell transplantation (HSCT) has the unique ability to modulate the immune system with healthy stem cells to "reset" the immune response. It has shown significant success in treating certain severe autoimmune diseases like multiple sclerosis and systemic sclerosis. Mesenchymal stem cells (MSCs) induce the production of T regulatory cells, a type of immune cell whose function is to protect the body against immunological self-attack. Autoimmune disease progression can be slowed down, reversed, or even stopped using stem cell therapy. The patient's age, the severity of their condition, and the length of the disease all affect how well they respond to treatment. To completely grasp the potential of stem cell therapy for autoimmune illnesses, more study is necessary.

(g) Tolerogenic Therapies: Research is ongoing into therapies that induce immune tolerance, where the immune system becomes less reactive to self-antigens. This includes oral and nasal tolerance induction and peptide-based therapies.

(h) Nanomedicine: Nanoparticles and nanocarriers are being explored to deliver targeted treatments to affected tissues, reducing systemic side effects of medications.

(i) Personalized Medicine: Advancements in genomics and precision medicine are allowing for more tailored treatment approaches, identifying specific genetic markers and immune pathways to guide therapy decisions.

(j) Complementary Therapies: Approaches like dietary modifications, probiotics, and lifestyle changes are being investigated to complement traditional treatments, aiming to manage symptoms and improve overall well-being.

It's important to note that while these therapies hold promise, not all are widely available or appropriate for every autoimmune disorder. Treatment decisions should be made in consultation with healthcare providers who can consider the specific condition, its severity, and the patient's individual needs and risks [73] (Table 5).

Table 5 Recent therapies for Autoimmune Diseases [73, 74]

S. No	Autoimmune disease	Recent therapies
1	Rheumatoid arthritis	JAK Inhibitors (e.g., Tofacitinib), Biologics (e.g., Adalimumab, Rituximab)
2	Lupus	Belimumab (targeting B cells), Benlysta (monoclonal antibody)
3	Multiple sclerosis	Ocrelizumab (B cell therapy), Fingolimod (Sphingosine-1-Phosphate modulator)
4	Inflammatory bowel disease	Vedolizumab (integrin receptor antagonist), Ustekinumab (IL-12/IL-23 inhibitor)
5	Psoriasis	IL-17 Inhibitors (e.g., Secukinumab), IL-23 Inhibitors (e.g., Risankizumab)
6	Type 1 diabetes	Immunomodulatory therapies in development, Beta-cell replacement therapy (under research)
7	Multiple myeloma (cancer with autoimmune aspects)	CAR-T Cell Therapy, Proteasome Inhibitors

7 Discussion and Conclusion

Autoimmune disorders are instances in which the immune system targets healthy cells, tissues, or organs, causing damage to numerous organs and tissues throughout the body. They are a serious source of worry for world health. The incidence of autoimmune diseases varies between people and geographical locations. Environmental variables, genetic predisposition, and immune system dysregulation all play a role in the development of these illnesses. Autoimmune disorders are becoming increasingly widespread, with rheumatoid arthritis, systemic lupus erythematosus, multiple sclerosis, type 1 diabetes, and celiac disease being the most regularly reported. Autoimmune diseases are a group of disorders where the immune system mistakenly targets and attacks the body's own cells and tissues. In recent years, significant progress has been made in understanding the epidemiology, pathogenesis, and prevalence rates of autoimmune diseases. This discussion will delve into these recent insights. Recent studies have shed light on the epidemiology of autoimmune diseases. It is now evident that these conditions are more prevalent than previously believed. The global burden of autoimmune diseases has been on the rise, with an increasing incidence across various populations. This trend may partly be attributed to improved diagnostic techniques and heightened awareness among healthcare providers. Furthermore, gender disparities have become increasingly apparent. Many autoimmune diseases, such as systemic lupus erythematosus (SLE) and rheumatoid arthritis (RA), disproportionately affect women. This gender bias raises important questions about the role of hormonal and genetic factors in disease susceptibility. Additionally, geographical variations in autoimmune disease incidence have been observed, suggesting environmental factors may contribute significantly to their development. Advancements in immunology have provided valuable insights into the pathogenesis of autoimmune diseases. One key discovery is the role of genetic predisposition. Genome-wide association studies (GWAS) have identified specific genetic variants associated with various autoimmune conditions. These findings underscore the hereditary component of autoimmune diseases, although multiple genes are typically involved, and their interactions are complex. Furthermore, the microbiome has emerged as a crucial player in autoimmune disease pathogenesis. The gut microbiota, in particular, has been linked to immune system regulation. Dysbiosis, an imbalance in the gut microbiome composition, may trigger or exacerbate autoimmune responses. This newfound understanding has opened doors to potential therapeutic interventions targeting the microbiome. Recent data have revealed a higher prevalence rate of autoimmune diseases than previously estimated. Conditions such as multiple sclerosis, type 1 diabetes, and celiac disease are now recognized as more widespread than initially believed. Improved awareness and diagnostic tools have led to earlier detection, enabling timely intervention and management. It is worth noting that the prevalence of autoimmune diseases varies among different conditions. Some, like Hashimoto's thyroiditis, exhibit a notably high prevalence, while others, such as systemic sclerosis, are less common. The reasons behind these disparities may include genetic predisposition, environmental factors, and differences in diagnostic criteria. In conclusion, recent insights into autoimmune diseases have illuminated various aspects of these complex disorders. Epidemiological data highlight the increasing global burden, gender disparities, and geographical variations, underscoring the need for improved awareness and tailored healthcare strategies. Pathogenesis studies have revealed genetic predispositions and the critical role of the microbiome, offering potential targets for therapeutic interventions. The recalibrated prevalence rates emphasize the importance of early diagnosis and effective management to mitigate the impact of autoimmune diseases on individuals and society as a whole. Continued research and collaboration between clinicians, geneticists, immunologists, and epidemiologists will be essential in further unraveling the mysteries of autoimmune diseases and developing more effective treatments.

References

1. Sasikala K, Kumari MR (2022) An account on promising alternative system of medicine to boost immunity. Plant Sci Today 9(sp2):47–50
2. Arango MT, Shoenfeld Y, Cervera R, Anaya JM. Infection and autoimmune diseases. InAutoimmunity: from bench to bedside [Internet] 2013 Jul 18. El Rosario University Press
3. Wang L, Wang FS, Gershwin ME (2015) Human autoimmune diseases: a comprehensive update. J Intern Med 278(4):369–395
4. Angum F, Khan T, Kaler J, Siddiqui L, Hussain A. The prevalence of autoimmune disorders in women: a narrative review. Cureus. 2020 May 13;12(5).
5. Smith DA, Germolec DR (1999) Introduction to immunology and autoimmunity. Environ Health Perspect 107(suppl 5):661–665
6. Jacobson DL, Gange SJ, Rose NR, Graham NM (1997) Epidemiology and estimated population burden of selected autoimmune diseases in the United States. Clin Immunol Immunopathol 84(3):223–243

7. Eaton WW, Rose NR, Kalaydjian A, Pedersen MG, Mortensen PB (2007) Epidemiology of autoimmune diseases in Denmark. J Autoimmun 29(1):1–9
8. Wahren-Herlenius M, Dörner T (2013) Immunopathogenic mechanisms of systemic autoimmune disease. The Lancet 382(9894):819–831
9. Milo R, Kahana E (2010) Multiple sclerosis: geoepidemiology, genetics and the environment. Autoimmun Rev 9(5):A387–A394
10. Rees F, Doherty M, Grainge M, Davenport G, Lanyon P, Zhang W (2016) The incidence and prevalence of systemic lupus erythematosus in the UK, 1999–2012. Ann Rheum Dis 75(1):136–141
11. Leung PS, Wang J, Naiyanetr P, Kenny TP, Lam KS, Kurth MJ, Gershwin ME (2013) Environment and primary biliary cirrhosis: electrophilic drugs and the induction of AMA. J Autoimmun 1(41):79–86
12. Fugger L, Jensen LT, Rossjohn J (2020) Challenges, progress, and prospects of developing therapies to treat autoimmune diseases. Cell 181(1):63–80
13. Lerner A, Jeremias P, Matthias T (2015) The world incidence and prevalence of autoimmune diseases is increasing. Int J Celiac Dis. 3(4):151–155
14. Ngo ST, Steyn FJ, McCombe PA (2014) Gender differences in autoimmune disease. Front Neuroendocrinol 35(3):347–369
15. Cooper GS, Bynum ML, Somers EC (2009) Recent insights in the epidemiology of autoimmune diseases: improved prevalence estimates and understanding of clustering of diseases. J Autoimmun 33(3–4):197–207
16. Singh AK, Tripathi A, Singh KK, Choudhary P, Vashist PC (2021) Artificial itelligence in medicine. In: Machine learning and the internet of medical things in healthcare. Academic Press (2021), pp 67–87
17. Rosenblum MD, Remedios KA, Abbas AK (2015) Mechanisms of human autoimmunity. J Clin Investig 125(6):2228–2233
18. Theofilopoulos AN, Kono DH, Baccala R (2017) The multiple pathways to autoimmunity. Nat Immunol 18(7):716–724
19. Rothschild BM, Turner KR, DeLuca MA (1988) Symmetrical erosive peripheral polyarthritis in the Late Archaic period of Alabama. Science 241(4872):1498–1501
20. Lee DM, Weinblatt ME (2001) Rheumatoid arthritis. Lancet (London, England) 358(9285):903–911. https://doi.org/10.1016/S0140-6736(01)06075-5
21. Smolen JS, Aletaha D, Barton A, Burmester GR, Emery P, Firestein GS, Kavanaugh A, McInnes IB, Solomon DH, Strand V, Yamamoto K (2018) Rheumatoid arthritis. Nature reviews. Dis Primers 418001
22. Firestein GS, McInnes IB (2017) Immunopathogenesis of rheumatoid arthritis. Immunity 46(2):183–196
23. Deane KD, Holers VM (2021) Rheumatoid arthritis pathogenesis, prediction, and prevention: an emerging paradigm shift. Arthritis Rheumatol 73(2):181–193
24. Safiri S, Kolahi AA, Hoy D, Smith E, Bettampadi D, Mansournia MA, Almasi-Hashiani A, Ashrafi-Asgarabad A, Moradi-Lakeh M, Qorbani M, Collins G (2019) Global, regional and national burden of rheumatoid arthritis 1990–2017: a systematic analysis of the Global Burden of Disease study 2017. Ann Rheum Dis 78(11):1463–1471
25. Tian J, Zhang D, Yao X, Huang Y, Lu Q (2023) Global epidemiology of systemic lupus erythematosus: a comprehensive systematic analysis and modelling study. Ann Rheum Dis 82(3):351–356
26. Pons-Estel GJ, Alarcón GS, Scofield L, Reinlib L, Cooper GS (2010) Understanding the epidemiology and progression of systemic lupus erythematosus. In: Seminars in arthritis and rheumatism, vol 39, no 4. WB Saunders, pp 257–268
27. Stojan G, Petri M (2018) Epidemiology of systemic lupus erythematosus: an update. Curr Opin Rheumatol 30(2):144
28. Demirkaya E, Sahin S, Romano M, Zhou Q, Aksentijevich I (2020) New horizons in the genetic etiology of systemic lupus erythematosus and lupus-like disease: monogenic lupus and beyond. J Clin Med 9(3):712

29. Malaviya AN, Singh RR, Singh YN, Kapoor SK, Kumar A (1993) Prevalence of systemic lupus erythematosus in India. Lupus 2(2):115–118
30. Karlinger K, Györke T, Makö E, Mester Á, Tarján Z (2000) The epidemiology and the pathogenesis of inflammatory bowel disease. Eur J Radiol 35(3):154–167
31. Alatab S, Sepanlou SG, Ikuta K, Vahedi H, Bisignano C, Safiri S, Sadeghi A, Nixon MR, Abdoli A, Abolhassani H, Alipour V (2020) The global, regional, and national burden of inflammatory bowel disease in 195 countries and territories, 1990–2017: a systematic analysis for the Global Burden of Disease Study 2017. Lancet Gastroenterol Hepatol 5(1):17–30
32. Hanauer SB (2006) Inflammatory bowel disease: epidemiology, pathogenesis, and therapeutic opportunities. Inflammatory bowel diseases, 12(suppl_1):S3–9
33. Heydarpour P, Khoshkish S, Abtahi S, Moradi-Lakeh M, Sahraian MA (2015) Multiple sclerosis epidemiology in Middle East and North Africa: a systematic review and meta-analysis. Neuroepidemiology 44(4):232–244
34. Walton C, King R, Rechtman L, Kaye W, Leray E, Marrie RA, Robertson N, La Rocca N, Uitdehaag B, van Der Mei I, Wallin M (2020) Rising prevalence of multiple sclerosis worldwide: insights from the Atlas of MS. Mult Scler J 26(14):1816–1821
35. Goodin DS (2009) The causal cascade to multiple sclerosis: a model for MS pathogenesis. PLoS ONE 4(2):e4565
36. Mobasseri M, Shirmohammadi M, Amiri T, Vahed N, Fard HH, Ghojazadeh M (2020) Prevalence and incidence of type 1 diabetes in the world: a systematic review and meta-analysis. Health Promot Perspect 10(2):98
37. American Diabetes Association (2010) Diagnosis and classification of diabetes mellitus. Diabetes care, 33(Supplement_1):S62–9
38. Kumar K, Uttekar PS (2009) What country has the most type 1 diabetics? diabetes health center/diabetes a-z list/
39. Echeverri AF, Tobón GJ (2013) Autoimmune diabetes mellitus (Type 1A). In: Autoimmunity: from bench to bedside [Internet]. El Rosario University Press
40. Janka HU, Michaelis D (2002) Epidemiology of diabetes mellitus: prevalence, incidence, pathogenesis, and prognosis. Zeitschrift fur arztlicheFortbildung und Qualitatssicherung. 96(3):159–165
41. Kakleas K, Soldatou A, Karachaliou F, Karavanaki K (2015) Associated autoimmune diseases in children and adolescents with type 1 diabetes mellitus (T1DM). Autoimmun Rev 14(9):781–797
42. Gvazava IG, Rogovaya OS, Borisov MA, Vorotelyak EA, Vasiliev AV (2018) Pathogenesis of type 1 diabetes mellitus and rodent experimental models. ActaNaturae (англоязычнаяверсия), 10(1 (36)):24–33
43. Van Doorn PA, Ruts L, Jacobs BC (2008) Clinical features, pathogenesis, and treatment of Guillain-Barré syndrome. Lancet Neurol 7(10):939–950
44. Van den Berg B, Walgaard C, Drenthen J, Fokke C, Jacobs BC, Van Doorn PA (2014) Guillain-Barré syndrome: pathogenesis, diagnosis, treatment and prognosis. Nat Rev Neurol 10(8):469–482
45. Kuwabara S (2004) Guillain-Barré syndrome: epidemiology, pathophysiology and management. Drugs 64:597–610
46. Newman HN (1999) Attrition, eruption, and the periodontium. J Dent Res 78(3):730–734
47. Chiò A, Cocito D, Bottacchi E, Buffa C, Leone M, Plano F, Mutani R, Calvo A (2007) Idiopathic chronic inflammatory demyelinating polyneuropathy: an epidemiological study in Italy. J Neurol Neurosurg Psychiatry 78(12):1349–1353
48. Seymour GJ, Whyte GJ, Powell RN (1986) Chemiluminescence in the assessment of polymorphonuclear leukocyte function in chronic inflammatory periodontal disease. J Oral Pathol Med 15(3):125–131
49. Machado AS, De Sousa AE, Andrade F, Vieira-Coelho M (2022) Multiple inpatient admissions for cannabis-induced psychotic disorder-sociodemographic, clinical and treatment evaluation. Eur Psychiatry 65(S1):S792-

50. Parisi R, Iskandar IY, Kontopantelis E, Augustin M, Griffiths CE, Ashcroft DM (2020) National, regional, and worldwide epidemiology of psoriasis: systematic analysis and modelling study. BMJ 28:369
51. Armstrong AW, Read C (2020) Pathophysiology, clinical presentation, and treatment of psoriasis: a review. JAMA 323(19):1945–1960
52. Boehncke WH (2015) Etiology and pathogenesis of psoriasis. Rheum Dis Clin 41(4):665–675
53. Wémeau JL, Klein M, Sadoul JL, Briet C, Vélayoudom-Céphise FL (2018) Graves' disease: introduction, epidemiology, endogenous and environmental pathogenic factors. In: Annalesd'endocrinologie, vol 79, no 6. Elsevier Masson, pp 599–607
54. Antonelli A, Fazzi P, Fallahi P, Ferrari SM, Ferrannini E (2006) Prevalence of hypothyroidism and Graves disease in sarcoidosis. Chest 130(2):526–532
55. Hu X, Chen Y, Shen Y, Tian R, Sheng Y, Que H (2022) Global prevalence and epidemiological trends of Hashimoto's thyroiditis in adults: a systematic review and meta-analysis. Front Public Health 13(10):1020709
56. Ragusa F, Fallahi P, Elia G, Gonnella D, Paparo SR, Giusti C, Churilov LP, Ferrari SM, Antonelli A (2019) Hashimotos' thyroiditis: epidemiology, pathogenesis, clinic and therapy. Best Pract Res Clin Endocrinol Metab 33(6):101367
57. Mocellin R, Walterfang M, Velakoulis D (2007) Hashimoto's encephalopathy: epidemiology, pathogenesis and management. CNS Drugs 21:799–811
58. Dresser L, Wlodarski R, Rezania K, Soliven B (2021) Myasthenia gravis: epidemiology, pathophysiology and clinical manifestations. J Clin Med 10(11):2235
59. McGrogan A, Sneddon S, De Vries CS (2010) The incidence of myasthenia gravis: a systematic literature review. Neuroepidemiology 34(3):171–183
60. Hoch W, McConville J, Helms S, Newsom-Davis J, Melms A, Vincent A (2001) Auto-antibodies to the receptor tyrosine kinase MuSK in patients with myasthenia gravis without acetylcholine receptor antibodies. Nat Med 7(3):365–368
61. Higuchi O, Hamuro J, Motomura M, Yamanashi Y (2011) Autoantibodies to low-density lipoprotein receptor–related protein 4 in myasthenia gravis. Ann Neurol 69(2):418–422
62. Pevzner A, Schoser B, Peters K, Cosma NC, Karakatsani A, Schalke B, Melms A, Kröger S (2012) Anti-LRP4 autoantibodies in AChR-and MuSK-antibody-negative myasthenia gravis. J Neurol 259:427–435
63. Zhang B, Shen C, Bealmear B, Ragheb S, Xiong WC, Lewis RA, Lisak RP, Mei L (2014) Autoantibodies to agrin in myasthenia gravis patients. PLoS ONE 9(3):e91816
64. Bubuioc AM, Kudebayeva A, Turuspekova S, Lisnic V, Leone MA (2021) The epidemiology of myasthenia gravis. J Med Life 14(1):7
65. Xi D, Lin H, Shah AA (2022) Overview of autoimmune liver disease: prevalence, risk factors, and role of autoantibodies. Clin Liver Dis 20(4):111
66. Francque S, Vonghia L, Ramon A, Michielsen P (2012) Epidemiology and treatment of autoimmune hepatitis. In: Hepatic medicine: evidence and research, pp 1–10
67. Czaja AJ, Manns MP (2010) Advances in the diagnosis, pathogenesis, and management of autoimmune hepatitis. Gastroenterology 139(1):58–72
68. Liberal R, Longhi MS, Mieli-Vergani G, Vergani D (2011) Pathogenesis of autoimmune hepatitis. Best Pract Res Clin Gastroenterol 25(6):653–664
69. Osio-Salido E, Manapat-Reyes H (2010) Epidemiology of systemic lupus erythematosus in Asia. Lupus 19(12):1365–1373
70. Plebani M, Pittoni M, Celadin M, Bernardi D, Mion MM (2009) Recent advances in diagnostic technologies for autoimmune diseases. Autoimmun Rev 8(3):238–243
71. Davidson A, Diamond B (2020) General features of autoimmune disease. In: The autoimmune diseases. Academic Press, pp 17–44
72. Rosato E, Pisarri S, Salsano F (2010) Current strategies for the treatment of autoimmune diseases. J Biol Regul Homeost Agents 24(3):251–259

73. Jung SM, Kim WU (2022) Targeted immunotherapy for autoimmune disease. Immune Netw. 22(1):e9
74. Granit V, Benatar M, Kurtoglu M et al (2023) Safety and clinical activity of autologous RNA chimeric antigen receptor T-cell therapy in myasthenia gravis (MG-001): a prospective, multicentre, open-label, non-randomised phase 1b/2a study. Lancet Neurol. https://doi.org/10.1016/PIIS1474-4422(23)00194-1

AI in Diagnosis and Prognosis

The Role of Artificial Intelligence and Machine Learning in Autoimmune Disorders

Faizan Siddiqui, Danish Aslam, Khushnuma Tanveer, and Mohamed Soudy

Abstract The immune system of an organism responds to threats from outside the body. Autoimmunity in immunology is the system of an organism's immune responses against its healthy cells, tissues, and other typical body parts. Therefore, a disorder known as an autoimmune illness results from an inappropriate immune reaction to a healthy bodily function. The science of developing computers with intelligence that both mimics and exceeds that of humans is known as artificial intelligence (AI). Programs having AI capabilities can contextualize and analyze data to deliver information or automatically initiate operations without the need for human intervention. Furthermore, AI can be attained through machine learning. This branch of AI applies to learning to make ever-better judgments using algorithms to discover patterns and acquire insights from data automatically. In this chapter, we present the role of AI and machine learning to analyze how autoimmunity behaves in conditions like autoimmune diseases. Moreover, we also discussed the impact of employing machine learning techniques to optimize precision medicine for patients.

Keywords Autoimmunity · Artificial intelligence · Image analysis · Immune disorders · Precision medicine

F. Siddiqui
International Medical Faculty, Osh State University, Osh City, Kyrgyzstan

D. Aslam · K. Tanveer
Department of Computer Science, Jamia Millia Islamia, New Delhi, India
e-mail: danish2101125@st.jmi.ac.in

M. Soudy (✉)
Bioinformatics Program, Faculty of Computer Science and Information, Ain Shams University, Cairo, Egypt
e-mail: mohmedsoudy2009@gmail.com

K. Raza and S. Singh (eds.), *Artificial Intelligence and Autoimmune Diseases*, Studies in Computational Intelligence 1133, https://doi.org/10.1007/978-981-99-9029-0_3

1 Introduction

The use of machine learning and deep learning in autoimmune disorders is a rapidly growing field of research, as it has the potential to revolutionize the diagnosis and treatment of these conditions. Machine learning is a subfield of Artificial Intelligence (AI) that uses algorithms to learn from data and make predictions. Deep learning, on the other hand, is a subset of machine learning that uses neural networks to process data. Both methods have been used in various applications related to autoimmune disorders, such as diagnosis, prognosis, drug discovery, and treatment optimization [1]. In terms of diagnosis, machine learning algorithms are used to analyze medical images or patient data to identify patterns associated with autoimmune disorders. For example, researchers utilized deep learning algorithms to analyze Magnetic Resonance Imaging (MRI) scans for Multiple Sclerosis (MS) and Rheumatoid Arthritis (RA) [2, 3]. The results showed that deep learning was able to detect MS and RA with high accuracy. Similarly, machine learning algorithms have been used to diagnose Systemic Lupus Erythematosus (SLE) by analyzing patient data such as age, gender, race/ethnicity, laboratory test results, and medical history [4, 5].

In terms of prognosis, machine learning algorithms are used to predict the course of an autoimmune disorder over time. For example, researchers utilized machine learning algorithms to predict how RA patients will respond to certain treatments based on their clinical features. Similarly, deep learning algorithms have been used to predict which patients with SLE are at risk for developing complications such as organ damage or stroke [6].

In terms of drug discovery and treatment optimization for autoimmune disorders, both machine learning and deep learning were utilized to identify new drugs or optimize existing treatments. For example, researchers have applied machine learning techniques such as random forest to identify novel drugs for RA that could target specific pathways involved in the disease progression [7]. Similarly, deep neural networks have been used to optimize existing treatments for MS by predicting which drugs would be most effective at reducing disease symptoms [7].

Overall, the use of machine learning and deep learning in autoimmune disorders has great potential for improving diagnostic accuracy and optimizing treatments for these conditions. In this chapter, we will go through the AI approaches used for diagnosis, and prognosis, and AI in treatment and drug discovery. Moreover, we will discuss the main workflow of the prediction of drug-induced autoimmune diseases utilizing autoimmune drug data and research databases as shown in Fig. 1.

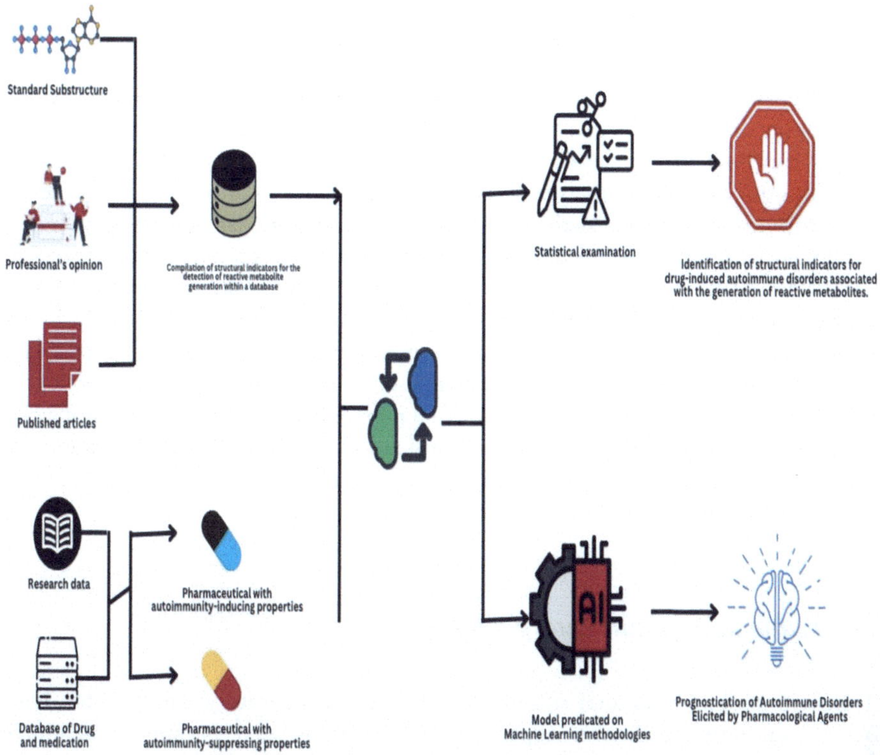

Fig. 1 Schematic representation of the methodology employed for the prediction of drug-induced autoimmune diseases utilizing autoimmune drug data and research databases

2 Literature Review

2.1 AI Approaches for the Diagnosis and Prognosis

In the diagnosis of autoimmune diseases, AI, models, and algorithms have emerged as extremely useful tools, particularly in the domains of image analysis, data from laboratory interpretation, and systems for clinical decision support [8]. In addition, the incorporation of AI with electronic health records (EHR), wearable devices, and patient-generated data has increased the scope of disease evaluation [9]. The following examples illustrate specific AI applications in the diagnosis of autoimmune diseases.

2.2 Image Analysis

AI-based assessment of images has shown great promise in making diagnoses of autoimmune diseases, especially rheumatoid arthritis and dermatological conditions such as psoriasis and systemic lupus erythematosus. In rheumatoid arthritis, AI algorithms are capable of analyzing radiographic images of afflicted joints to identify identifying indications such as joint erosions and synovial hypertrophy. Using methods such as deep learning and machine learning on huge amounts of radiographic image data, AI models may be trained to identify and measure these pathological features, thereby aiding in the precise diagnosis of RA [10]. Similarly, AI algorithms can analyze depictions of skin lesions in dermatological autoimmune diseases such as psoriasis and SLE to recognize particular patterns and evaluate disease prevalence. The training of deep learning models on vast databases of dermoscopic or histopathological images enables the automatic identification of disease-specific characteristics. This aids dermatologists in diagnosing these conditions and developing the most suitable treatment plans [11].

2.3 Laboratory Data Interpretation

AI algorithms play a crucial role in the analysis of laboratory data for the diagnosis of autoimmune disease, especially in conditions such as multiple sclerosis and neuromyelitis optica (NMO). AI models can analyze MRI images to detect and measure brain and spinal cord lesions in these diseases [12]. By employing machine learning techniques, these models can recognize patterns and structural abnormalities that aid in differentiating autoimmune neurological disorders [13]. In addition, AI-based evaluation of serological indicators such as autoantibodies aids in the diagnosis of autoimmune diseases. For instance, AI models can analyze patient-specific autoantibody profiles and clinical data to predict disease activity and assess the risk of organ involvement in systemic lupus erythematosus. Using machine learning algorithms, these models provide personalized predictions and facilitate clinical decision-making [14].

2.4 Clinical Decision Support Systems

AI-powered medical decision support systems help in the diagnosis of autoimmune disorders by providing essential support to doctors and nurses. By incorporating data from patients, scientific research, and AI algorithms, these systems provide suggestions based on evidence to enhance diagnostic precision [15]. It aids in processing

EHR data, such as patient history, symptoms, and laboratory results, to generate diagnostic hypotheses, recommend appropriate testing, and facilitate differential diagnosis. Moreover, clinical decision support systems powered by AI may analyze longitudinal patient data, such as the progression of the disease, response to treatment, and adverse reactions to refine and enhance the diagnostic procedure [16]. These systems continually gain insight from new data, enabling recommendations to be updated and contributing to the timely and individualized diagnosis of autoimmune diseases [17].

2.5 *Integration of Electronic Health Records, Wearable Technologies, and Patient-Generated Data*

The incorporation of AI with electronic health records, wearable devices, and patient-generated data enables a comprehensive evaluation of autoimmune diseases. Using EHR data, AI algorithms can uncover latent trends, connections, and risk factors associated with autoimmune diseases [18]. By utilizing Natural Language Processing (NLP) techniques, AI can extract pertinent information from unstructured clinical notes, thereby facilitating accurate diagnosis and prognosis. In addition, wearable devices, such as smartwatches and biosensors, acquire physiological data in real time, such as heart rate, temperature, and activity levels [19]. In conjunction with contextual information, AI algorithms can analyze this data to detect disease flares, predict symptom exacerbation, and optimize treatment. Using AI techniques, patient-generated data, such as symptom diaries and self-reported outcomes, can be analyzed to enhance disease monitoring and assist in diagnosis [20]. AI applications in the diagnosis of autoimmune diseases include image analysis, interpretation of laboratory data, and clinical decision support systems, among others [21]. These applications demonstrate the potential of AI to improve diagnostic accuracy, facilitate personalized medical care, and enable comprehensive disease assessment. As AI continues to advance, its integration with healthcare systems is likely to improve the efficiency and efficacy of diagnosing autoimmune diseases, ultimately leading to better patient outcomes [22]. AI has shown promise in medical diagnosis, but it should always be utilized alongside clinical experience. AI should be used to improve healthcare professionals' diagnoses while preserving human judgment and personalized patient care. The list of various AI-based applications for human disease is listed in Table 1.

3 AI Approaches in Treatment and Drug Discovery

In recent years, the role of AI in the treatment and drug discovery of autoimmune diseases has become increasingly prominent. Autoimmune diseases occur when the body's immune system mistakenly attacks its healthy cells and tissues. Through the

Table 1 A summary of current AI-based tools and their applications in autoimmune diseases

Disease	AI-Based tools	Application	References
Cancer diagnosis	ER APP, Breast Cancer (Visiopharm A/S); Kaiku Health (Kaiku Oy); Transpara (ScreenPoint Medical BV); ColonFlag (Medial EarlySign Inc.); GI Genius (Medtronic Inc. (parent company: Medtronic plc.))	AI was used to utilize the data of cancer biomarkers, scan multiple biopsies, uncover trends, and detect, classify, and forecast illnesses using sophisticated algorithms and machine learning	[23]
Cardiovascular disease assessment	Bay Labs, Caption HealthZebra Medical Vision, Arterys LLC, Aidoc	Medical pictures, ECGs, and genetic data may be used for AI to diagnose cardiovascular disorders. Risk factors, cardiac illnesses, including heart attacks and strokes may be predicted using machine learning algorithms	[24]
Neurological disorder diagnosis	Icometrix, BrainScope, Mindstrong Health, Aidlab, Synchron, Neural Analytics, Viz.ai	Alzheimer's, Parkinson's, and multiple sclerosis may be diagnosed using AI. AI systems are used to find biomarkers and trends in brain scans, genetic data, and patient complaints	[25]
Dermatological diagnosis	DermAI, MetaOptima, SkinVision, VUNO	AI-powered systems were used to detect skin cancers like melanoma. AI systems may help doctors detect skin lesions by analyzing photos and comparing them to large databases	[26]
Pulmonary disease detection	Subtle Medical, Quantib, RadLogics, Lunit, VIDA Diagnostics, Aidful, Enlitic, Butterfly Network	AI can diagnose asthma, COPD, and pneumonia. Lung function tests, medical pictures, and patient information may be used by machine learning algorithms to diagnose respiratory disorders	[27]
Genetic disease identification	FDNA, Sophia Genetics, Deep Genomics, Diploid, Genoox, Fabric Genomics, Blueprint Genetics	AI systems are used to discover genetic abnormalities and illness risks by analyzing DNA sequencing and genomic profiles. AI can diagnose hereditary disorders by comparing genome variants to genetic markers	[28]

(continued)

Table 1 (continued)

Disease	AI-Based tools	Application	References
Ophthalmic disease diagnosis	IDx-DR, RetinAI Medical, Visulytix, Eyenuk Inc, ZEISS, NovaSight, Google DeepMind	AI is used to identify diabetic retinopathy and age-related macular degeneration. AI algorithms may help ophthalmologists diagnose and treat anomalies in retinal pictures	[29]
Mental health assessment	Woebot, Ginger, Talkspace, SilverCloud Health, Lantern, Cogito Corporation, X2AI, Taliaz, AiCure, Cerebri	AI technologies were used to diagnose depression, anxiety, and bipolar illness by analyzing voice, text, and facial expressions. Natural language processing and sentiment analysis algorithms may identify mental health trends and indications for early intervention and personalized therapy	[30]
Rare disease diagnosis	FDNA (now part of Invitae corporation), Mendelian, RD-Connect, Deep 6 AI, SOPHiA Genetics, Congenica, Genomenon, Fabric Genomics, Diploid, N-of-One (part of Qiagen)	Patient symptoms, genetic data, and medical literature may help AI diagnose uncommon illnesses. Machine learning algorithms may help doctors detect rare diseases	[31]

integration of AI, significant advancements have been made in improving diagnosis, personalizing treatment plans, and accelerating the discovery of effective therapies for these complex conditions. Moreover, AI has the potential to significantly impact the treatment of autoimmune diseases in several ways. For Predictive Analytics, AI algorithms can be trained on patient data to develop predictive models that estimate disease progression, treatment response, and potential complications. These models can help healthcare providers make informed decisions regarding personalized treatment plans and identify high-risk patients who require closer monitoring. For Precision Medicine, AI can facilitate precision medicine approaches by analyzing individual patient characteristics, such as genetic profiles, lifestyle factors, and medical history, to develop personalized treatment strategies. This can lead to more targeted and effective interventions, minimizing adverse effects and optimizing outcomes. For Treatment Optimization, AI algorithms can continuously analyze patient data, treatment outcomes, and real-time monitoring data to optimize treatment protocols. By considering multiple variables and adjusting treatment plans in real time, AI can help healthcare providers make data-driven decisions and improve patient outcomes. It is important to note that while AI holds great promise, they are not meant to replace healthcare professionals. Instead, they are tools that can augment their capabilities, improve decision-making processes, and enhance patient care in the context of autoimmune diseases and other complex medical conditions.

3.1 Predictive Analytics for Disease Progression and Treatment Response

In several studies associated with inflammatory bowel diseases, machine learning-based methods such as Random Forest and Support Vector Machine (SVM) were implemented to predict response to treatment, disease risk, and disease severity [32]. Notably, in a study associated with Type 1 diabetes, a machine learning-based fTPM approach for the diagnosis and monitoring of Type 1 Diabetes Mellitus (T1DM) was presented. The study focused on assessing the physical state of Red Blood Cell (RBC) membranes, which undergo alterations in T1DM and serve as an indicator for disease progression. The researchers observed increasing fluidification of RBC membranes as the disease progressed, along with the formation of microdomains exhibiting different fluidity. Sub-micrometric fluidity maps showed a widening of the fluidity spectrum and a consistent increase in the fluid region. Based on these findings, a diagnostic system was developed to measure variations in a measurable quantity induced by the disease [33]. Additionally, various novel methods/hybrid models based on Neural Networks, and Support Vector Regression have been used for studying disease progression and autoimmune diseases.

3.2 Precision Medicine for Disease Progression and Treatment Response

In the case of rheumatoid arthritis, the treatment selection process primarily relies on trial and error, despite the availability of various targeted biological and conventional therapies. This highlights the existence of a "precision gap" in the field of rheumatic diseases, which indicates the factors hindering the advancement and adoption of precision medicine approaches [34]. Notably, in a study associated with Systemic Sclerosis, a machine learning approach was employed to identify pathways that were down-regulated by treatment. Genes demonstrating a significant decrease after treatment were utilized as positive examples in an SVM classifier, while genes exhibiting no evidence of differential expression served as negative examples. By learning the connectivity patterns of differentially expressed genes in a skin network, the classifier ranked all genes in the genome. The top-ranked genes held great relevance to treatment response, even if they were missed due to small sample sizes or undetectable changes at the mRNA level. In summary, the integration of machine learning in this framework enabled a more comprehensive and nuanced understanding of treatment response, allowing for the identification of key pathways, potential therapeutic targets, and the exploration of alternative therapies for patients who do not respond to initial treatments. This approach enhances the precision and individualization of treatment strategies, paving the way for more effective and tailored precision medicine interventions [35].

3.3 Treatment Optimization for Autoimmune Diseases

In autoimmune diseases, such as rheumatoid arthritis, personalized and precise medicine holds promise. Current treatment approaches often involve trial and error, leading to suboptimal outcomes and increased healthcare costs. Implementing a precision medicine approach based on patients' biological profiles could enhance treatment responsiveness [36]. Machine learning algorithms have demonstrated the ability to predict treatment response using demographic and clinical data, achieving high accuracy with Area Under the ROC Curve (AUC) up to 0.84 [37, 38]. Additionally, machine learning techniques have been employed to forecast the need for treatment escalation, identifying patients who may require more powerful medications. Omics data, including genetic and microbiome information, offer valuable insights for predicting treatment response. Random forest models utilizing gut microbiome data achieved an AUC of 0.84 in identifying methotrexate (MTX) responders while incorporating transcriptomics data reached an AUC of 0.78 for MTX response prediction [39, 40]. Notably, omics data appear more beneficial in predicting response to second or third-line biological disease-modifying antirheumatic drugs (bDMARDs) compared to MTX [41, 42].

Incorporating imaging data, such as ultrasound images, can further enhance response prediction. Scoring systems based on the severity of synovitis, tenosynovitis, and enthesitis on ultrasound images have been developed to assess treatment response, enabling the identification of patient clusters with significantly different treatment outcomes [43]. The use of virtual patient models and AI-enhanced Quantitative Systems Pharmacology (QSP) allows for the prediction of drug efficacy and optimization of treatment regimens for autoimmune and inflammatory diseases [44]. These models help in selecting dosing regimens, administration schemes, and clinical endpoints to improve the effectiveness of the drug. Additionally, the identification of biomarkers through machine learning analysis aids in patient stratification and monitoring during treatment, further optimizing the therapeutic approach. Overall, these methods contribute to the optimization of drug therapies in the context of autoimmune and inflammatory diseases [44].

3.4 AI Approaches for Target Identification

The identification of suitable therapeutic targets for autoimmune and inflammatory diseases (AIDs) can be enhanced through AID modeling combined with AI-powered computational analyses. By conducting comprehensive multi-omics molecular profiling of patients, these models facilitate patient stratification into homogeneous subgroups [45]. Moreover, they shed light on dysregulated pro-inflammatory pathways and generate hypotheses regarding potential therapeutic targets and candidate biomarkers, aiding in patient stratification and monitoring during treatment. AID models provide valuable insights into the rational design of combination therapies that target independent pro-inflammatory pathways associated with various immune compartments contributing to AID pathophysiology [46]. These immune compartments encompass pro-inflammatory signals originating from tissues, innate immune mechanisms, T lymphocyte activation, autoantibodies, and B cell activation, as well as soluble mediators involved in immune cross-talk.

By integrating multi-omics data and leveraging AI algorithms, AID modeling optimizes the identification of therapeutic targets for AIDs. This approach allows for a more personalized and precise treatment strategy by identifying combinations of therapies that effectively target distinct aspects of the disease pathology. Ultimately, AID modeling plays a vital role in advancing precision medicine for AIDs, leading to improved patient outcomes [47]. Despite significant investments and extensive preclinical research, there is a significant discrepancy between the number of promising lead compounds and the limited number of approved drugs. A major contributing factor to this issue is the inadequate predictive validity of animal models of multiple sclerosis (MS) in translating pathogenic mechanisms into safe and effective treatments for patients. This concerning situation has led to criticism regarding the relevance of current animal models used in preclinical research and has sparked a call for the enhancement of these models [48].

4 AI Approaches for Optimization of Drug Candidates and Repurposing Existing Drugs

Machine learning techniques were utilized to predict the risk of drug-induced autoimmune diseases [49]. Their approach involves analyzing structural alerts, which are specific molecular features associated with adverse drug reactions, as well as considering the daily dose of the drug. By training a machine learning model on a dataset of known drug-induced autoimmune diseases, the researchers aim to develop a predictive model that can assess the potential risk of these adverse events based on the structural properties of the drug and its dosage. This approach holds the potential to enhance the evaluation of the safety profile of new drugs and guide the drug development process, reducing the occurrence of autoimmune adverse reactions. In a study, a model was employed to identify potential drug candidates for repurposing [50]. The model utilized a methodology involving data collection and integration, followed by the evaluation and selection of candidate drugs based on predefined criteria. Through this approach, promising drug candidates were identified for treating these diseases. The findings of the study highlight the potential of drug repurposing as a strategy to enhance treatment options for rheumatic autoimmune inflammatory diseases, offering new avenues for improving patient outcomes in this challenging therapeutic area. The study utilizes machine learning approaches that capitalize on network medicine concepts. These approaches aim to replicate the intricate interactions between drugs and diseases. One specific tool mentioned is deepDR [51], which integrates various networks such as drug-side effect, drug-target, drug-disease, and multiple drug-drug networks. In this tool, an autoencoder is employed to learn drug features from these networks. These learned features are then utilized to predict approved drugs for neurodegenerative diseases. The study highlights the potential of machine learning in overcoming limitations associated with a lack of mechanistic understanding of complex diseases, as demonstrated in the context of neurodegenerative diseases.

5 Challenges and Future Directions

Despite the considerable promise shown by AI and machine learning in the realm of autoimmune disease research, some challenges require attention and resolution. To achieve optimal performance, AI models need the use of comprehensive and high-quality datasets, including both a substantial volume and superior standards. Ensuring the accessibility of databases related to rare autoimmune diseases is a significant challenge. The issue of interpretability becomes relevant when examining black-box AI models since their ability to provide predictions is hindered by the challenge of understanding the underlying biological processes. The significance of developing interpretable AI models lies in its contribution to the pursuit of comprehending disease processes. The incorporation of AI in the healthcare sector requires the development of ethical and regulatory structures to adequately address issues related to patient privacy, transparency, and accountability. The use of AI and machine learning techniques in the realm of autoimmune disease research has ushered in a new era of investigation and progress. The technologies listed above have the potential to significantly transform the detection, treatment, and management of autoimmune diseases, therefore improving the general health and well-being of many individuals worldwide. Despite the presence of enduring challenges, the field of AI holds promise for ongoing progress as a result of the relentless attempts undertaken by researchers, medical professionals, and individuals participating in research and cooperative initiatives.

6 Conclusion

The use of machine learning and deep learning in autoimmune disorders is a rapidly growing field of research, as it has the potential to revolutionize the diagnosis and treatment of these conditions. Incorporating different omics and clinical data may lead to better results in both prognosis and treatment of autoimmune diseases. AI has proven its potential in improving diagnosis, personalizing treatment plans, and accelerating the discovery of effective therapies. Through predictive analytics, precision medicine, and treatment optimization, AI empowers healthcare providers to make informed decisions, develop personalized treatment strategies, and optimize patient outcomes. Additionally, AI plays a crucial role in drug discovery by identifying potential targets, optimizing drug candidates, and uncovering repurposing opportunities. By leveraging AI's capabilities, the field of autoimmune diseases can benefit from enhanced precision medicine approaches and optimized drug therapies. AI serves as a powerful tool in the fight against autoimmune diseases, offering new possibilities for improved patient care and outcomes.

References

1. Stafford IS, Kellermann M, Mossotto E, Beattie RM, MacArthur BD, Ennis S (2020) A systematic review of the applications of artificial intelligence and machine learning in autoimmune diseases. NPJ Digital Med 3(1):30
2. Momtazmanesh S, Nowroozi A, Rezaei N (2022) Artificial intelligence in rheumatoid arthritis: current status and future perspectives: a state-of-the-art review. Rheumatol Therapy 9(5):1249–1304
3. Bonacchi R, Filippi M, Rocca MA (2022) Role of artificial intelligence in MS clinical practice. NeuroImage: Clinical 103065
4. Yaung KN, Yeo JG, Kumar P, Wasser M, Chew M, Ravelli A, Law AHN et al (2023) Artificial intelligence and high-dimensional technologies in the theragnosis of systemic lupus erythematous. Lancet Rheumatol 5(3):e151–e165
5. Zhou Y, Wang M, Zhao S, Yan Y (2022) Machine learning for diagnosis of systemic lupus erythematosus: a systematic review and meta-analysis. Computat Intell Neurosci (2022)
6. Vodencarevic A, Tascilar K, Hartmann F, Reiser M, Hueber AJ, Haschka J, Bayat S et al (2021) Advanced machine learning for predicting individual risk of flares in rheumatoid arthritis patients tapering biologic drugs. Arthritis Res Ther 23(1): 1–8
7. Kalweit M, Walker UA, Finckh A, Müller R, Kalweit G, Scherer A, Boedecker J, Hügle T (2021) Personalized prediction of disease activity in patients with rheumatoid arthritis using an adaptive deep neural network. PLoS ONE 16(6):e0252289
8. Raza K, Singh NK (2021) A tour of unsupervised deep learning for medical image analysis current medical imaging. Bentham Sci 17(9):1059–1077. https://doi.org/10.2174/1573405617666210127154257
9. Ahn JC, Connell A, Simonetto DA, Hughes C, Shah VH (2021) Application of artificial intelligence for the diagnosis and treatment of liver diseases. Hepatol Baltim Md 73(6):2546–2563. https://doi.org/10.1002/hep.31603
10. Chen H, Sung JJY (2021) Potentials of AI in medical image analysis in gastroenterology and hepatology. J Gastroenterol Hepatol 36(1):31–38. https://doi.org/10.1111/jgh.15327
11. Christou CD, Tsoulfas G (2021) Challenges and opportunities in the application of artificial intelligence in gastroenterology and hepatology. World J Gastroenterol 27(37):6191–6223. https://doi.org/10.3748/wjg.v27.i37.6191
12. Siddiqui MF et al (2022) Computational intelligence: a step forward in cancer biomarker discovery and therapeutic target prediction. In: Oncology KR (ed) Computational intelligence. Studies in computational intelligence, vol 1016. Singapore: Springer Singapore, pp 233–250. https://doi.org/10.1007/978-981-16-9221-5_14.
13. Khalifa A, Obeid JS, Erno J, Rockey DC (2023) The role of artificial intelligence in hepatology research and practice. Curr Opin Gastroenterol 39(3):175–180. https://doi.org/10.1097/MOG.0000000000000926
14. Krittanawong C, Zhang H, Wang Z, Aydar M, Kitai T (2017) Artificial intelligence in precision cardiovascular medicine. J Am Coll Cardiol 69(21):2657–2664. https://doi.org/10.1016/j.jacc.2017.03.571

15. Magrabi F et al (2019) Artificial intelligence in clinical decision support: challenges for evaluating AI and practical implications. Yearb Med Inform 28(1):128–134. https://doi.org/10.1055/s-0039-1677903
16. Garcia-Vidal C, Sanjuan G, Puerta-Alcalde P, Moreno-García E, Soriano A (2019) Artificial intelligence to support clinical decision-making processes. EBioMedicine 46:27–29. https://doi.org/10.1016/j.ebiom.2019.07.019
17. Shaikh F et al (2021) Artificial intelligence-based clinical decision support systems using advanced medical imaging and radiomics. Curr Probl Diagn Radiol 50(2):262–267. https://doi.org/10.1067/j.cpradiol.2020.05.006
18. Wong GL-H, Yuen P-C, Ma AJ, Chan AW-H, Leung HH-W, Wong VW-S (2021) Artificial intelligence in prediction of non-alcoholic fatty liver disease and fibrosis. J Gastroenterol Hepatol 36(3):543–550. https://doi.org/10.1111/jgh.15385
19. Siddiqui MF et al (2023) Leveraging healthcare system with nature-inspired computing techniques: an overview and future perspective. In: Raza K (ed) Nature-inspired intelligent computing techniques in bioinformatics. Studies in computational intelligence, vol 1066. Singapore: Springer Nature Singapore, pp 19–42. https://doi.org/10.1007/978-981-19-6379-7_2
20. Su T-H, Wu C-H, Kao J-H (2021) Artificial intelligence in precision medicine in hepatology. J Gastroenterol Hepatol 36(3):569–580. https://doi.org/10.1111/jgh.15415
21. Qazi, S, Iqbal N, Raza K (2022) Fuzzy logic-based hybrid models for clinical decision support systems in cancer. In: Computational intelligence in oncology. Studies in computational intelligence (SCI), vol 1016. Springer, pp 1–13. https://doi.org/10.1007/978-981-16-9221-5_12
22. Le Berre C et al (2020) Application of artificial intelligence to gastroenterology and hepatology. Gastroenterology 158(1):76-94.e2. https://doi.org/10.1053/j.gastro.2019.08.058
23. Mitsala A, Tsalikidis C, Pitiakoudis M, Simopoulos C, Tsaroucha AK (2021) Artificial intelligence in colorectal cancer screening, diagnosis and treatment. A new era. Curr. Oncol. Tor. Ont 28(3):1581–1607. https://doi.org/10.3390/curroncol28030149
24. Siontis KC, Noseworthy PA, Attia ZI, Friedman PA (2021) Artificial intelligence-enhanced electrocardiography in cardiovascular disease management. Nat Rev Cardiol 18(7):465–478. https://doi.org/10.1038/s41569-020-00503-2
25. Patel UK et al (2021) Artificial intelligence as an emerging technology in the current care of neurological disorders. J Neurol 268(5):1623–1642. https://doi.org/10.1007/s00415-019-09518-3
26. Young AT, Xiong M, Pfau J, Keiser MJ, Wei ML (2020) Artificial intelligence in dermatology: a primer. J Invest Dermatol 140(8):1504–1512. https://doi.org/10.1016/j.jid.2020.02.026
27. Hong L, Cheng X, Zheng D (2021) Application of artificial intelligence in emergency nursing of patients with chronic obstructive pulmonary disease. Contrast Media Mol Imaging 2021:6423398. https://doi.org/10.1155/2021/6423398
28. James KN, Phadke S, Wong TC, Chowdhury S (2023) Artificial intelligence in the genetic diagnosis of rare disease. Clin Lab Med 43(1):127–143. https://doi.org/10.1016/j.cll.2022.09.023
29. Li J-PO et al (2021) Digital technology, tele-medicine and artificial intelligence in ophthalmology: a global perspective. Prog Retin Eye Res 82:100900. https://doi.org/10.1016/j.preteyeres.2020.100900
30. Fiske A, Henningsen P, Buyx A (2019) Your robot therapist will see you now: ethical implications of embodied artificial intelligence in psychiatry, psychology, and psychotherapy. J Med Internet Res 21(5):e13216. https://doi.org/10.2196/13216
31. Noll R et al (2022) Conception, development and validation of classification methods for coding support of rare diseases using artificial intelligence. Stud Health Technol Inform 295:422–425. https://doi.org/10.3233/SHTI220755
32. Stafford IS, Kellermann M, Mossotto E et al (2020) A systematic review of the applications of artificial intelligence and machine learning in autoimmune diseases. npj Digit Med 3, 30. https://doi.org/10.1038/s41746-020-0229-3

33. Maulucci G et al (2017) Phase separation of the plasma membrane in human red blood cells as a potential tool for diagnosis and progression monitoring of type 1 diabetes mellitus. PLoS ONE 12
34. Lin CMA, Cooles FAH, Isaacs JD (2022) Precision medicine: the precision gap in rheumatic disease. Nat Rev Rheumatol 18:725–733. https://doi.org/10.1038/s41584-022-00845-w
35. Taroni JN, Martyanov V, Mahoney JM, Whitfield ML (2017) A functional genomic meta-analysis of clinical trials in systemic sclerosis: toward precision medicine and combination therapy. J Invest Dermatol 137:1033–1041
36. Momtazmanesh S, Nowroozi A, Rezaei N (2022) Artificial intelligence in rheumatoid arthritis: current status and future perspectives: a state-of-the-art review. Rheumatol Ther 9:1249–1304. https://doi.org/10.1007/s40744-022-00475-4
37. Amin Shipa MR, Yeoh SA, Embleton-Thirsk A, Mukerjee D, Ehrenstein MR (2022) The synergistic efficacy of hydroxychloroquine with methotrexate is accompanied by increased erythrocyte mean corpuscular volume. Rheumatology (Oxford) 61(2):787–793
38. Westerlind H, Maciejewski M, Frisell T, Jelinsky SA, Ziemek D, Askling J (2021) What is the persistence to methotrexate in rheumatoid arthritis, and does machine learning outperform hypothesis-based approaches to its prediction? ACR Open Rheumatol. 3:457–463
39. Artacho A, Isaac S, Nayak R, Flor-Duro A, Alexander M, Koo I, Manasson J, Smith PB, Rosenthal P, Homsi Y et al (2021) The pretreatment gut microbiome is associated with lack of response to methotrexate in new-onset rheumatoid arthritis. Arthritis Rheumatol 73:931–942
40. Plant D, Maciejewski M, Smith S, Nair N, Hyrich K, Ziemek D, Barton A, Verstappen S (2019) Maximising therapeutic utility in rheumatoid arthritis consortium tRSG. Profiling of gene expression biomarkers as a classifier of methotrexate nonresponse in patients with rheumatoid arthritis. Arthritis Rheumatol 71:678–84
41. Tao W, Concepcion AN, Vianen M, Marijnissen ACA, Lafeber F, Radstake T, Pandit A (2021) Multiomics and machine learning accurately predict clinical response to adalimumab and etanercept therapy in patients with rheumatoid arthritis. Arthritis Rheumatol 73:212–222
42. Kim KJ, Kim M, Adamopoulos IE, Tagkopoulos I (2019) Compendium of synovial signatures identifies pathologic characteristics for predicting treatment response in rheumatoid arthritis patients. Clin Immunol 202:1–10
43. Kato M, Ikeda K, Sugiyama T, Tanaka S, Iida K, Suga K, Nishimura N, Mimura N, Kasuya T, Kumagai T et al (2021) Associations of ultrasound-based inflammation patterns with peripheral innate lymphoid cell populations, serum cytokines/chemokines, and treatment response to methotrexate in rheumatoid arthritis and spondyloarthritis. PLoS ONE 16:e0252116
44. Moingeon P (2023) Artificial intelligence-driven drug development against autoimmune diseases. Trends Pharmacol Sci 31:S0165–6147(23)00088–3. https://doi.org/10.1016/j.tips.2023.04.005. Epub ahead of print. PMID: 37268540
45. Desvaux E, Aussy A, Hubert S, Keime-Guibert F, Blesius A, Soret P, Guedj M, Pers JO, Laigle L, Moingeon P (2022) Model-based computational precision medicine to develop combination therapies for autoimmune diseases. Expert Rev Clin Immunol. 18(1):47–56. https://doi.org/10.1080/1744666X.2022.2012452. Epub 2021 Dec 13. PMID: 34842494
46. Aghamiri SS, Amin R, Helikar T (2022) Recent applications of quantitative systems pharmacology and machine learning models across diseases. J Pharmacokinet Pharmacodyn 49(1):19–37. https://doi.org/10.1007/s10928-021-09790-9. Epub 2021 Oct 20. PMID: 34671863; PMCID: PMC8528185.
47. Zhang T, Androulakis IP, Bonate P, Cheng L, Helikar T, Parikh J, Rackauckas C, Subramanian K, Cho CR (2022) Working Group. Two heads are better than one: current landscape of integrating QSP and machine learning: An ISoP QSP SIG white paper by the working group on the integration of quantitative systems pharmacology and machine learning. J Pharmacokinet Pharmacodyn. 49(1):5–18. https://doi.org/10.1007/s10928-022-09805-z. Epub 2022 Feb 1. PMID: 35103884; PMCID: PMC8837505
48. Hart BA, Luchicchi A, Schenk GJ, Killestein J, Geurts JJG (2021) Multiple sclerosis and drug discovery: a work of translation. EBioMedicine. 68:103392. https://doi.org/10.1016/j.ebiom.2021.103392. Epub 2021 May 24. PMID: 34044219; PMCID: PMC8245896

49. Wu Y, Zhu J, Fu P, Tong W, Hong H, Chen M (2021) Machine learning for predicting risk of drug-induced autoimmune diseases by structural alerts and daily dose. Int J Environ Res Public Health 18(13):7139. https://doi.org/10.3390/ijerph18137139.PMID:34281077;PMCID:PMC8296890
50. Kingsmore KM, Grammer AC, Lipsky PE (2020) Drug repurposing to improve treatment of rheumatic autoimmune inflammatory diseases. Nat Rev Rheumatol 16:32–52. https://doi.org/10.1038/s41584-019-0337-0
51. Zeng X et al (2019) deepDR: a network-based deep learning approach to in silico drug repositioning, Bioinformatics 35(24):5191–5198. https://doi.org/10.1093/bioinformatics/btz418

Autoimmune Autonomic Disorder: AI-Based Diagnosis and Prognosis

Ritu Karwasra, Sneha Sharma, Isha Sharma, and Shiv Kant Sharma

Abstract Autoimmune Autonomic Disorders (AAD) are a group of rare conditions that affect the autonomic nervous system, leading to a wide range of debilitating symptoms. Timely and accurate diagnosis is crucial for effective management and treatment. This article explores the application of artificial intelligence (AI) in the diagnosis and prognosis of AAD, presenting an innovative approach to improve patient care. AI-based diagnostic tools have shown promising results in identifying AAD by analysing various clinical data sources, including patient histories, laboratory tests, and autonomic function tests. Machine learning algorithms, such as deep neural networks and support vector machines, can efficiently process large datasets and extract valuable patterns and features that might escape human detection. These AI models can assist clinicians in making more precise and timelier AAD diagnoses. Furthermore, AI can also aid in the prognosis of AAD by predicting disease progression and treatment outcomes. This article highlights the potential of AI in revolutionizing the diagnosis and prognosis of AAD, ultimately leading to improved patient outcomes and a better understanding of these complex autoimmune disorders. However, further research and clinical validation are necessary to fully integrate AI-based tools into routine medical practice for AAD management.

Keywords Autoimmune disorders · Artificial intelligence · Prognosis · Machine learning

R. Karwasra
Central Council for Research in Unani Medicine, Ministry of Ayush, Government of India, New Delhi 110058, India

S. Sharma · I. Sharma · S. K. Sharma (✉)
Department of Pharmaceutical Sciences, Gurugram University, Gurugram 122003, India
e-mail: shivkantvats@gmail.com

K. Raza and S. Singh (eds.), *Artificial Intelligence and Autoimmune Diseases*, Studies in Computational Intelligence 1133, https://doi.org/10.1007/978-981-99-9029-0_4

1 Introduction

Autoimmune diseases, initially identified by Ian Mackay and Macfarlane Burnet in 1963, occur when an organism's immune system fails to tolerate its own cells and tissues, leading to an abnormal immune response involving lymphocytes and antibodies [1]. This results in tissue damage and dysfunction in the targeted organs or body systems, which can range from systemic to affecting specific areas such as the endocrine, gastrointestinal, liver, rheumatological, and neurological systems [2]. Autoimmune diseases are chronic, multifactorial conditions. The progression of autoimmune diseases is influenced by three aspects: immune system dysregulation, environmental conditions, and genetic predisposition. The diagnosis and prognosis of autoimmune disease are uncertain because of the variety of onset and development. Defects in pathways that lead to a loss of self-tolerance are the root cause of an inherited propensity for autoimmunity [3]. Further immune system dysregulation, in both the innate and adaptive immune systems, leads to the development of autoimmune disorders [4]. Self-reactive lymphocytes can be induced by external antigens, microbial antigens, and cytokine dysregulation [5]. Further upsetting the immune system's balance is the possibility of T and B cells becoming hyperactive as well as changes in the time and property of their response. Since different studies have varying illustrations of diseases, therefore there is no comprehensive list. It is challenging to determine the prevalence of autoimmune disorders [6, 7]. According to reports, the prevalence rate for all autoimmune illnesses ranges from 4.5% to 9.4%.

1.1 Artificial Intelligence

The study of techniques to mimic intelligent human behaviours, including making judgements in the face of ambiguity, is known as artificial intelligence (AI). Both AI are distinct from conventional statistical techniques in that they prioritize categorization and prediction from high-dimensional data over inference. Combined clinical and "omic" data have limited value without interpretive techniques. AI and machine learning algorithms can find therapeutically useful patterns within a wealth of data [8], thereby filling a gap in the market. Using these data to categorize patients has implications for their care, including risk assessment for autoimmune diseases, diagnosis, initial and continuing management, monitoring, therapy response, and prognosis.

AI is commonly traced back to the introduction of the term "robot" by Karel Capek in his 1921 play, "R.U.R." Isaac Asimov further popularized it in mid-twentieth-century science fiction. Artificial intelligence (AI) is widely attributed to its origins in the concept of robots, popularized by Karel Capek in his 1921 play, "R.U.R." The term "robot," spelt as "robota" in Czech, originally referred to biosynthetic machines used as forced labour in a factory. Isaac Asimov later popularized the term "robot" in mid-twentieth-century science fiction. However, the concept of humanoid automata dates back to ancient China in the third century, when engineer Yan Shi presented a human-shaped mechanical figure to Emperor Mu of Zhou, constructed from leather, wood, and artificial organs [9].

AI techniques are highly effective in diagnosing various diseases, significantly enhancing medical services, improving patient outcomes, and reducing costs. These models extend beyond automation, involving patients, families [10, 11], and healthcare professionals in data generation, recommendations, and collaborative evaluation.

AI has emerged as a transformative force in healthcare, revolutionizing the industry in numerous ways. One of its most significant impacts lies in its ability to enhance diagnosis and treatment. AI algorithms can analyse vast amounts of patient data, including medical records, images, and genetic information, to identify patterns and anomalies that may be imperceptible to human practitioners. This not only accelerates the diagnostic process but also improves accuracy, reducing misdiagnoses and enabling earlier intervention. Moreover, AI-driven predictive analytics plays a pivotal role in disease prevention and management. Machine learning models can forecast disease outbreaks, identify at-risk populations, and recommend personalized interventions to improve patient outcomes. Wearable devices and remote monitoring systems equipped with AI can continuously track vital signs, providing real-time data to healthcare professionals, and enabling timely interventions, especially for chronic conditions [12].

AI-powered robotics and automation are transforming surgery and patient care. Robots can perform precise, minimally invasive surgeries with greater precision than human hands, reducing recovery times and complications. AI also streamlines administrative tasks, such as billing and appointment scheduling, allowing healthcare providers to allocate more time to patient care. Drug discovery and development benefit immensely from AI, as it can analyse vast datasets to identify potential drug candidates, predict their efficacy, and optimize clinical trial designs. This expedites the development of new treatments, potentially saving lives and reducing costs. However, the deployment of AI in healthcare also raises important ethical and privacy concerns. Safeguarding patient data, ensuring transparency in AI algorithms, and maintaining the human touch in healthcare delivery remain critical challenges. Nevertheless, the growing importance of AI in healthcare is undeniable, offering the promise of more accurate diagnoses, personalized treatments, and improved patient outcomes in a field where every moment counts.

Researchers have employed a range of AI-based techniques, including machine and deep learning models, for the early detection of diseases like skin, liver, heart, Alzheimer's, and more. Previous studies have presented various methods such as the Boltzmann machine, K-nearest neighbour (kNN), support vector machine (SVM), decision tree, logistic regression, fuzzy logic, and artificial neural network (ANN), along with their respective accuracies for disease diagnosis. To gain a comprehensive understanding of how AI aids in disease diagnosis and prediction, it is crucial to grasp the utility and suitability of diverse techniques like SVM, kNN, Naïve Bayes, Decision Tree, Ada Boost, Random Forest, K-Mean clustering, Recurrent Neural Network (RNN), Convolutional Neural Networks (CNN), Deep-CNN, Generative

Adversarial Networks (GAN), Long Short-Term Memory (LSTM), and numerous others across various disease detection systems [13].

1.2 AI Evolution

Intuitive Surgical, an American company, developed a surgical system known as Da Vinci, named in homage to the renowned historical figure. This system received FDA approval in 2000 and has since seen over 5,000 units deployed worldwide. The Da Vinci surgical systems are instrumental in conducting intricate surgeries through minimally invasive techniques, offering surgeons the ability to control them from a console. These systems find frequent application in procedures such as prostatectomies and gynecologic surgeries and are now being adopted for cardiac valve repair as well.

The evolution of robots took an intriguing turn with the "Flute Player," a remarkable mechanical creation conceived in the eighteenth century by French inventor Jacques de Vaucanson. This innovative "automaton" was designed to play the flute and boasted a repertoire of 12 songs. Fast forward two centuries to 1948, and William Gray Walter gained fame for crafting the first electronic autonomous robot, which he named "Machina Speculatrix." Walter's objective was to illustrate the functioning of the brain, and his work revealed that connections among a limited number of "brain cells" could give rise to highly complex behaviours.

The Perceptron model had a profound impact on the development of neural networks and connection mechanisms, enabling the creation of recognition systems based on "neurons." This pioneering work continues to be a relevant and frequently discussed topic in introductory AI courses today. In 1960, the perceptron algorithm was taken a step further when it was implemented in physical hardware known as the "Mark 1 Perceptron." This artificial brain consisted of an array of perceptrons connected to a camera, representing a significant advancement in the field [14].

In subsequent years, computers began tackling complex mathematical problems, capturing the interest of the U.S. Department of Defense. Following a period of slowdowns in the 1980s, a new era of progress commenced, marked by the application of logistic data mining and medical diagnosis. This era witnessed the development of instruments with increasingly powerful computational capabilities. This newfound computational power enabled significant milestones, including IBM's victory over the world chess champion, Gary Kasparov, on May 11, 1997.

Today, AI is recognized as a field of engineering that introduces innovative concepts and solutions to address intricate challenges. With the ongoing advancements in computing speed, capacity, and software programming, the prospect of computers attaining human-level intelligence remains a possibility. It is important to acknowledge the substantial contribution of contemporary cybernetics to the evolution of AI [15].

2 AI-Based Diagnosis of Different Autoimmune Diseases

A set of diseases known as autoimmune disorders are brought on by the immune system targeting the body's healthy cells and tissues. They can affect different parts of the body, including joints, muscles, skin, and internal organs. Autoimmune diseases are challenging to diagnose, as their symptoms can be vague and often overlap with other conditions. Therefore, the development of accurate diagnostic tools is essential for early detection and effective treatment of autoimmune diseases.

The diagnosis of autoimmune illnesses has shown potential when using AI. AI systems can examine a lot of patient data and find trends that can lead to an autoimmune condition. This can assist physicians in making accurate diagnoses and developing personalized treatment plans for patients [4]. A framework for the disease detection system is shown in Fig. 1. In this article, we will discuss the potential applications of AI in the diagnosis of autoimmune diseases, the challenges faced by AI-based diagnosis, and the future direction of research in this field.

2.1 Applications of AI in Autoimmune Disease Diagnosis

Analysing electronic medical records (EMRs) is one way that AI is used to diagnose autoimmune diseases. Patient's medical histories, test findings, and imaging studies are all included in EMRs. These data can be examined by AI algorithms, which can also recognize trends that can lead to the existence of an autoimmune disease. For instance, researchers at Stanford University examined the EMRs of patients with rheumatoid arthritis (RA) using machine learning algorithms. The algorithm was likely to accurately identify people with RA and identify those who were at

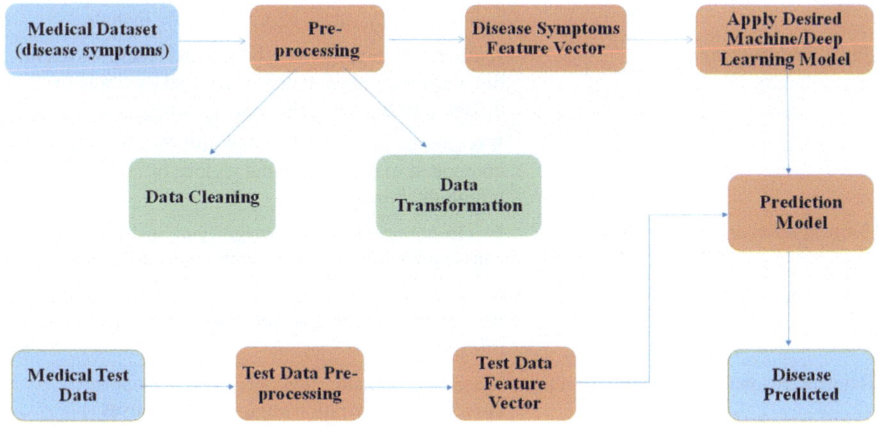

Fig. 1 Framework for disease detection system [12]

risk of getting the condition. Similar to this, a study that appeared in the journal Arthritis Research & Therapy examined the EMRs of people who had systemic lupus erythematosus (SLE). The algorithm was able to accurately identify patients with SLE and foretell which patients were most likely to experience serious organ damage. The study of imaging investigations, such as X-rays, CT scans, and MRIs, is another aspect that AI is used in the diagnosis of autoimmune disorders. AI systems can examine these pictures and look for patterns that can show the existence of an autoimmune disease. For example, a study published in the journal Annals of Rheumatic Diseases used deep learning algorithms to analyse MRI scans of patients with RA. The algorithm was able to predict disease activity with high accuracy, and also identify patients who were likely to respond to treatment. Similarly, a study published in the journal Arthritis Care & Research used deep learning algorithms to analyse X-ray images of patients with RA. The algorithm was able to predict disease progression with high accuracy, and also identify patients who were likely to respond to treatment [16]. Various medical imaging types have been listed in Table 1.

Table 1 Medical imaging types with their respective descriptions [17, 18]

Medical imaging types	Description
Radiographic imaging	Radiographic imaging is utilized in the ionizing of electromagnetic radiation, for example, X-beams to see objects
DEXA	It is likewise called Dual X-beam Absorptiometry or bone densitometry which is utilized for osteoporosis tests
Computed tomography (CT)	Computed tomography examination utilizes an immense measure of ionizing radiation related to a PC to make pictures of delicate and hard tissues
Magnetic resonance imaging	Magnetic resonance imaging (MRI) filtering is a clinical examination that utilizes excellent magnet and radiofrequency waves to create a body picture
Ultrasound imaging	It utilizes high-recurrence broadband sound waves in the megahertz range that are reflected by tissue to differing degrees to deliver 3D pictures
Bone scan	It is an imaging procedure that utilizes a radioactive compound to distinguish the regions of mending within the bone
Electron microscopy	Electron microscopy is a magnifying instrument that can amplify tiny subtleties with high settling power
Nuclear medicine	Nuclear medication on the entire incorporates both the finding and treatment of infections utilizing atomic properties
Magnetic resonance angiography scans	Magnetic resonance angiography represents an attractive reverberation angiogram that gives exceptionally itemized pictures of the veins in the body

Biomarkers are biological markers that can be measured and analysed to help diagnose autoimmune diseases. AI algorithms can analyse biomarker data and identify patterns that may indicate the presence of an autoimmune disease. For instance, a study published in the journal Clinical and Experimental Rheumatology used machine learning algorithms to analyse gene expression data from blood samples of patients with SLE. The algorithm was able to identify biomarkers that could differentiate between different subtypes of SLE with high accuracy. Similarly, a study published in the journal Nature Communications used machine learning algorithms to analyse gene expression data from blood samples of patients with RA. The algorithm was able to identify biomarkers that could predict disease activity with high accuracy, and also identify patients who were likely to respond to treatment [19].

3 AI-Based Prognosis of Different Autoimmune Diseases

The goal of prognosis is to assess the equipment's current health status (known as degradation assessment [DA]) and forecast when it will fail in the future (known as remaining useful life [RUL]) in order to serve as the foundation for subsequent predictive maintenance. The industry is very concerned about the vital equipment's operational state because a sudden breakdown or shutdown might result in significant financial losses and even put the operators' lives in danger. According to literature statistics, there are four main categories for prediction approaches: physics-based, statistics-based, data-driven, and hybrid methods. Physics-based techniques frequently rely on dynamic modelling to assess the system's dynamic response and rate of deterioration in response to a specific input, such as stimulation [20], the finite element model [21], etc. Physics-based methods call for precise mathematical models and knowledge of the particular system, which is challenging to apply to intricate mechanical machinery. The RUL of equipment is frequently assumed by statistically based methods to follow an empirical distribution, such as a Weibull distribution [22]. It is of little consequence that statistically based approaches require data in order to update the empirical distribution's parameters to fit the device's deterioration process, which is in fact data-dependent. To determine the pattern of present equipment degradation, data-driven approaches extract the characteristics of the device degradation process from past run-to-failure data. The hybrid methods are created by combining the aforementioned three techniques, giving them relevant advantages. Figure 2 represents the relationship between monitoring, prognosis, diagnosis, and health management.

3.1 Applications of AI in Autoimmune Disease Prognosis

In recent years, the potential for using AI in the prognosis of many autoimmune disorders has risen significantly:

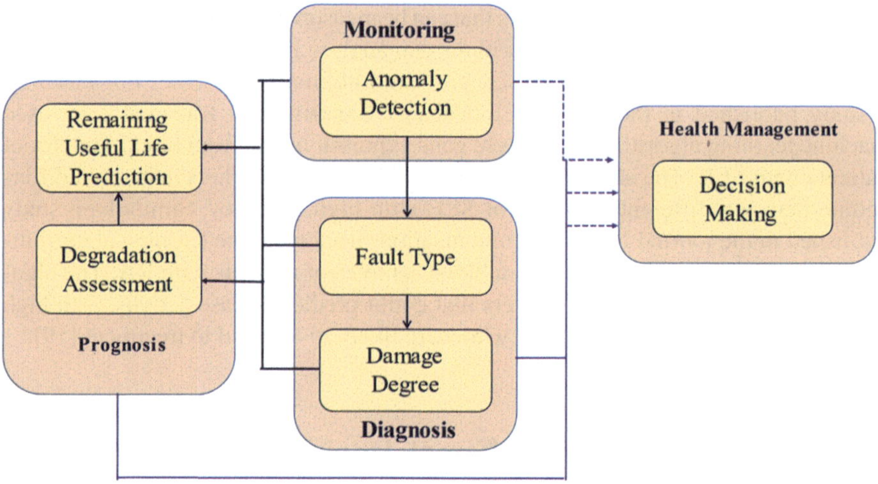

Fig. 2 Relationship between monitoring, prognosis, diagnosis, and health management [23]

AI-based investigation of patient heterogeneity by Establishing AIIDs models and target identification for autoimmune diseases. Recent studies in AIIDs have used a variety of AI-based modelling techniques based on molecular profiling information [24]. The discovery of clinically meaningful genetic or digital biomarkers will be essential for classifying and monitoring patients in terms of prognosis, therapeutic response, and safety risks in order to expedite precision medicine approaches to AIIDs employing AI [25]. It is possible to map all the genes or proteins that are either up- or down-regulated in comparison to healthy controls for each distinct patient cluster by first identifying homogenous patient clusters [26]. A wide range of patient data, including genetic information, medical imaging, electronic health records, and even data from wearable devices, have been analysed using AI algorithms. AI can find intricate patterns and correlations in these datasets by using machine learning techniques, which makes it possible to forecast disease outcomes for autoimmune patients in a more precise and individualized way. Early identification and diagnosis of autoimmune illnesses can be facilitated by AI-based prognostic models, allowing for prompt intervention and therapy.

These AI systems may also continually track the course of a disease, giving doctors real-time information on a patient's condition and assisting them in modifying treatment plans as necessary. Furthermore, AI's capacity to identify latent biomarkers and therapeutic targets opens up new possibilities for the creation of innovative, focused treatments. The application of AI in healthcare to the prognosis of autoimmune diseases has the capacity to significantly enhance patient care and management as the field develops (Table 2).

Table 2 Healthcare applications and their purpose [27, 28]

S. no.	Healthcare applications	Purpose
1	Analysis and disease identification	Machine and deep learning play a crucial role in healthcare, particularly in identifying and analysing challenging-to-diagnose diseases
2	Drug development	The initial stage of drug discovery can greatly benefit from machine and deep learning. AI can identify patterns in data without making predictions, which is highly advantageous
3	Digital health records	Maintaining and managing vital health records is a lengthy and costly process, but it has played a crucial role in facilitating data access
4	Medical trials	Machine and deep learning, utilizing analytical analysis, are the foundation for identifying potential clinical trial candidates. Researchers can narrow down their selection from a vast array of data sources
5	Outbreak prediction	Machine and deep learning techniques are employed to monitor and forecast global outbreaks, helping predict epidemics
6	Medical imaging diagnostics	AI methods are proving to be more extensive and efficient in their ability to comprehend a growing array of data sources from various medical images

4 Challenges in AI-Based Diagnosis of Autoimmune Diseases

The calibre of the data utilized to train AI algorithms determines their accuracy. Predictions and diagnoses can be incorrect as a result of erroneous or inadequate data. Therefore, it is crucial to make sure that the data utilized to train AI algorithms is precise and complete. However, collecting high-quality data can be challenging, particularly for autoimmune diseases, as their symptoms can be vague and overlap with other conditions. Additionally, different physicians may use different terminology to describe the same symptoms, making it difficult to aggregate data from multiple sources. AI algorithms can generate large amounts of data, making it challenging for physicians to interpret the results. It is essential to develop user-friendly interfaces that can present the results in a meaningful and understandable way. Additionally, AI algorithms are also capable of spotting trends that can point to the existence of an autoimmune disease, but they cannot provide a definitive diagnosis. Therefore, it is important to ensure that physicians are involved in the diagnostic process and can provide their expertise in interpreting the results.

Autoimmune diseases are rare conditions, and collecting data on them can be challenging. This can limit the availability of data for training AI algorithms and may lead to overfitting, where the algorithm is trained to recognize patterns in the data that are specific to the training set, but may not generalize to new data. To overcome this challenge, it may be necessary to collaborate with multiple institutions to aggregate data and develop larger datasets for training AI algorithms. AI-based diagnosis and prognosis of autoimmune diseases raises several ethical considerations, particularly around privacy and data security. Patient data must be protected and stored securely, and patients must be informed of how their data will be used. Additionally, AI algorithms might be biased, especially if they were trained on data that was not representative of the whole population. It is crucial to make sure that AI algorithms are created and verified on a variety of datasets in order to meet this difficulty.

Finally, AI-based diagnosis of autoimmune diseases must be integrated into clinical practice to be effective. Physicians must be trained on how to use AI algorithms and interpret the results. Additionally, it can also be essential to create new workflows and processes to integrate AI-based diagnosis into clinical practice. Compliance with healthcare regulations and standards is essential for AI applications in medical diagnosis and prognosis. Addressing these challenges will be critical to realizing the full potential of AI in improving the prognosis and treatment of autoimmune diseases.

5 Role of AI in Different Autoimmune Diseases

5.1 AI in Addison's Disease

AI can aid in the diagnosis and treatment of Addison's disease in several ways. A rare disorder known as Addison's disease is when the adrenal glands fail to produce adequate cortisol and aldosterone. AI can help in the diagnosis and management of Addison's disease in several ways [29, 30]. The symptoms of Addison's disease can be non-specific, making it challenging to diagnose. However, AI algorithms can help in examining patient information, including medical history, symptoms, and lab results, to find trends that can point to the presence of Addison's disease. AI algorithms can evaluate blood samples, for instance, to find low cortisol levels and high ACTH levels, which may signify Addison's ailments. AI software can also examine a patient's symptoms to identify non-specific symptoms, such as fatigue and weight loss, that may be indicative of Addison's disease. AI algorithms can help to differentiate Addison's disease from other conditions that have similar symptoms. For example, AI algorithms can analyse patient data to distinguish between Addison's disease and primary adrenal insufficiency, which is another condition that affects the adrenal glands [31].

AI algorithms can help to determine the appropriate treatment for patients with Addison's disease. For example, these algorithms can analyse patient data to determine the appropriate dose of glucocorticoids, which are the primary treatment for Addison's disease. Additionally, these can analyse patient data to identify potential drug interactions or side effects, which can help to optimize treatment regimens. It can aid in the forecast of Addison's disease progression and the identification of patients who could be more susceptible to complications. AI algorithms, for instance, can examine patient data to identify risk factors for adrenal crisis, which is a life-threatening complication of Addison's disease. These algorithms can assist in personalizing therapy for patients with Addison's disease based on their individual characteristics. For example, AI algorithms can analyse patient data to find genetic variations that may impact treatment response or predict the likelihood of disease progression. In conclusion, AI has an important place in the diagnosis and treatment of Addison's disease. By analysing patient data, AI algorithms can observe patterns and predict outcomes, leading to improved diagnosis and personalized treatment plans. However, AI should be utilized as a tool to assist clinical decision-making and not as a replacement for clinical expertise [32].

AI-based prognosis in Addison's disease involves the use of AI algorithms and machine learning techniques to analyse medical data and predict the disease's progression, outcomes, and response to treatment. These systems gather and consolidate vast amounts of medical data related to Addison's disease. This data may include patient records, symptoms, laboratory results, imaging scans, and treatment history. It preprocesses the collected data, ensuring it is in a suitable format for analysis. This step may involve data cleaning, normalization, and feature extraction to identify relevant patterns and correlations. AI employs various machine learning models to analyse the preprocessed data. These models can be classified into different types, such as regression, decision trees, support vector machines, or deep learning neural networks. AI algorithms identify the most relevant features or variables that contribute to predicting the disease's prognosis. These features could be certain symptoms, lab values, or patient characteristics. Training and Validation: The AI model is trained on a subset of the data, and its performance is validated using another subset. The goal is to optimize the model's accuracy and generalizability. Once the AI model is trained and validated, it can be used to make prognostic predictions for new patients with Addison's disease. By inputting a patient's data into the model, it can estimate the likelihood of certain outcomes or disease progression over time.

Benefits of AI-based prognosis in Addison's disease are that it can help identify early signs of disease progression, allowing for timely intervention and management. By analysing a patient's specific data, AI can recommend tailored treatment plans based on predicted outcomes. AI can process vast amounts of data quickly and identify patterns that may be challenging for human clinicians to notice, potentially leading to more accurate prognostic assessments. However, it is crucial to recognize that AI-based predictions are not infallible, and they should always be used in conjunction with medical expertise. AI systems can integrate data from various sources, such as electronic health records, wearable devices, and patient-reported data, to provide a comprehensive view of the patient's health status. This holistic approach can aid in more accurate prognosis and treatment decisions. AI-powered tools can empower patients with Addison's disease by providing them with real-time insights into their condition. Patients can monitor their symptoms, medication adherence, and lifestyle factors more effectively, leading to improved self-management. AI can support telemedicine by enabling remote monitoring of Addison's disease patients. This is particularly beneficial for patients in remote areas or those who have difficulty accessing healthcare facilities regularly [33].

5.2 AI in Rheumatoid Arthritis

AI can play a significant role in the diagnosis, treatment, and management of rheumatoid arthritis (RA) through various means. RA, a chronic autoimmune ailment primarily impacting the joints and resulting in tissue inflammation and damage, can benefit from AI's contributions [34, 35]. The symptoms of RA can vary in severity, making it challenging to diagnose and manage. AI algorithms possess the capability to assess patient information, encompassing medical records, symptoms, and imaging findings, to detect patterns that could suggest the existence of rheumatoid arthritis. One example involves AI's capability to examine joint X-rays or ultrasounds to detect inflammation or structural damage to the joints. Additionally, AI systems are able to evaluate patient symptoms to identify non-specific symptoms, such as fatigue and stiffness, that may be indicative of rheumatoid arthritis. These algorithms can help to differentiate rheumatoid arthritis from other conditions that have similar symptoms. For instance, AI algorithms can examine patient information to distinguish between rheumatoid arthritis and osteoarthritis, which is another condition that affects the joints [36].

AI algorithms are valuable tools in tailoring treatments for patients with rheumatoid arthritis. They can analyse patient data to prescribe suitable doses of disease-modifying antirheumatic drugs (DMARDs), the mainstay of treatment. Moreover, AI can identify potential drug interactions and adverse effects by analysing patient data., which can help to optimize treatment regimens. These can help to predict the progression of rheumatoid arthritis and identify patients who may be at increased risk of complications. For example, AI algorithms can analyse patient data to identify risk factors for joint damage, which is a common complication of rheumatoid arthritis. It plays a key role in customizing treatment for rheumatoid arthritis patients by considering their unique attributes. They can examine patient data to detect genetic differences that affect treatment outcomes and forecast disease advancement. Furthermore, AI algorithms can assess patient data to unveil insights, monitor disease activity, and adjust treatment plans accordingly. It is valuable in tracking disease progression by evaluating data sourced from electronic health records (EHRs), encompassing imagery, lab results, medication records, and clinical notes. This aids in early identifying disease advancement, facilitating swift intervention and enhanced results. In conclusion, AI significantly contributes to diagnosing, treating, and managing rheumatoid arthritis. Through data analysis, AI detects trends, forecasts outcomes, and tailors treatment strategies, elevating diagnosis and disease control. Nonetheless, AI should be a supplementary tool to clinical judgement and not a substitute for medical expertise [37]. A comparison of various RA diseases in terms of diagnosis, personalized medicine, image analysis, monitoring, and prognosis is presented in Table 3.

Table 3 Comparison of various RA diseases in terms of diagnosis, personalized medicine, image analysis, monitoring, prognosis

Factor	Rheumatoid arthritis (RA)	Juvenile idiopathic arthritis (JIA)	Psoriatic arthritis (PsA)
Diagnosis	Clinical symptoms, blood tests (RF, CCP), imaging (X-rays, MRI)	Clinical symptoms, blood tests, imaging, joint fluid analysis	Clinical symptoms, blood tests, imaging (X-rays, MRI)
Personalized medicine	Tailored medication based on disease activity, genetics, and patient response	Individualized treatment plans considering age, subtype, and response	Treatment may be personalized based on disease severity and comorbidities
Image analysis	X-rays, MRIs, and ultrasounds to monitor joint damage	Imaging used to assess joint inflammation and damage	Imaging helps evaluate joint involvement
Monitoring	Regular check-ups, assessment of disease activity (DAS28), tracking joint damage progression	Regular check-ups, assessment of disease activity (JADAS), joint examinations	Regular check-ups, assessment of disease activity, monitoring for skin and nail involvement
Prognosis	Variable; depends on disease severity, early diagnosis, and response to treatment	Variable; prognosis can improve with early diagnosis and effective therapy	Variable; depends on disease severity and response to treatment

Given the amount of information accessible in EHRs, there are more variable treatment and outcome trajectories linked to diverse patient comorbidities, drugs, and other factors than a human, even a skilled doctor, can employ. Clinical data analysis has made use of a variety of machine learning approaches, such as Cox proportional hazards regression, random forests, and LASSO (least absolute shrinkage and selection operator). However, these algorithms are typically not appropriate for predicting outcomes based on EHR data because of data points between patients, enormous amounts of missing data, and highly variable dimensions with time-dependent interactions. Deep learning, a branch of artificial intelligence, has revolutionized computer vision in clinical applications, such as picture data for melanoma, retinopathy, metastatic breast cancer, and other biomedical and healthcare domains, and earned countless victories. A large number of EHR-related datasets are being subjected to deep learning, similar to the application of technology to any new industry, there are both potential and difficulties. A healthcare provider could tailor existing treatment options to align with a patient's future well-being with the aim of altering the progression of their medical conditions. However, achieving this level of customization would necessitate advanced modelling and comprehensive patient data. If artificial intelligence models had the capability to predict future patient outcomes, they might offer valuable support to both healthcare professionals and patients by enabling the anticipation of treatment results and the simulation of potential outcomes across different treatment scenarios. The objective of this research is to determine the accuracy of an artificial intelligence system in predicting the disease activity status of a patient with rheumatoid arthritis (RA) before their upcoming clinical appointment [38].

5.3 AI in Systemic Lupus Erythematosus

Systemic lupus erythematosus (SLE) diagnosis and treatment are two areas where AI can be helpful. The body's various organs and systems are affected by the complicated autoimmune disease known as SLE. The symptoms of SLE can be diverse and non-specific, making it challenging to diagnose and manage. In order to find patterns that can point to the presence of SLE, AI algorithms can assess patient data such as medical history, symptoms, laboratory test results, and imaging results. For instance, AI algorithms can examine blood tests to find the existence of SLE-specific autoantibodies like anti-dsDNA and anti-Smith. Additionally, AI algorithms can analyse patient symptoms to find non-specific symptoms, such as joint pain and rash, that may be indicative of SLE. AI algorithms can help to differentiate SLE from other conditions that have similar symptoms. To differentiate between SLE and other autoimmune disorders like rheumatoid arthritis and systemic sclerosis, for instance, AI systems can examine patient data.

AI algorithms can analyse patient data to identify potential drugs AI algorithms can assist in choosing the best course of treatment for SLE patients. For instance, AI algorithms can examine patient information to calculate the proper dosage of immunosuppressive medications, which are the mainstay of SLE treatment. Additionally, AI algorithms can also examine patient data to find possible medication candidate's interactions or side effects, which can help to optimize treatment regimens [39]. AI algorithms can aid in predicting the course of SLE and detecting people who could be more susceptible to problems. AI algorithms, for instance, can examine patient data to identify risk factors for renal involvement, which is a common complication of SLE.

Based on their unique traits, AI systems may assist to tailor treatment for SLE patients. AI systems, for instance, can examine patient data to find genetic variants that may affect how well a patient responds to treatment or indicate the risk that a disease will worsen. AI systems can also examine patient data to track ailments activity and modify treatment strategies as necessary. By examining information from the patient's EHR, such as imaging, laboratory test results, prescription use, and clinical notes, AI techniques can assist in tracking the evolution of the disease. With fast action and better results, this can aid in the early detection of illness progression. In conclusion, AI can be extremely useful in the identification, management, and therapy of SLE. AI systems can better diagnose and manage diseases by analysing patient data to find patterns, forecast outcomes, and personalize treatment strategies. However, AI should be used as an appliance for medical decision-making and not as a replacement for clinical expertise [40]. The management of lupus nephritis and the assessment of patient prognosis depend on accurate pathological classification and the use of acute and chronic pathological indicators. The most accurate forecasting power is available from renal biopsy. However, in some situations, supplemental instruments are still necessary for clinicians.

5.4 AI in Multiple Sclerosis

The diagnosis and treatment of multiple sclerosis (MS) could be improved by AI. Inflammation, destruction of the myelin sheath, and a variety of neurological symptoms are all indications of MS, a chronic inflammatory condition that affects the central nervous system [42]. AI can be applied to MS patients to enhance diagnosis, anticipate disease progression, and personalize management approaches.

MS can be challenging to diagnose, especially in the early stages when symptoms can be vague and non-specific. AI algorithms can examine patient information, such as medical history, clinical examination, imaging, and laboratory tests, to find patterns that may indicate the presence of MS. AI can analyse MRI scans and other imaging tests to detect changes in the brain and spinal cord that are characteristic of MS. AI algorithms can also analyse cerebrospinal fluid (CSF) samples to identify the presence of biomarkers associated with MS. AI algorithms can predict disease progression in MS patients by analysing longitudinal patient data, such as MRI scans, laboratory tests, and clinical notes. These algorithms can find patterns and trends that may indicate a worsening of symptoms, disease activity, or the need for treatment escalation. Predictive analytics can help clinicians intervene early before irreversible damage occurs, and optimize treatment plans based on individual patient characteristics [43]. These algorithms have the capability to analyse a variety of patient data, including genetic markers, demographic details, and past treatment records. This analysis can be used to create personalized treatment strategies for individuals with MS. One significant advantage of this approach is the identification of patient subgroups that exhibit distinct responses to various treatments. AI can play a crucial role in enhancing therapy optimization, minimizing adverse effects, and ultimately enhancing patient outcomes. For instance, AI-powered algorithms can effectively determine the subset of patients that are more likely to positively respond to disease-modifying therapies. These therapies are designed to slow down the progression of the disease in MS patients. AI can help to automate the analysis of MRI scans and other imaging tests in MS. AI algorithms can segment lesions, quantify changes in brain volume, and identify regions of interest that may be indicative of disease activity. Image analysis can help to standardize and automate the assessment of disease severity, reducing inter-rater variability, and improving accuracy [44].

AI can be used to remotely monitor MS patients and collect real-time data on disease activity, symptoms, and management response. Remote monitoring can improve patient outcomes, reduce healthcare costs, and enhance patient engagement. For example, AI-powered wearable devices can monitor gait, balance, and mobility in MS patients, providing clinicians with objective measures of disease severity. In conclusion, AI has the potential to transform the diagnosis and management of MS. AI can help to identify early disease markers, predict disease progression, personalize treatment plans, and automate image analysis. While AI is not a substitute for clinical expertise, it has the potential to elevate clinical decision-making, enhance patient outcomes, and lower healthcare expenses [45]. There is currently no technique to predict the likelihood of a recurrence of MS. We created a clinical tool for estimating the likelihood of an MS relapse using EHR data that is easily accessible at the point of care [46].

5.5 AI in Sjogren's Disease

Sjogren's disease is a chronic autoimmune disorder that affects the exocrine glands, resulting in dryness of the mouth, eyes, and other mucous membranes. It can also affect other organs, such as the kidneys, lungs, and joints. AI can be utilized to improve the prognosis, monitoring, and treatment of Sjogren's disease [47, 48].

Sjogren's disease can be challenging to diagnose, as the symptoms can be nonspecific and overlap with other autoimmune diseases. AI algorithms have the capability to examine patient information, including medical records, clinical evaluations, medical imaging, and lab results, with the purpose of detecting specific patterns that could potentially suggest the existence of Sjogren's disease.AI can analyse salivary gland biopsies to detect the presence of lymphocytic infiltrates, which are characteristic of Sjogren's disease. AI can also analyse blood tests to identify biomarkers associated with Sjogren's disease [49]. AI algorithms have the capability to assess patient information, including genetic indicators, demographic details, and past therapies, in order to tailor treatment approaches for individuals with Sjogren's disease. By identifying patient subgroups that respond differently to treatment, AI can help to optimize therapy, reduce side effects, and improve outcomes. As an illustration, AI algorithms possess the capability to detect individuals who are likely to exhibit positive reactions to immunosuppressive treatments. These interventions can effectively diminish inflammation and hinder organ deterioration in cases of Sjogren's disease.

It can help automate the analysis of imaging tests, such as salivary gland ultrasound, in Sjogren's disease. AI algorithms can segment salivary gland tissue, quantify changes in glandular structure and function, and identify regions of interest that may be indicative of disease activity. Image analysis can help to standardize and automate the assessment of disease severity, reducing inter-rater variability, and improving accuracy [50]. AI algorithms can predict disease progression in Sjogren's disease patients by examining longitudinal individual data, like imaging tests, laboratory tests, and clinical notes. These factors can determine patterns and trends which may indicate a worsening of symptoms, disease activity, or the need for treatment escalation. Predictive analytics can help clinicians intervene early, before irreversible damage occurs, and optimize treatment plans based on individual patient characteristics. AI has the potential to be employed for remote monitoring of individuals with Sjogren's disease, enabling the collection of real-time information regarding disease activity, symptoms, and the effectiveness of treatments. This approach to remote monitoring holds the promise of enhancing patient outcomes, lowering healthcare expenses, and fostering greater patient involvement. For example, AI-powered wearable devices can monitor dryness of the mouth and eyes in Sjogren's disease patients, providing clinicians with objective measures of disease severity [51].

AI possesses the capability to revolutionize the diagnosis and treatment of Sjögren's disease. AI can help to identify early disease markers, personalize treatment plans, automate image analysis, predict disease progression, and remotely monitor patients. Although AI cannot replace clinical expertise, it has the potential to augment clinical decision-making, enhance patient outcomes, and lower healthcare expenses. Identifying risk factors capable of anticipating the onset and outlook of non-Hodgkin's lymphoma (NHL) presents a formidable challenge. Nevertheless, individuals at an elevated risk of encountering this complication exhibit specific clinical and serological attributes that set them apart. Over the previous decade, investigations concentrating on heightened B-cell activity, indicative of lymphoproliferation linked with pSS, have unveiled certain biological and molecular elements influencing disease advancement and lymphoma expansion. These findings propose potential markers for gauging the emergence and prognosis of lymphoma [52, 53].

5.6 AI in Insulin-Dependent Diabetes Mellitus

Type 1 diabetes is a lasting autoimmune condition marked by the decomposition of insulin-producing beta cells within the pancreas. AI can be used to improve the treatment of type 1 diabetes by predicting blood sugar levels, optimizing insulin dosing, and identifying risk factors for complications [29, 30]. AI algorithms have the capability to process data from continuous glucose monitoring (CGM) devices, which provide real-time measurements of blood sugar levels, to predict future blood glucose levels. These predictions can be used to adjust insulin dosing and prevent hypoglycemia or hyperglycemia. AI algorithms can also identify patterns and trends in blood glucose levels, such as nocturnal hypoglycemia, that may not be detected by traditional blood glucose monitoring.

AI can be used to automate insulin dosing based on CGM data, in a process called closed-loop insulin delivery or artificial pancreas. AI algorithms can predict blood glucose levels and adjust insulin delivery in real-time, without the need for manual intervention. Closed-loop insulin delivery can enhance glycemic management, minimize the likelihood of hypoglycemia, and ameliorate the quality of life for individuals with type 1 diabetes. AI algorithms can examine patient data, including genetic markers, demographic details, and treatment records, to individualize treatment strategies for individuals with type 1 diabetes. By identifying distinct patient subsets with varied responses to insulin therapy, AI can contribute to refining insulin dosages, diminishing adverse effects, and advancing outcomes. For instance, AI algorithms can predict patients prone to complications., such as diabetic retinopathy or nephropathy, and provide early interventions to prevent or delay their onset

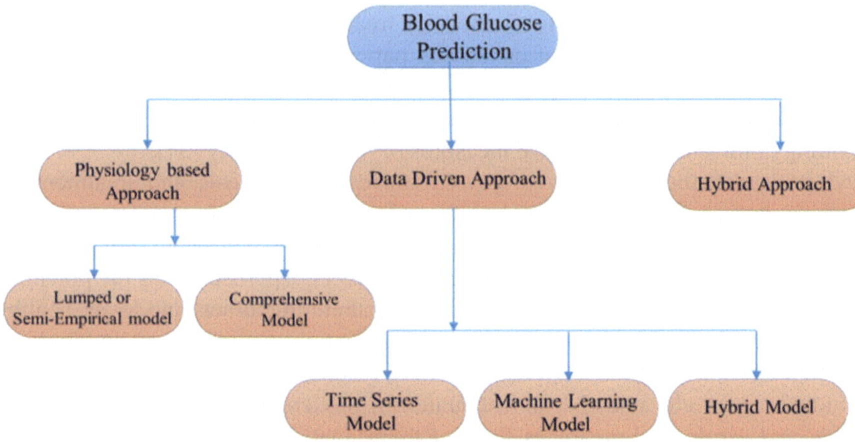

Fig. 3 Blood glucose prediction approach [54]

[31]. AI algorithms have the capacity to anticipate blood glucose levels in type 1 diabetes patients through the analysis of longitudinal patient data, including continuous glucose monitoring (CGM) data, insulin administration, and dietary intake. These algorithms can recognize patterns and trends that might suggest deteriorating glycemic management or the necessity for an escalated treatment approach. Predictive analytics can help clinicians intervene early, before severe hyperglycemia or ketoacidosis occurs, and optimize treatment plans based on individual patient characteristics. Various AI-based approaches for blood glucose prediction are shown in Fig. 3.

AI-driven chatbots and mobile apps can assist in educating and involving individuals with type 1 diabetes in their self-care efforts. These tools can provide personalized feedback and support based on CGM data and insulin dosing, help patients to set goals and track progress, and connect patients with peer support networks. Patient education and engagement can improve self-care behaviours, reduce diabetes-related distress, and enhance treatment adherence.

In summary, AI holds the promise of revolutionizing type 1 diabetes management by foreseeing blood glucose levels, refining insulin dosage, and recognizing complications and risk factors [32]. AI can help to personalize treatment plans, automate insulin delivery, predict glycemic trends, and enhance patient education and engagement. While AI is not a substitute for clinical expertise, it has the capability to improve clinical decision-making, enhance patient outcomes, and lower healthcare expenses.

It has been demonstrated that bolus insulin calculators are useful in aiding in the treatment of the condition. This section describes our proposed R4 model-based temporal CBR system for insulin bolus recommendations. First, we decide how the cases for T1DM bolus are modelled and the attributes needed to describe a case. The development and adaptation of each R4 model step to deal with temporal information is then described [55, 56].

6 Future Perspectives

AI is a promptly developing field with promising applications in healthcare. Despite the challenges, AI-based diagnosis and prognosis of autoimmune diseases have the potential to revolutionize the field of rheumatology. Future research should focus on addressing the challenges outlined above and developing AI algorithms that can accurately diagnose autoimmune diseases and predict patient outcomes. One area of research is the development of AI algorithms that can integrate multiple types of data, such as imaging studies, EMRs, and biomarkers. By analysing multiple types of data, AI algorithms may be able to identify patterns that are not apparent when analysing individual types of data.

Additionally, future studies should concentrate on creating AI programmes that can predict treatment outcomes. By analysing patient data, AI algorithms may be able to identify which treatments are likely to be helpful for certain patients by analysing patient data, resulting in personalized treatment plans and better patient outcomes. Finally, it is essential to involve patients and physicians in the development of AI-based diagnosis tools. Patients and physicians can provide valuable feedback on the usability and effectiveness of AI algorithms, ensuring that they are developed in a way that is clinically applicable and patient-centred [57].

7 Conclusion

AI represents a broad domain encompassing data, algorithms, analytics, deep learning, neural networks, and insights, continually evolving to meet the healthcare industry's demands and benefit patients. As per the study results, AI plays a crucial role in healthcare, especially in illness detection. AI-based diagnosis of autoimmune diseases has the potential to improve patient outcomes and revolutionize the field of rheumatology. However, there are several challenges that must be addressed, including data quality, interpreting results, limited data availability, ethical considerations, and integration with clinical practice. Thus, much work is required to train the AI-based systems so that there will be an increase in the accuracy to predict the methods for diagnosing diseases. Future research should focus on developing AI algorithms that can integrate multiple types of data, predict treatment outcomes, and involve patients and physicians in the development process.

References

1. Araki Y, Mimura T (2017) The histone modification code in the pathogenesis of autoimmune diseases. Mediat Inflam 2017
2. Ngo ST, Steyn FJ, McCombe PA (2014) Gender differences in autoimmune disease. Front Neuroendocrinol 35(3):347–369
3. Goodnow CC, Sprent J, de St Groth BF, Vinuesa CG (2005) Cellular and genetic mechanisms of self tolerance and autoimmunity. Nature 435(7042):590–597
4. Stafford IS, Kellermann M, Mossotto E, Beattie RM, MacArthur BD, Ennis S (2020) A systematic review of the applications of artificial intelligence and machine learning in autoimmune diseases. NPJ Digit Med 3(1):30
5. Kuchroo VK, Ohashi PS, Sartor RB, Vinuesa CG (2012) Dysregulation of immune homeostasis in autoimmune diseases. Nat Med 18(1):42–47
6. Cooper GS, Bynum ML, Somers EC (2009) Recent insights in the epidemiology of autoimmune diseases: improved prevalence estimates and understanding of clustering of diseases. J Autoimmun 33(3–4):197–207
7. Hayter SM, Cook MC (2012) Updated assessment of the prevalence, spectrum and case definition of autoimmune disease. Autoimmun Rev 11(10):754–765
8. Jiang F, Jiang Y, Zhi H, Dong Y, Li H, Ma S, Wang Y, Dong Q, Shen H, Wang Y (2017) Artificial intelligence in healthcare: past, present and future. Stroke Vascul Neurol 2(4)
9. Needham J (2004) Science and civilisation in China: Volume 7, the social background, part 2, general conclusions and reflections. Cambridge University Press
10. Musleh MM, Alajrami E, Khalil AJ, Abu-Nasser BS, Barhoom AM, Naser SA (2019) Predicting liver patients using artificial neural network. Int J Acad Inf Syst Res (IJAISR) 3(10)
11. Dabowsa NI, Amaitik NM, Maatuk AM, Aljawarneh SA (2017) A hybrid intelligent system for skin disease diagnosis. In: 2017 international conference on engineering and technology (ICET) 2017. IEEE, pp 1–6
12. Kumar Y, Koul A, Singla R, Ijaz MF (2022) Artificial intelligence in disease diagnosis: a systematic literature review, synthesizing framework and future research agenda. J Ambient Intell Humaniz Comput 13:1–28
13. Owais M, Arsalan M, Choi J, Mahmood T, Park KR (2019) Artificial intelligence-based classification of multiple gastrointestinal diseases using endoscopy videos for clinical diagnosis. J Clin Med 8(7):986
14. Hay JC, Martin FC, Wightman CW (1960) The mark-1 perceptron-design and performance. In: Proceedings of the institute of radio engineers 1960, vol 48, No 3, pp 398–399
15. Wiener N (1948) Cybernetics: control and communication in the animal and the machine. Wiley
16. Tsakalidou VN, Mitsou P, Papakostas GA (2022) Computer vision in autoimmune diseases diagnosis—Current status and perspectives. In: Computational vision and bio-inspired computing: proceedings of ICCVBIC 2021 2022. Springer Singapore, Singapore, pp 571–586
17. Tian C, Yu M, Shan L, Wu Y, Zhang T, Bi B, Zhang F, Zhang Q, Liu D, Wang W, Yuan Z (2019) Radiography of direct drive double shell targets with hard x-rays generated by a short pulse laser. Nucl Fusion 59(4):046012
18. Yang J, Min BJ, Kang J (2020) A feasibility study of LYSO-GAPD detector for DEXA applications. J Instrum 15(05):P05017
19. Bhattacharya S, Sengupta S (2018) Application of data mining techniques in autoimmune diseases research and treatment. In: Machine learning and IoT 2018. CRC Press, pp 113–131
20. Berri PC, Dalla Vedova MD, Mainini L (2019) Real-time fault detection and prognostics for aircraft actuation systems. In: AIAA Scitech 2019 Forum 2019, p 2210
21. Bartram GW, Mahadevan S (2023) Integrating heterogeneous information in diagnosis and prognosis. In: 54th AIAA/ASME/ASCE/AHS/ASC Structure,Structure Dynamics ,and Materials Conference, 2023, p 1941

22. Ali JB, Chebel-Morello B, Saidi L, Malinowski S, Fnaiech F (2015) Accurate bearing remaining useful life prediction based on Weibull distribution and artificial neural network. Mech Syst Signal Process 56:150–172
23. Zhao Z, Wu J, Li T, Sun C, Yan R, Chen X (2021) Challenges and opportunities of AI-enabled monitoring, diagnosis and prognosis: a review. Chinese J Mech Engin 34(1):1–29
24. Barturen G, Beretta L, Cervera R, Van Vollenhoven R, Alarcón-Riquelme ME (2018) Moving towards a molecular taxonomy of autoimmune rheumatic diseases. Nat Rev Rheumatol 14(2):75–93
25. Laigle L (2023) Biomarkers for autoimmune diseases: current status and new perspective.Expert Rev. Clin Immunol 19:305–314
26. Moingeon P, Kuenemann M, Guedj M (2022) Artificial intelligence-enhanced drug design and development: toward a computational precision medicine. Drug Discov Today 27(1):215–222
27. Memon MH, Li JP, Haq AU, Memon MH, Zhou W (2019) Breast cancer detection in the IOT health environment using modified recursive feature selection. Wireless Commun Mobile Comput 2019:1–9
28. Braun LW, Martins MA, Romanini J, Rados PV, Martins MD, Carrard VC (2021) Continuing education activities improve dentists' self-efficacy to manage oral mucosal lesions and oral cancer. Eur J Dent Educ 25(1):28–34
29. Neto RA, de Carvalho JF (2014) Diagnosis and classification of Addison's disease (autoimmune adrenalitis). Autoimmun Rev 13(4–5):408–411
30. Betterle C, Morlin L (2011) Autoimmune Addison's disease. Pediatric adrenal diseases. 20:161–172
31. Bratland E, Husebye ES (2011) Cellular immunity and immunopathology in autoimmune Addison's disease. Mol Cell Endocrinol 336(1–2):180–190
32. Falorni A, Brozzetti A, Torre DL, Tortoioli C, Gambelunghe G (2008) Association of genetic polymorphisms and autoimmune Addison's disease. Expert Rev Clin Immunol 4(4):441–456
33. Lathan P, Thompson AL (2018) Management of hypoadrenocorticism (Addison's disease) in dogs. Veterin Med: Res Rep 9:1
34. Hügle M, Omoumi P, van Laar JM, Boedecker J, Hügle T (2020) Applied machine learning and artificial intelligence in rheumatology. Rheumatol Adv Pract 4(1):rkaa005
35. Kothari S, Gionfrida L, Bharath AA, Abraham S (2019) Artificial intelligence (AI) and rheumatology: a potential partnership. Rheumatology 58(11):1894–1895
36. Momtazmanesh S, Nowroozi A, Rezaei N (2022) Artificial intelligence in rheumatoid arthritis: current status and future perspectives: a state-of-the-art review. Rheumatol Therapy. 9(5):1249–1304
37. Demoruelle MK, Deane KD (2012) Treatment strategies in early rheumatoid arthritis and prevention of rheumatoid arthritis. Curr Rheumatol Rep 14:472–480
38. Norgeot B, Glicksberg BS, Trupin L, Lituiev D, Gianfrancesco M, Oskotsky B, Schmajuk G, Yazdany J, Butte AJ (2019) Assessment of a deep learning model based on electronic health record data to forecast clinical outcomes in patients with rheumatoid arthritis. JAMA Netw Open 2(3):e190606
39. Sawada T, Fujimori D, Yamamoto Y (2019) Systemic lupus erythematosus and immunodeficiency. Immunol Med 42(1):1–9
40. Lutton JD, Winston R, Rodman TC (2004) Multiple sclerosis: etiological mechanisms and future directions. Exp Biol Med 229(1):12–20
41. Tang Y, Zhang W, Zhu M, Zheng L, Xie L, Yao Z, Zhang H, Cao D, Lu B (2018) Lupus nephritis pathology prediction with clinical indices. Sci Rep 8(1):10231
42. Barile B, Ashtari P, Stamile C, Marzullo A, Maes F, Durand-Dubief F, Van Huffel S, Sappey-Marinier D (2022) Classification of multiple sclerosis clinical profiles using machine learning and grey matter connectome. Front Robot AI 9:926255
43. Arani LA, Hosseini A, Asadi F, Masoud SA, Nazemi E (2018) Intelligent computer systems for multiple sclerosis diagnosis: a systematic review of reasoning techniques and methods. Acta Inf Med 26(4):258

44. Cunha B, Madureira A, Gonçalves L (2023) A review on artificial intelligence applications for multiple sclerosis evaluation and diagnosis. In: Innovations in bio-inspired computing and applications: proceedings of the 13th international conference on innovations in bio-inspired computing and applications (IBICA 2022) Held during December 15–17, 2022. Springer Nature Switzerland, Cham, pp 373–381
45. Maggi P, Fartaria MJ, Jorge J, La Rosa F, Absinta M, Sati P, Meuli R, Du Pasquier R, Reich DS, Cuadra MB, Granziera C (2020) CVSnet: a machine learning approach for automated central vein sign assessment in multiple sclerosis. NMR Biomed 33(5):e4283
46. Ahuja Y, Kim N, Liang L, Cai T, Dahal K, Seyok T, Lin C, Finan S, Liao K, Savovoa G, Chitnis T (2021) Leveraging electronic health records data to predict multiple sclerosis disease activity. Ann Clin Translat Neurol 8(4):800–810
47. Foulquier N, Redou P, Le Gal C, Rouvière B, Pers JO, Saraux A (2018) Pathogenesis-based treatments in primary Sjogren's syndrome using artificial intelligence and advanced machine learning techniques: a systematic literature review. Hum Vaccin Immunother 14(11):2553–2558
48. Chiorini JA, Cihakova D, Ouellette CE, Caturegli P (2009) Sjögren syndrome: advances in the pathogenesis from animal models. J Autoimmun 33(3–4):190–196
49. Kelly AL, Nelson RJ, Sara R, Alberto S (2022) Sjögren syndrome: new insights in the pathogenesis and role of nuclear medicine. J Clin Med 11(17):5227
50. Fox RI, Howell FV, Bone RC, Michelson PE (1984) Primary Sjogren syndrome: clinical and immunopathologic features. In: Seminars in arthritis and rheumatism, vol 14, No 2. WB Saunders, pp 77–105
51. Randell RL, Lieberman SM (2021) Unique aspects of pediatric Sjögren disease. Rheum Dis Clin 47(4):707–723
52. Papageorgiou A, Voulgarelis M, Tzioufas AG (2015) Clinical picture, outcome and predictive factors of lymphoma in Sjögren syndrome. Autoimmun Rev 14(7):641–649
53. Baldini C, Ferro F, Luciano N, Bombardieri S, Grossi E (2018) Artificial neural networks help to identify disease subsets and to predict lymphoma in primary Sjögren's syndrome. Clin Exp Rheumatol 36(Suppl 112):S137–S144
54. Woldaregay AZ, Årsand E, Botsis T, Albers D, Mamykina L, Hartvigsen G (2019) Data-driven blood glucose pattern classification and anomalies detection: machine-learning applications in type 1 diabetes. J Med Internet Res 21(5):e11030
55. Brown D, Aldea A, Harrison R, Martin C, Bayley I (2018) Temporal case-based reasoning for type 1 diabetes mellitus bolus insulin decision support. Artif Intell Med 85:28–42
56. Herrero P, Georgiou P, Oliver N, Johnston DG, Toumazou C (2012) A bio-inspired glucose controller based on pancreatic β-cell physiology. J Diabetes Sci Technol 6(3):606–616
57. Fritzler MJ, Mahler M (2021) Precision medicine as an approach to autoimmune diseases. In: Precision medicine and artificial intelligence. Academic, pp. 39–63

Detection of Rheumatoid Arthritis Using CNN by Transfer Learning

Afroj Alam, Muhammad Kalamuddin Ahamad, K. O. Mohammed Aarif, and Taushif Anwar

Abstract Rheumatoid arthritis (RA) represents a long-term autoimmune condition marked by joint inflammation, resulting in discomfort and distortions of the joint structure. Early and accurate detection of RA plays a pivotal role in managing the disease and preventing irreversible joint damage. In this study, we propose a novel approach for detecting Rheumatoid Arthritis through the utilization of Convolutional Neural Networks (CNN) employing transfer learning. Our methodology leverages pre-trained CNN architectures to extract hierarchical features from medical images, particularly X-ray images of affected joints. Transfer learning enables the model to capitalize on the knowledge learned from large and diverse datasets, enhancing its ability to discriminate between healthy and RA-affected joints even with limited labeled data. Fine-tuning of the pre-trained model is performed to adapt the network to the specific characteristics of RA-related features. We present a comprehensive evaluation of our approach using a dataset consisting of X-ray images from both RA patients and healthy individuals. The experimental results showcase the effectiveness of our CNN-based transfer learning method in accurately detecting RA. The outcomes of this research have significant implications for early diagnosis and management of RA. By harnessing the power of deep learning and transfer learning, our approach contributes to the development of a non-invasive and efficient tool for RA detection, which can aid healthcare practitioners in making informed decisions and improving patient outcomes.

A. Alam (✉) · M. K. Ahamad
Department of Computer Application, Integral University, Lucknow, U.P, India
e-mail: alamafroj@student.iul.ac.in; mohdkalam@iul.ac.in

A. Alam
Department of CSE, School of Engineering Presidency University, Bangalore, India

K. O. Mohammed Aarif
Department of ECE, School of Engineering, Presidency University, Bangalore, India

T. Anwar
Department of Computer Science and Engineering, Koneru Lakshmaiah Education Foundation, Vaddeswaram 522302, India

K. Raza and S. Singh (eds.), *Artificial Intelligence and Autoimmune Diseases*, Studies in Computational Intelligence 1133, https://doi.org/10.1007/978-981-99-9029-0_5

Keywords Artificial intelligence · Deep learning · Rheumatoid arthritis · Convolutional neural network

1 Introduction

Rheumatoid Arthritis (RA) stands as a significant and complex autoimmune disorder that affects millions of individuals worldwide. Characterized by chronic inflammation primarily targeting the synovial joints, RA often leads to progressive joint destruction, functional impairment, and reduced quality of life for those afflicted. This condition is not only physically debilitating but also poses considerable challenges to healthcare systems due to its chronic nature and associated comorbidities. The etiology of RA involves a combination of genetic predisposition, environmental triggers, and dysregulated immune responses. The immune system's attack on healthy joint tissues results in synovial membrane inflammation, leading to the release of inflammatory mediators that further perpetuate joint damage. Over time, this inflammatory process can lead to cartilage erosion, bone destruction, and joint deformities, significantly impacting an individual's mobility and overall well-being. Clinically, RA manifests as joint pain, swelling, stiffness, and reduced range of motion. Its systemic nature may also give rise to extra-articular manifestations, affecting organs such as the skin, heart, lungs, and blood vessels. The disease course is heterogeneous, with periods of exacerbation and remission, often making its diagnosis and management intricate tasks. Early diagnosis and intervention are crucial for mitigating the adverse effects of RA. Prompt and appropriate treatment can help alleviate symptoms, control inflammation, and slow down joint damage progression. The landscape of RA management has evolved significantly with the advent of disease-modifying antirheumatic drugs (DMARDs) and biologic therapies, which have shown efficacy in controlling disease activity and improving patients' quality of life. The diagnosis of RA involves a combination of clinical assessment, laboratory tests, and medical imaging. Radiographs, magnetic resonance imaging (MRI), and ultrasound are essential tools for visualizing joint damage and assessing disease severity Sugiyama et al. [1]. However, the interpretation of these imaging modalities requires expertise and consideration of various factors, such as disease duration, patient demographics, and clinical presentation. Progress in the field of medical technology and artificial intelligence has introduced fresh possibilities for enhancing the precision and effectiveness of diagnosing RA Källberg et al. [2]. Researchers are investigating automated methods of analyzing images, including machine learning and deep learning, to aid in interpreting medical images and identifying early signs of RA-induced alterations. Notably, the recent strides in deep learning, especially Convolutional Neural Networks (CNNs), have brought about a transformative impact on the domain of medical image analysis. CNNs have demonstrated remarkable performance in various medical image interpretation tasks, including disease detection and classification. Transfer learning, a variant of CNNs, exploits pre-trained models on large and diverse datasets to extract high-level features from images, enabling their application to specific diagnostic tasks with limited available data [15].

In this paper, we present a novel approach for the early detection of RA using a CNN-based transfer learning framework. By harnessing the power of deep learning and transfer learning, our proposed method seeks to enhance the accuracy and efficiency of RA detection through the analysis of X-ray images of affected joints. The primary goal is to create a robust and automated tool that can assist healthcare practitioners in swiftly and accurately identifying RA cases. Our contribution lies in the integration of two essential components: the architectural advancements of CNNs and the domain adaptation capabilities of transfer learning. By capitalizing on these cutting-edge technologies, we aim to address the challenges associated with RA diagnosis, such as the complexities of image interpretation and the limited availability of annotated data. Through rigorous experimentation and evaluation, we demonstrate the efficacy of our approach in distinguishing between healthy and RA-affected joints, thereby providing a significant advancement in the field of medical image analysis for early RA detection.

The remainder of the paper is organized as follows: Sect. 2 provides an overview of related work in the domains of rheumatoid arthritis diagnosis and CNN-based image analysis. Section 3 presents the methodology, detailing the architectural aspects of our CNN model and the principles of transfer learning employed. Section 4 describes the experimental setup, including dataset characteristics, evaluation metrics, and results, and discussions are presented, followed by conclusions and potential future research directions in Sect. 5. Through this work, we endeavor to contribute to the growing body of research at the intersection of deep learning and medical diagnostics, specifically targeting the early detection of RA.

2 Literature Review

The majority of the research related to grading the severity of rheumatoid arthritis focuses on locating finger joints or detecting bone deterioration within a collection of X-ray images. Finger joint space assessment is the primary focus of current research on individuals with rheumatoid arthritis. Compared to autoimmune diseases like rheumatoid arthritis, degenerative, non-inflammatory osteoarthritis has more current research. An accuracy of 66.71% is achieved when Nikseresht et al. [3] utilize a deep Siamese CNN for prediction of RA disease. With a CNN used on X-ray pictures of hip joints, Xue et al. [4] accurately identify osteoarthritis with 92.8% accuracy. This approach surpasses manual measurements and exhibits resilience in the face of noise, rotation, and changes in joint size.

Recently, Mehveen et al. [5] in their study address the need for efficient identification and diagnosis of "rheumatoid arthritis," a chronic inflammatory condition affecting joints and tissues. The research employs image processing and a CNN to develop an intelligent system for identifying "rheumatoid arthritis" in hand images, particularly during pre-diagnostic stages. The system consists of two main components. The first part involves image processing, encompassing steps like pre-processing, image segmentation, and Gabor filter-based feature extraction. In the second phase, these extracted features are input into a neural convolutional network that classifies whether the displayed hands are healthy or arthritic. The CNN algorithm conducts classification using both normal and abnormal hand images. The experiments achieved an identification rate of 83.5% when using the same number of photos as in the test set. This research demonstrates the potential of combining image processing and CNN techniques to create an intelligent system for identifying "rheumatoid arthritis" in-hand images. Chung-Ming et al. in [6] employed 214 images of non-septic arthritis and 64 images of septic arthritis obtained through grayscale and Power Doppler ultrasound. They utilized a deep learning-based vision transformer (ViT) for feature extraction from the images, followed by machine learning classifiers with ten-fold cross-validation to classify septic arthritis. The results indicated that using support vector machines, grey-scale, and Power Doppler features achieved accuracies of 86% and 91%, with area under the curve (AUC) values of 0.90 and 0.92, respectively. The combination of both feature sets yielded the highest accuracy (92%) and AUC (0.92). This approach represents the first computer-aided diagnosis (CAD) system using deep learning for septic arthritis diagnosis in knee ultrasound images. Pre-trained ViT improved accuracy and computational efficiency compared to convolutional neural networks. Fahim et al. [7] introduce a deep learning framework designed to identify inaccurately segmented regions on object boundaries, aiming to enhance segmentation quality assessment and control. The method employs a CNN to learn features associated with object boundaries, enabling the pinpointing of specific locations with segmentation errors. The identified error locations can be used to facilitate interactive image segmentation. The framework was tested on two benchmark datasets. Significantly, it attained mean sensitivity rates of 0.95 and 0.92, accompanied by mean positive predictive values of 0.78 and 0.91, when identifying erroneous surface regions in knee cartilage and calf muscle segmentation, respectively. The trial highlighted the method's capacity for automated identification of flawed surface regions within medical image segmentation, thereby enhancing the assessment of segmentation quality. Sakaria et al. [8], aimed to enhance RA diagnosis and conducted research using five distinct machine learning models. The study aimed to identify the most effective approach for diagnosing RA by comparing the accuracy of these algorithms. The process entails two primary stages: image processing and algorithm-driven prediction. In image processing, techniques are applied to optimize the uploaded image, eliminating false negatives and improving image quality for better input into the subsequent phase. The second step involves using the most efficient machine learning model for processing the image, resulting in an impressive 98% prediction accuracy, a notable improvement compared to existing research in the field. Sundaramurthy et al. [9] focus on medical disorder classification related to RA using Ensemble methods. They gathered real-time information from a rheumatology center, comprising 1000 patient records, among which 750 profiles showed signs of RA while 250 profiles were unaffected. The dataset offers complexity in classification due to its multiple numerical attributes. The research employs three ensemble methods: support vector machine (SVM), AdaBoost, and random sub-space. These techniques use k-NN and Random Forest as reference points for classification. The classification procedure entails employing tenfold cross-validation and assessing performance using metrics like accuracy, precision, and ROC. The investigation contrasts these metric outcomes with those obtained from baseline algorithms and various ensemble classifiers to gauge their efficacy.

Makino et al. in [10] suggest using machine learning for joint recognition in X-ray images. The proposed system involves four steps: conversion, training, validation, and feedback. The system's effectiveness was evaluated using X-ray images of patients with rheumatoid arthritis. The findings indicate the importance of having sufficient accurate data to enhance accuracy. The study suggests that incorporating revised data from doctors as feedback into the training system is a more effective approach for improving accuracy. Even Sana et al. [11] employed various supervised machine-learning algorithms to analyze and compare their performance. The input for these classifiers consists of gene sequence feature vectors, categorized as either positive or negative. The evaluation of the classifiers is based on their accuracy and f1-scores, providing insights into their effectiveness in handling RA-related gene sequence data. In their work presented in [12], Padki and S. Selvam directed their attention toward the early anticipation of rheumatoid arthritis through the utilization of a machine learning method, specifically employing an SVM. Their approach centers on the HLA-DRB4 gene sequence and the rate of genetic mutations. This technique aims to predict the disease early by comparing DNA nucleotide mutations in the HLA-DRB4 gene, a key candidate gene associated with rheumatoid arthritis. The mutation rate is calculated by comparing these mutations with mutated gene samples. Based on the computed mutation rate, individuals with high risk may be recommended to undergo a rheumatoid arthritis susceptibility test. By applying SVM with a linear kernel on gene data, this approach significantly improves the likelihood of early disease prediction. Such early prediction could be highly beneficial for healthcare professionals and the general population, potentially preventing individuals from experiencing severe pain and impaired quality of life associated with rheumatoid arthritis. An overview of current developments in machine learning techniques for the diagnosis and prognosis of Alzheimer's disease (AD) is given in this review paper. The authors go over numerous machine learning methods that have been applied to analyze neuroimaging, genetic, and clinical data in AD research, including deep learning, random forests, and support vector machines. The report also identifies the difficulties and restrictions associated with applying machine learning to AD research and makes recommendations for future lines of investigation Khan et al. [13]. Overall, these studies demonstrate the potential of machine learning and image processing techniques to enhance the diagnosis, prediction, and assessment of rheumatoid arthritis, ultimately contributing to better patient care and outcomes. While the mentioned studies utilize innovative machine-learning techniques and image processing for diagnosing and assessing RA, there are several potential limitations and demerits associated with these methods. Meanwhile, addressing these limitations requires careful consideration of data collection, preprocessing, model selection, validation, and ongoing monitoring. It's essential to strike a balance between the benefits of using machine learning techniques and the potential challenges and pitfalls associated with their implementation in the medical field. So CNNs via transfer learning offer several advantages that can help mitigate or overcome some of the limitations mentioned when applying machine learning techniques to medical diagnosis and assessment, particularly for conditions like RA.

3 Data and Methodology

In this section, we elucidate the methodology employed for the comprehensive analysis of RA utilizing the provided dataset. Our approach encompasses data collection, preprocessing, and transfer learn pre-trained CNN models for knee joint detection and KL grading, ensuring a robust framework for our investigation.

3.1 Dataset Description

The dataset under examination contains knee X-ray images, serving a dual purpose: knee joint detection and knee KL grading [14]. Knee osteoarthritis, characterized by the degeneration of articular cartilage and associated structural changes, is the focal point of our study. The dataset's relevance is underscored by its potential to aid in both diagnostic and prognostic endeavors.

3.2 Data Collection and Source

The knee X-ray images were acquired from the Kaggle repository, renowned for its meticulous data curation and adherence to diagnostic standards. To ensure a comprehensive portrayal of knee osteoarthritis, the dataset encompasses a range of severity levels, including the following KL grading descriptions as shown in Fig. 1.

Grade 0 (Healthy): Images of knees displaying no indications of degeneration or abnormalities in the joint.

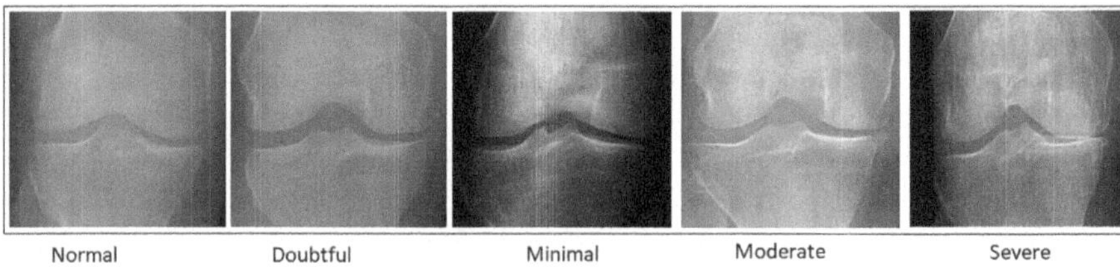

Fig. 1 Exemplary images of our selected dataset with the severity grading

Grade 1 (Doubtful): Images illustrating uncertain joint narrowing, potentially accompanied by the presence of osteophytic lipping.

Grade 2 (Minimal): Images showcasing clear evidence of osteophytes along with possible narrowing of the joint space.

Grade 3 (Moderate): Images presenting multiple osteophytes, distinct joint space narrowing, and mild sclerosis.

Grade 4 (Severe): Images featuring prominent osteophytes, significant joint narrowing, and severe sclerosis.

3.3 Data Preprocessing

A meticulous data preprocessing pipeline was established to ensure the quality and reliability of the dataset. This involved the removal of duplicate, corrupted, or low-quality images, bolstering the dataset's integrity. Image augmentation techniques were also employed to enhance dataset diversity and minimize overfitting, thereby fortifying the robustness of subsequent analyses. For knee joint detection, a specialized CNN architecture was transferred and learned to accurately identify knee joint regions within the X-ray images. The CNN was trained on a subset of the dataset with meticulously annotated knee joint bounding boxes. The model's performance was rigorously evaluated and the KL grading was approached as a multi-class classification task. Model training involved optimizing categorical cross-entropy loss and employing transfer learning techniques for enhanced performance.

3.4 Transfer Learning Procedure for Detection of Rheumatoid Arthritis Using CNN

Transfer learning stands as a potent strategy that utilizes insights acquired from one task to enhance the performance of another interconnected task. In our investigation concentrated on identifying RA through the application of CNNs, transfer learning assumes a pivotal role in elevating the model's efficiency and efficacy. This procedure (Fig. 2) allows us to benefit from the pre-trained knowledge of a CNN model while adapting it to our specific RA detection task.

Selection of Pre-trained Model: We begin by selecting a suitable pre-trained CNN model that has demonstrated exceptional performance on a large and diverse image dataset. The choice of architecture is influenced by its ability to capture relevant features, such as textures and structures, from medical images. For our study, a pre-trained model like AlexNet, GoogleNet, MobileNet, SqueezeNet, and Xecption is chosen due to their established track record in image classification tasks.

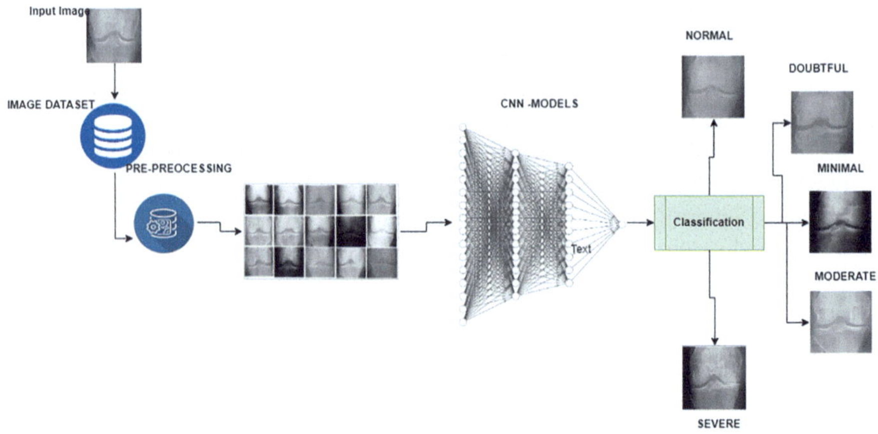

Fig. 2 CNN layered architecture for rheumatoid arthritis detection

Feature Extraction: In the transfer learning process, we retain the convolutional layers of the selected pre-trained model. These layers act as feature extractors that can identify high-level patterns and features in the input images. By utilizing these layers, the model can capture important information from our knee X-ray images related to RA characteristics, even though the model was trained initially on a different dataset.

Reconfiguration of Fully Connected Layers: The pre-trained model's original fully connected layers are tailored to match the number of classes in our RA detection task. For our purpose, we configure the final layers to have two output neurons: one representing the presence of RA and the other representing the absence of RA.

Fine-Tuning and Training: To adapt the pre-trained model to the specific nuances of our RA detection task, we initiate the process of fine-tuning. This involves training the reconfigured model on our RA-enriched subset of the knee X-ray dataset. During fine-tuning, the model learns to extract features that are particularly relevant to detecting RA-associated patterns, such as joint deformities and abnormalities.

Regularization and Hyperparameter Tuning: To prevent overfitting and enhance the generalization capabilities of the model, regularization techniques such as dropout and weight decay are applied. Additionally, hyperparameters such as learning rate, batch size, and optimizer settings are fine-tuned through systematic experimentation, employing methods like grid search and cross-validation.

4 Experimental Analysis and Discussion

The primary objective of our study was to evaluate the performance of these models in accurately detecting RA from knee X-ray images. Table 1 presents a comparison of different CNN models' performance under various conditions, denoted by the ratios of healthy (WOPP—Without Overlapping Positive Pairs) and affected (WPP—With Positive Pairs) cases. The models evaluated include AlexNet, GoogleNet, SqueezeNet, MobileNet, and Xception. In general, across all models, the introduction of positive pairs leads to improved performance compared to the conditions without overlapping positive pairs. This suggests that incorporating positive pair samples enhances the models' ability to discriminate between healthy and affected cases. Among the models tested, Xception consistently achieves the highest accuracy in both WOPP and WPP conditions, followed closely by GoogleNet. This indicates that Xception and GoogleNet possess strong feature extraction capabilities that are effective for classifying cases of interest. While all models exhibit an improvement in accuracy with the inclusion of positive pairs, the extent of improvement varies. Xception consistently shows the largest accuracy improvement when moving from WOPP to WPP conditions, followed by GoogleNet. The trend in accuracy improvement remains relatively consistent across different ratios of healthy to affected cases (9:1, 8:2, and 7:3). This suggests that the evaluated models are robust to changes in class distribution and maintain their effectiveness in distinguishing between the classes. Table 1 highlights the positive impact of introducing positive pairs on the performance of CNN models for the task of classification between healthy and affected cases.

The experimental results demonstrate varying performance across different CNN models. This highlights the importance of selecting an appropriate architecture for the specific task of RA detection. The achieved results demonstrate the potential of CNN models for RA detection from knee X-ray images. Such tools could assist healthcare professionals in early and accurate diagnosis, leading to timely interventions and improved patient outcomes. Additional exploration might involve delving into ensemble techniques that amalgamate the advantages of various models to enhance

Table 1 Analysis of preprocessing and augmentation in the accuracy of CNN models (WOPP: With Our Preprocessing and Augmentation; WPP: With Preprocessing and Augmentation)

CNN models	Class distribution ratio					
	9:1		8:2		7:3	
Condition	WOPP	WPP	WOPP	WPP	WOPP	WPP
AlexNet	86.11	90.71	84.90	89.5	83.9	88.5
GoogleNet	87.27	91.97	86.06	90.76	85.06	89.76
SqueezeNet	84.21	89.12	83.00	87.91	82.00	86.91
MobileNet	85.96	89.74	84.75	88.53	83.75	87.53
Xecption	88.56	92.74	87.35	91.53	86.35	90.53

overall performance. Moreover, model interpretability techniques could be employed to gain insights into the features and regions influencing the models' predictions. The experimental analysis reveals the viability of utilizing various pre-trained CNN models for the detection of Rheumatoid Arthritis from knee X-ray images. The choice of model should be guided by the trade-offs between accuracy, computational efficiency, and deployment considerations. The study underscores the potential of leveraging advanced technology in the domain of medical image analysis, fostering advancements in RA diagnosis and patient care.

Figure 3 provides a comprehensive analysis of different CNN models' performance across various class distribution ratios (9:1, 8:2, 7:3) for four distinct epochs. Across all CNN models, there is a consistent pattern where higher accuracy is achieved when the dataset has a higher proportion of healthy cases (lower percentage of affected cases). This is evident for each class distribution ratio (9:1, 8:2, 7:3) and across all conditions (10, 30, 60, and 80). Among the evaluated CNN models (AlexNet, GoogleNet, SqueezeNet, MobileNet, Xception), Xception consistently performs the best, achieving the highest accuracy across most conditions and class distribution ratios. GoogleNet and MobileNet also exhibit competitive performance, while AlexNet and SqueezeNet generally achieve lower accuracies. As the affected cases become the majority class, accuracy tends to decrease for all models. This highlights the challenge of class imbalance in the dataset and its impact on classification performance. Notably, for some models and conditions, the accuracy increases as the proportion of healthy cases increases (e.g., AlexNet at 80 epochs). This might indicate potential overfitting, where the model becomes too specialized in recognizing one class and struggles with the minority class. Figures 4 and 5 underscore the importance of class distribution in the accuracy of CNN models for classification tasks. Xception emerges as the top-performing model, demonstrating consistent accuracy across different conditions and class distribution ratios. It's evident that class imbalance poses challenges, with higher proportions of the affected class leading to decreased accuracy across all models. These insights shed light on the interplay between class distribution, model performance, and potential overfitting.

5 Conclusion

This study introduces a groundbreaking approach to the early detection of Rheumatoid Arthritis (RA) by harnessing the capabilities of CNNs and transfer learning. By exploiting the wealth of knowledge embedded in pre-trained CNN architectures and fine-tuning them to capture RA-specific features, our methodology demonstrates remarkable accuracy in discerning between healthy joints and those afflicted by RA, even when confronted with limited labeled data. The comprehensive evaluation of our approach using a diverse dataset of X-ray images underscores its effectiveness in the precise identification of Rheumatoid Arthritis. This advancement holds profound implications for the field of healthcare, offering a non-invasive and efficient solution for early diagnosis and management of the condition. Through the synergy of

Fig. 3 Comprehensive analysis of different CNN models' performance across various class distribution ratios

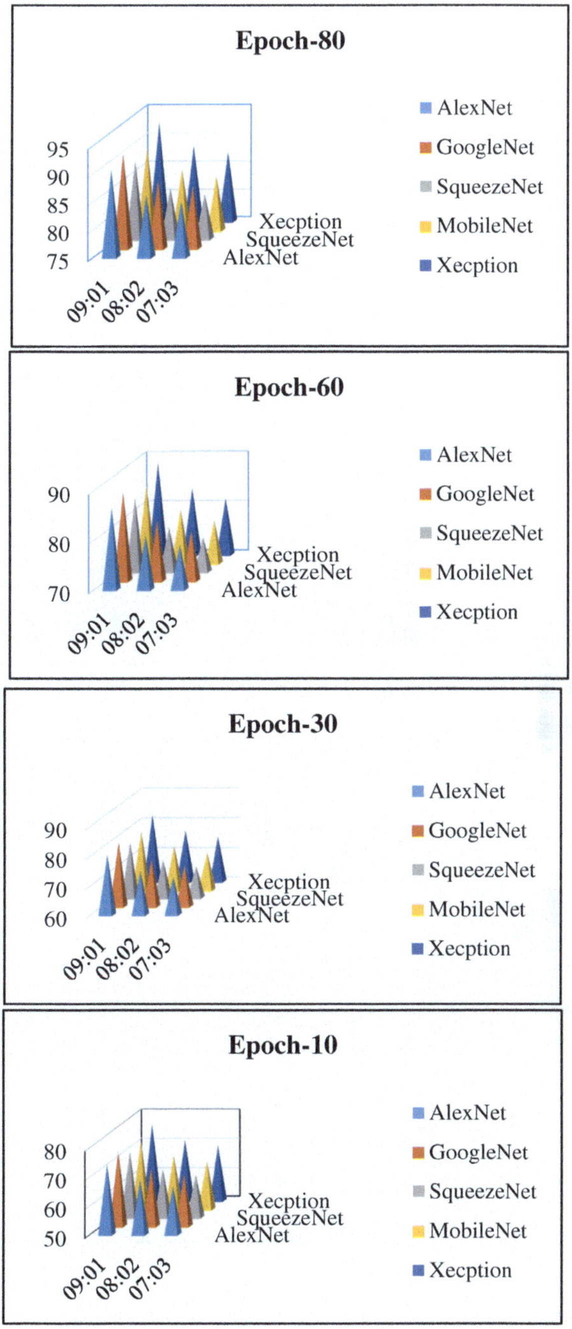

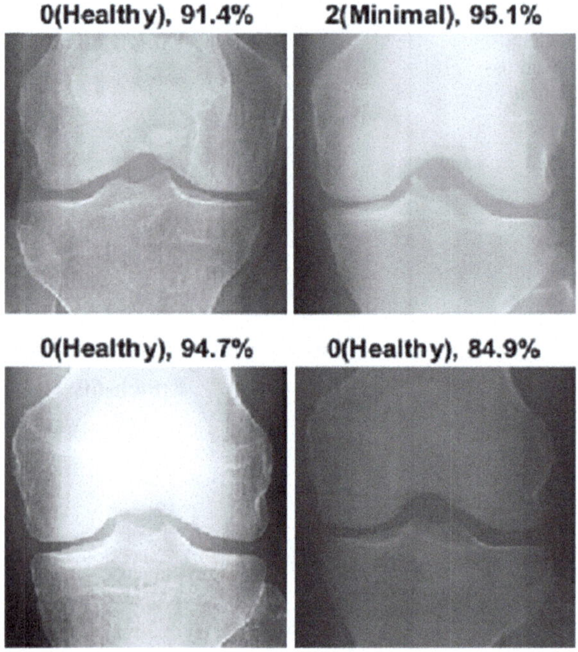

Fig. 4 Classification results of random classes with their accuracy

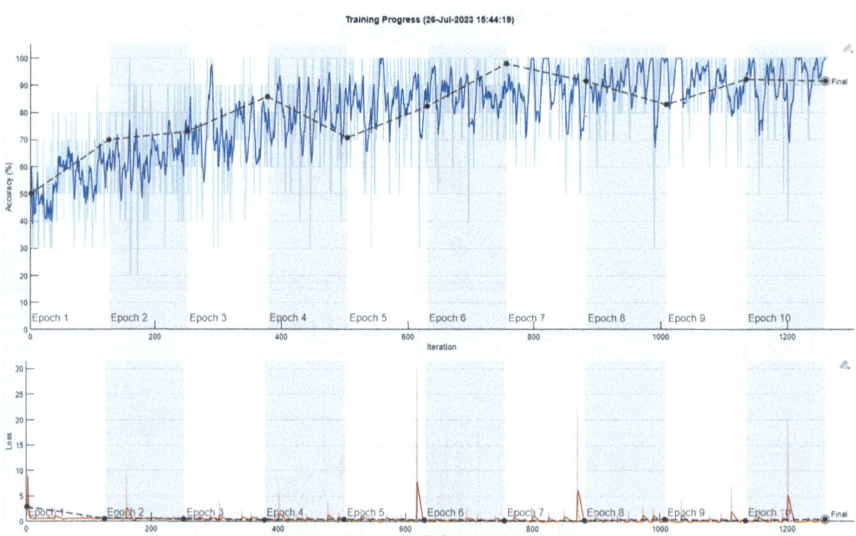

Fig. 5 Loss function and accuracy attained w.r.t. number of iterations

deep learning and transfer learning models, healthcare practitioners are empowered with a valuable tool to facilitate timely interventions, informed decision-making, and ultimately, improved patient outcomes in the realm of Rheumatoid Arthritis care.

References

1. Sugiyama D, Nishimura K, Tamaki K, Tsuji G, Nakazawa T, Morinobu A, Kumagai S (2010) Impact of smoking as a risk factor for developing rheumatoid arthritis: a meta-analysis of observational studies. Ann Rheum Dis 69(01):70–81
2. Källberg H, Ding B, Padyukov L, Bengtsson C, Rönnelid J, Klareskog L, EIRA Study Group (2011) Smoking is a major preventable risk factor for rheumatoid arthritis: estimations of risks after various exposures to cigarette smoke. Ann Rrheum Diseases 70(3):508–511
3. Nikseresht A, Hajipour B, Pishva N, Mohammadi HA (2022) Using artificial intelligence to make sustainable development decisions considering VUCA: a systematic literature review and bibliometric analysis. Environ Sci Pollut Res 29(28):42509–42538
4. Xue Y, Zhang R, Deng Y, Chen K, Jiang T (2017) A preliminary examination of the diagnostic value of deep learning in hip osteoarthritis. PloS One 12(6):e0178992
5. Khatoon MM, Singh BRN, Harshita MS, Sreeja K, Reddy SS, Latha JS (2023) Automated diagnosis of "rheumatoid arthritis" based on CNN. In: 2023 international conference on advances in computing, communication and applied informatics (ACCAI), Chennai, India, pp 1–5. https://doi.org/10.1109/ACCAI58221.2023.10200053
6. Lo C-M, Lai K-L (2023) Deep learning-based assessment of knee septic arthritis using transformer features in sonographic modalities. Comput Methods Programs Biomed 237:107575. ISSN 0169–2607. https://doi.org/10.1016/j.cmpb.2023.107575.
7. Zaman FA, Zhang L, Zhang H, Sonka M, Wu X (2023) Segmentation quality assessment by automated detection of erroneous surface regions in medical images. Comput Biol Med 164:107324. ISSN 0010-4825. https://doi.org/10.1016/j.compbiomed.2023.107324
8. Sakaria S, Jain S, Rana MK (2023) Rheumatoid arthritis predictor using ML techniques and explainable AI. In: 2023 international conference on distributed computing and electrical circuits and electronics (ICDCECE), Ballar, India, pp 1–7. https://doi.org/10.1109/ICDCECE57866.2023.10150759
9. Sundaramurthy SC, Kshirsagar P (2020) Prediction and classification of rheumatoid arthritis using ensemble machine learning approaches. In: 2020 international conference on decision aid sciences and application (DASA), Sakheer, Bahrain, pp 17–21. https://doi.org/10.1109/DASA51403.2020.9317253
10. Makino K, Koyama K, Hioki Y, Haro H, Terada H (2020) Recognition system of positions of joints of hands in an X-ray photograph to develop an automatic evaluation system for rheumatoid arthritis using machine learning. In: 2020 13th international conference on human system interaction (HSI), Tokyo, Japan, pp 216–221. https://doi.org/10.1109/HSI49210.2020.9142640
11. Sana A, Khawaja SA, Farooq M (2021) Rheumatoid arthritis genes classification using ML classifiers. In: 2021 international conference on innovative computing (ICIC), Lahore, Pakistan, pp 1–6. https://doi.org/10.1109/ICIC53490.2021.9693009
12. Padki P, Selvam S (2023) Prediction of rheumatoid arthritis susceptibility using gene mutation rate. In: 2023 international conference on advances in electronics, communication, computing andintelligent information systems (ICAECIS), Bangalore, India, pp 22–26. https://doi.org/10.1109/ICAECIS58353.2023.10170167
13. Khan A, Usman M (2015) Early diagnosis of Alzheimer's disease using machine learning techniques: a review paper. In: 2015 7th international joint conference on knowledge discovery, knowledge engineering and knowledge management (IC3K), vol 1. IEEE, pp 380–387

14. Chen P (2018) Knee osteoarthritis severity grading dataset. Mendeley data, V1. https://doi.org/10.17632/56rmx5bjcr.1
15. Raza K, Singh NK (2021) A tour of unsupervised deep learning for medical image analysis. Current Med Imaging 17(9):1059–1077. https://doi.org/10.2174/1573405617666210127154257

The Emerging Applications of Machine Learning in the Diagnosis of Multiple Sclerosis

Anshul Sharma, Nitin Sharma, Akshita Arora, and Richa Pal

Abstract A chronic autoimmune inflammatory condition called multiple sclerosis (MS) affects the central nervous system which can cause issues related to the brain, optic nerve, and spinal cord. Machine learning (ML) and artificial intelligence (AI)-based multiple sclerosis diagnosis is a rapidly growing field. Multiple sclerosis is a chronic immune system disorder that impacts the central nervous system over an extended period of time and manifests as a variety of symptoms, making it difficult to diagnose. AI and ML techniques have the ability to increase the accuracy and efficiency of MS diagnosis by examining vast quantities of medical information and recognizing patterns that may be challenging for humans to identify. This chapter reviews the current state of the art in AI and ML-based diagnosis of MS, including the use of imaging data, clinical data, and biomarkers. Additionally, it highlights the challenges and limitations of AI and ML in MS diagnosis, along with the potential future possibilities of research in this area.

Keywords Multiple sclerosis · Artificial intelligence · Machine learning · Diagnosis · Autoimmune disease

A. Sharma · N. Sharma (✉) · A. Arora · R. Pal
Department of Pharmaceutics, ISF College of Pharmacy, Ghal Kalan, GT Road, Moga, Punjab 142001, India
e-mail: sharma.nitin0909@gmail.com

A. Sharma
e-mail: anshul.sharma@pilani.bits-pilani.ac.in

A. Sharma
Department of Pharmacy, Birla Institute of Technology And Science, Pilani (BITS Pilani), Pilani, Rajasthan 333031, India

N. Sharma
Department of Pharmaceutics, Amity Institute of Pharmacy, Amity University, Uttar Pradesh, Sector-125, Noida 201303, India

K. Raza and S. Singh (eds.), *Artificial Intelligence and Autoimmune Diseases*, Studies in Computational Intelligence 1133, https://doi.org/10.1007/978-981-99-9029-0_6

1 Introduction

Multiple Sclerosis (MS) is a chronic autoimmune disease that has a major impact on the central nervous system (CNS). It is distinguished by damage to the protective covering (myelin sheath) of nerve fibers, leading to various symptoms such as muscle weakness, fatigue, mobility issues, and vision problems [1]. When the immune cells of the body target the neurological system, it leads to inflammation and ultimately results in nerve damage [2]. Plaques of localized primary demyelination and various types of neurodegenerations are brought on by MS and affect the brain, spinal cord, and white and grey matter [3]. A number of pathogenic processes, including demyelination, axonal degeneration, localized lymphocyte infiltration, and activation of microglia, contribute to the pathogenesis of MS [4]. When there's damage to the blood–brain barrier due to factors like stress, fibrinogens are deposited in the brain tissue. This leads to the activation of microglia, which are resident immune cells in the central nervous system. Activated microglia release inflammatory molecules such as cytokines and chemokines. These molecules attract immune cells like T cells and macrophages to the site of inflammation leading to myelin damage and neuroinflammation (Fig. 1). The exact causes of MS are still not entirely comprehended, but it is thought that a mix of hereditary as well as environmental factors contribute [5].

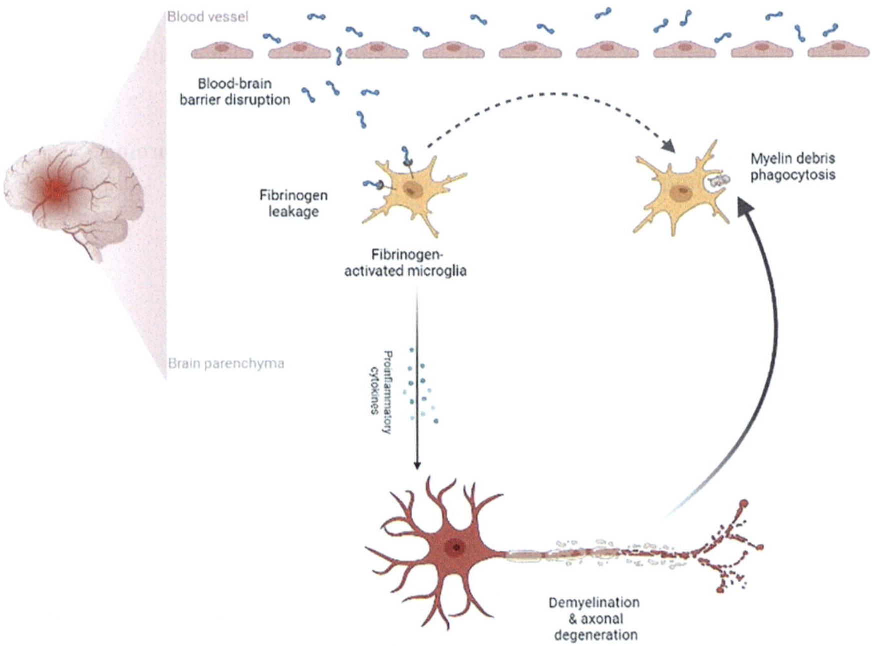

Fig. 1 Pathophysiology of multiple sclerosis

MS can be classified into several subtypes, depending on the severity and progression of symptoms. The most common form is relapsing–remitting MS, where symptoms come and go over time [6]. Secondary progressive MS is an advanced phase of relapsing–remitting MS that occurs later and where the disease progresses without remissions. Progressive relapsing MS is a rare form where symptoms progressively worsen from the onset of the disease without remission. It is estimated that globally there are 2.8 million individuals suffering from MS, which translates to a rate of 35.9 per 100,000 population [7]. Starting from 2013, the occurrence of MS has risen by 30% worldwide. Among the 75 countries that have reported their data, the yearly rate of MS diagnosis stands at 2.1 per 100,000 individuals [8]. Approximately 5% of people diagnosed with MS first experience symptoms during their childhood, which are usually indicative of the relapsing–remitting form of the disease [9].

Diagnosis of MS can be challenging, as symptoms may mimic other conditions, and there is no single test that can confirm the disease [10]. It is crucial to quickly recognize the indications and manifestations of MS as it enables individuals to get medical attention and plan accordingly. The majority of the time, it is impossible to forecast and accurately predict MS symptoms. Neurologists usually diagnose MS through a combination of medical history, physical and neurological examination, imaging tests, and examination of spinal fluid. When someone shows symptoms that suggest they may have MS, it is strongly advised to undergo an MRI scan, as almost all individuals with confirmed MS show abnormal brain scans on MRI and over 80% of patients with isolated symptoms later develop this disease also have abnormal MRI results [10].

Despite the fact that there is presently no cure for MS, there are a number of treatments that are available and can offer assistance and help control the disease's symptoms and slow down its progression [11]. These include disease-modifying drugs like dimethyl fumarate, glatiramer acetate, natalizumab, and fingolimod, among others that target the underlying causes of MS, and symptomatic treatments that relieve specific symptoms such as pain, spasticity, and fatigue [12]. Physical therapy and rehabilitation can also help improve mobility, balance, and coordination.

2 Current Challenges that AI Can Tackle in Diagnosis

The identification of the malfunctioning biological mechanism and its related degree is referred to as disease diagnosis. It is essential for developing a successful treatment strategy and guaranteeing patients' well-being. Integrated outputs from diagnosis are typically utilized in health management to determine the best logistical and maintenance choices for treating the disease. The fundamental component of AI-enabled diagnostics is using conventional ML or deep learning (DL) techniques to carry out the ultimate health management. The effectiveness and accuracy of diagnosis can be improved with the application of AI. Clinical analysis of medical information is a difficult cognitive task. This notion is true for both seasoned medical experts and junior doctors. The appropriate diagnosis is difficult to make because of the time constraints placed on medical experts [13]. The condition gets worse as a result of dynamic changes in the pathophysiology of the disease throughout time. However, a thorough diagnostic approach is essential to ensure prompt treatment and, as a result, achieve safe and efficient patient care [14].

The utilization of AI in the process of diagnosing a condition has become increasingly crucial. The implementation of AI in diagnosing a disease today is narrowed down to a specific task [15]. By continually analyzing fresh and current information, algorithms make predictions, consistently educate, and grow over a period of time. Algorithms gather information either through a variety of inputs and sources of knowledge. As a result, AI-enabled computers can store more information than humans, perhaps surpassing the human's capabilities for some medical activities [16]. The incorporation of AI into the modern technological infrastructure speeds up finding relevant medical information from many sources that is suitable for the patient's needs and the therapy method. Furthermore, AI produces results based on a bigger population rather than on individualized, personal perception, obtains the same outcomes when using the same medical data, and is not affected by context, mood, or time. AI has the capacity to make a contribution to the development of simple, inexpensive, and precise medical diagnostic tools to screen and identify patients for chronic diseases including cancer, tuberculosis, and multiple sclerosis [17, 18]. Additionally, AI solutions can considerably contribute to reducing the time and money associated with diagnostic procedures [19].

3 Overview of AI and ML Techniques

AI and ML are two fast-growing fields that have revolutionized the way we interact with technology. The more general idea of AI is that of computers performing things in a manner that we would deem "smart", while ML refers specifically to the use of algorithms to allow a computer to learn from data [20]. At the heart of ML lies the concept of mathematical models, or algorithms, that are trained on a large dataset and then used to make predictions or decisions. There are many different ML algorithms, ranging from simple linear regression to complex deep neural networks [21]. One of the simplest and most commonly used ML techniques is linear regression, which is used to predict a continuous output based on one or more input variables. Linear regression is one of the most popular and versatile statistical and ML methods, commonly utilized to identify a linear connection between one or more predictors [22].

Another popular ML technique is decision trees, which is a tree-like structure used to model decisions or relationships between values. In a decision tree, the algorithm starts at the root node and follows a series of judgments made depending on the values of the input variables until it reaches a leaf node that represents the final prediction [23].

Another important family of ML algorithms are neural networks, which draw inspiration from the design and operation of the human brain [24]. Neural networks are made up of layers of interconnected nodes, and they undergo training that involves processing massive amounts of data to identify patterns and make predictions [25]. There are numerous varieties of neural networks, including convolutional, recurrent, and feedforward networks [26]. Artificial neural networks have been used to solve issues as diverse as voice recognition, protein secondary structure prediction, categorizing cancer types, and gene prediction [27]. High processing rates and the capacity to learn a problem's solution from a series of examples are only two of the remarkable characteristics of neural networks [28].

Another technique known as "deep learning" which is a subfield of ML is focused on using neural networks with many layers, or deep networks, to solve complex problems. Deep learning has become a very popular area of research due to its ability to attain state-of-the-art outcomes or results in areas such as robotics, natural language processing, and speech and image recognition. Deep learning enables computational models to acquire various levels of abstract data representations by incorporating multiple layers of processing [29]. Another important area of ML is reinforcement learning, which is used to train agents to make decisions in an environment based on rewards and punishments. Reinforcement learning is used in many different applications, including game AI, robotics, and autonomous vehicles. Unsupervised learning is another type of ML, in which the algorithm is given a dataset without any labeled outputs, and it must find patterns and structure in the data on its own. One common unsupervised learning technique is clustering, in which the algorithm groups similar data points together. Another technique is dimensionality reduction, which is used to decrease the number of input variables while preserving as much of the original information as possible.

Among ML methods, supervised learning is the most prevalent approach and it is used to train the algorithm on a labeled dataset in order to make predictions. In supervised learning, the algorithm is given input/output pairs, and it must acquire an understanding of the connection between the inputs and outputs in order to make accurate predictions [30].

Today, AI is a thriving field with many practical applications in the area of active research. These technologies have revolutionized the healthcare industry in recent years. New advancements in AI studies have shown that using computers to aid in diagnosis can help detect diseases like MS at an earlier stage by analyzing medical images to classify, quantify, and identify patterns that indicate the presence of the disease. ML algorithms can be used to analyze various types of data related to MS, including magnetic resonance imaging (MRI) scans, patient symptoms, and demographic information [31]. The algorithms can learn from the data and develop predictive models to diagnose MS with a high degree of accuracy. For example, a convolutional neural network (CNN) can be trained to identify characteristic lesions in MRI scans that are indicative of MS [32]. This can help to reduce the time and resources required for manual review of images and increase the speed and accuracy of diagnoses. AI and ML have the potential to play a significant role in the diagnosis of MS. By automating tasks such as image analysis and decision-making, these technologies can improve the speed, accuracy, and efficiency of the diagnostic process. This can help to improve patient outcomes and reduce the burden on healthcare professionals.

4 Emerging Trends of AI and ML Used in MS Diagnosis

4.1 Imaging-Based Diagnosis

MS is a persistent neurological condition that significantly impacts the CNS, leading to a diverse array of symptoms that can differ in their presentation from one individual to another. The diagnosis of MS is typically done using a combination of clinical symptoms, imaging studies, and other tests [33]. However, the accurate and timely diagnosis of MS can be challenging, especially during the disease's early stages, when symptoms could be minor or non-specific [34].

Advancements in AI and ML can improve the accuracy and efficiency of MS diagnosis by using image-based analysis [35]. MRI is the most commonly used imaging technique for the diagnosis of MS, as it can provide detailed information about the brain and spinal cord [36]. However, the interpretation of MRI images can be time-consuming and subjective, and it requires specialized expertise.

AI and ML algorithms can be trained to analyze MRI images and identify patterns and anomalies that may be indicative of MS [37]. These algorithms can be trained on large datasets of MRI scans from both healthy individuals and patients with MS, allowing them to learn to differentiate between the two. By analyzing multiple MRI images of the same patient over time, AI and ML algorithms can also help identify changes in the brain or spinal cord that may indicate disease progression.

One key advantage of AI and ML in MS diagnosis is the possibility of reducing the cost and duration of diagnosis. With the help of AI and ML, radiologists and neurologists can quickly and accurately analyze MRI images, enabling earlier and more precise MS diagnosis [38]. This can be particularly important in cases where the diagnosis is uncertain or where symptoms are mild or non-specific. AI and ML can also help identify specific markers of disease progression that may be missed by human interpretation of MRI images [39]. For example, AI and ML can identify subtle changes in brain volume or lesion size that may be indicative of disease activity [40]. By detecting these changes earlier, physicians may be able to intervene with more effective treatments before irreversible damage occurs.

The utilization of AI and ML in diagnosing MS also presents certain difficulties. One major challenge is the need for large datasets of high-quality MRI images to train the algorithms [41]. This requires collaboration between institutions and the sharing of data, which can be complicated by issues of patient privacy and data ownership. The possibility of bias in the algorithms is another difficulty. AI and ML algorithms may be trained on datasets that do not accurately represent the diversity of the patient population, leading to biased results [42]. It is important to ensure that the datasets used to train the algorithms are diverse and representative of the patient population to ensure the accuracy and fairness of the results.

In conclusion, AI and ML have the potential to revolutionize the diagnosis and management of MS by improving the accuracy and efficiency of image-based analysis. With the ability to quickly and accurately analyze MRI images, AI and ML can aid in the early and accurate diagnosis of MS, identify markers of disease progression, and help guide treatment decisions [43]. However, certain challenges are also associated with the use of AI and ML, which include the need for large datasets and potential biases in the algorithms. It is important to continue to address these challenges and to work toward the development of safe and effective AI and ML tools for the diagnosis and management of MS.

4.1.1 Clinical Support

There are many different symptoms that can accompany MS making it challenging for doctors and radiologists to diagnose [10]. However, recent advances in AI and ML technology have enabled medical professionals to accurately diagnose and treat MS more effectively [44]. This section will explore how AI and ML are used to assist doctors and radiologists in making a diagnosis of MS.

One of the primary ways AI and ML are used to assist doctors in diagnosing MS is through the analysis of medical imaging data [45]. MRI is a commonly used imaging technique that can reveal areas of inflammation and demyelination in the brain and spinal cord, which are key indicators of MS. However, analyzing MRI images manually can be time-consuming and prone to errors. AI and ML algorithms can quickly and accurately analyze large sets of MRI images, flagging areas of concern and providing insights that can aid in the diagnosis of MS.

For example, researchers have created an AI system called DeepSCAN that can automatically detect and quantify MS lesions in MRI scans. DeepSCAN uses a deep learning algorithm to analyze MRI images and produce a quantitative map of MS lesions, which can assist radiologists in making a diagnosis of MS [46, 47]. This can help doctors and radiologists to make more accurate and timely diagnoses, resulting in earlier treatment and improved patient outcomes.

Researchers have also investigated the use of unsupervised machine learning techniques to classify MS subtypes based on pathological features using brain MRI scans. Their study applies unsupervised machine learning algorithms to analyze brain MRI scans obtained from previously published studies. The aim is to identify groups with similar features and classify MS subtypes based on these pathological features. The study demonstrates that unsupervised machine learning applied to MRI data can effectively classify MS subtypes based on pathological features. This approach has the potential to improve treatment stratification and enhance our understanding of the pathophysiological boundaries of MS subtypes. The findings of this study have significant clinical implications for the stratification and personalized treatment of MS patients [48].

Another way AI and ML are used to assist doctors in diagnosing MS is through the analysis of clinical data. MS has a varied symptomatology, with manifestations that can span a broad spectrum which includes fatigue, muscle weakness, and cognitive impairment. AI and ML algorithms can analyze large sets of clinical data to recognize patterns and trends that can aid in MS diagnosis. For example, researchers at the University of California, San Diego have developed an AI system called DIADEM

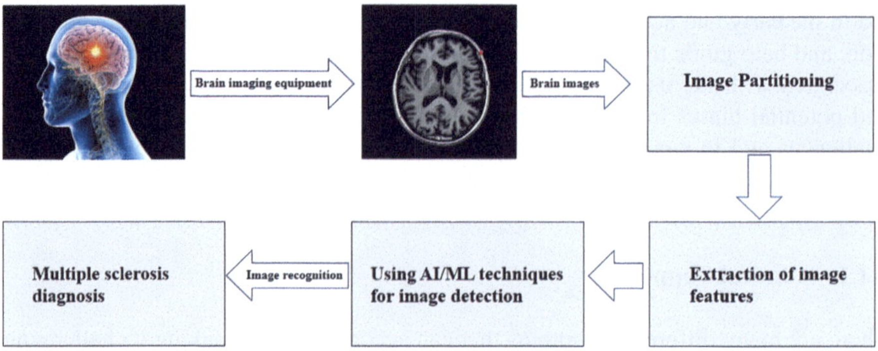

Fig. 2 The step-by-step process by which AI and ML operate in disease diagnosis

that uses machine learning algorithms to analyze clinical data and predict the likelihood of MS in patients with neurological symptoms [49, 50]. DIADEM uses a combination of demographic, clinical, and radiological data to generate a risk score that can aid doctors in making a diagnosis of MS. While DIADEM is still in development, it holds the potential to improve the accuracy and speed of MS diagnosis, which could lead to earlier treatment and better outcomes for patients. A brief explanation of how this works is illustrated in the flow chart Fig. 2.

In light of these findings, we can say that AI and ML technology has the potential to revolutionize the diagnosis and treatment of MS. By analyzing medical imaging and clinical data, AI and ML algorithms can assist doctors and radiologists in making more accurate and timely diagnoses of MS, as well as developing personalized treatment plans that are tailored to each individual patient's needs. We can anticipate even more inventive solutions as these technologies develop and will improve the lives of MS patients around the world. Table 1 highlights a selection of patents that showcase how AI and ML can be effectively harnessed in the domain of disease diagnosis.

5 Conclusion and Future Directions

A thorough diagnosis of the disease is necessary for successful planning, effective therapy, and patient safety. The broad and diverse field of AI, which is always expanding and evolving to satisfy the needs of the healthcare system and its clients, is made up of AI, ML, and DL. Despite significant developments in the last several years, reliable diagnostics of a disease still face a number of challenges that must be overcome and continually enhanced in order to efficiently manage new diseases. Even medical practitioners are aware of the challenges that need to be solved before illness may be recognized using AI. At the moment, even physicians do not completely depend on AI-based methods because they are unsure of their capacity to foresee diseases and their associated conditions. It takes a lot of work to train AI-based

Table 1 Recent patents on the use of AI and ML in MS diagnosis

Patents	Patent no.	Outcomes	References
System and method for risk assessment of MS	US20220293217A1	The sample isolated from the human body is subjected to DNA stretch analyses followed by the production of neuroactive compounds. Ultimately, utilizing the ML to generate the metabolic potential of these compounds and predict the disease severity	[51]
Automatic identification of subjects at risk of multiple sclerosis	US11272843B2	The embodiment includes use of a magnetic resonance imaging scanner to analyze the ailment. It particularly uses certain algorithms like central vein and paramagnetic algorithms to predict the diseased areas	[52]
miRNA fingerprint in the diagnosis of multiple sclerosis	US9187785B2	In this, the miRNA isolated from human body samples are subjected to certain procedures and mathematics along with ML methodologies are implemented for diagnosis of the severity of the disease	[53]
Method of predicting the severity of multiple sclerosis	US10506986B2	This describes a method for predicting the severity of multiple sclerosis in an individual using ML techniques. The method involves analyzing medical data from the patient, including MRI data and clinical information, to identify features that are indicative of MS severity	[54]

systems so that they can anticipate disease diagnosis techniques with greater accuracy. This is the demand of time that there is a need to make AI-based systems more accurate and reliable by new technologies. Therefore, in the coming future, research on AI should be undertaken while taking the problem noted before into account to create a partnership between AI and doctors that is mutually advantageous. It is advised to conduct additional research work in the area of AI and deep learning for disease diagnosis in order to analyze enormous amounts of medical information and data more quickly and reliably to produce satisfactory outcomes. The effectiveness of AI algorithms as a clinical support system for diagnosis, assisting physicians by offering an additional second opinion, should be further investigated in future studies.

References

1. Ciccarelli O, Barkhof F, Bodini B, De Stefano N, Golay X, Nicolay K et al (2014) Pathogenesis of multiple sclerosis: insights from molecular and metabolic imaging. Lancet Neurol 13(8):807–822
2. Dargahi N, Katsara M, Tselios T, Androutsou M-E, De Courten M, Matsoukas J et al (2017) Multiple sclerosis: immunopathology and treatment update. Brain Sci 7(7):78

3. Compston A, Coles A (2002) Multiple sclerosis. Lancet 359(9313):1221–1231
4. Brambilla R (2019) The contribution of astrocytes to the neuroinflammatory response in multiple sclerosis and experimental autoimmune encephalomyelitis. Acta Neuropathol 137(5):757–783
5. Ebers GC, Sadovnick AD, Risch NJ (1995) A genetic basis for familial aggregation in multiple sclerosis. Nature 377(6545):150–151
6. Filippi M, Bar-Or A, Piehl F, Preziosa P, Solari A, Vukusic S et al (2018) Multiple sclerosis. Nat Rev Dis Primers 4(1):1–27
7. Walton C, King R, Rechtman L, Kaye W, Leray E, Marrie RA, et al. Rising prevalence of multiple sclerosis worldwide: Insights from the Atlas of MS, third edition. Multiple Sclerosis Journal. 2020;26(14):1816–21.
8. Browne P, Chandraratna D, Angood C, Tremlett H, Baker C, Taylor BV et al (2014) Atlas of multiple sclerosis 2013: a growing global problem with widespread inequity. Neurology 83(11):1022–1024
9. Sharma A, Sharma N, Singh S, Dua K (2023) Review on theranostic and neuroprotective applications of nanotechnology in multiple sclerosis. J Drug Deliv Sci Technol 2023:104220
10. Brownlee WJ, Hardy TA, Fazekas F, Miller DH (2017) Diagnosis of multiple sclerosis: progress and challenges. The Lancet 389(10076):1336–1346
11. Damal K, Stoker E, Foley JF (2013) Optimizing therapeutics in the management of patients with multiple sclerosis: a review of drug efficacy, dosing, and mechanisms of action. Biol: Targets Therapy. 2013:247–58.
12. Wingerchuk DM, Carter JL (eds) (2014) Multiple sclerosis: current and emerging disease-modifying therapies and treatment strategies. Mayo clinic proceedings. Elsevier
13. Yadav MK, Ahmad S, Raza K, Kumar S, Eswaran M, Pasha KM (2023) Predictive modeling and therapeutic repurposing of natural compounds against the receptor-binding domain of SARS-CoV-2. J Biomol Struct Dyn 41(5):1527–1539
14. Behara K, Bhero E, Agee JT, Gonela V (2022) Artificial intelligence in medical diagnostics: a review from a South African context. Scientific African, p e01360
15. Sahu A, Qazi S, Raza K, Singh A, Verma S (2022) Machine learning-based approach for early diagnosis of breast cancer using biomarkers and gene expression profiles. In: Computational intelligence in oncology: applications in diagnosis, prognosis and therapeutics of cancers: Springer, pp 285–306
16. Kumar Y, Koul A, Singla R, Ijaz MF (2022) Artificial intelligence in disease diagnosis: a systematic literature review, synthesizing framework and future research agenda. J Ambient Intell Human Comput
17. Qazi S, Iqbal N, Raza K (2021) Machine learning in cancer diagnosis, prognosis and therapy. Artif Intell Data-Driven Med Diagnosis 3:103
18. Khan FN, Yousef M, Raza K (2022) Machine learning-based models in the diagnosis, prognosis and effective cancer therapeutics: current state-of-the-art. In: Computational intelligence in oncology: applications in diagnosis, prognosis and therapeutics of cancers. Springer, pp 19–54
19. Mirbabaie M, Stieglitz S, Frick NRJ (2021) Artificial intelligence in disease diagnostics: A critical review and classification on the current state of research guiding future direction. Heal Technol 11(4):693–731
20. Kaplan A, Haenlein M (2019) Siri, Siri, in my hand: Who's the fairest in the land? On the interpretations, illustrations, and implications of artificial intelligence. Bus Horiz 62(1):15–25
21. Yadav SS, Jadhav SM (2019) Deep convolutional neural network based medical image classification for disease diagnosis. J Big Data 6(1):1–18
22. Ramprasad R, Batra R, Pilania G, Mannodi-Kanakkithodi A, Kim C (2017) Machine learning in materials informatics: recent applications and prospects. npj Comput Mater 3(1):54.
23. Quinlan JR (1986) Induction of decision trees. Mach Learn 1:81–106
24. Cox DD, Dean T (2014) Neural networks and neuroscience-inspired computer vision. Curr Biol 24(18):R921–R929
25. French MN, Krajewski WF, Cuykendall RR (1992) Rainfall forecasting in space and time using a neural network. J Hydrol 137(1–4):1–31

26. Kriegeskorte N, Golan T (2019) Neural network models and deep learning. Curr Biol 29(7):R231–R236
27. Krogh A (2008) What are artificial neural networks? Nat Biotechnol 26(2):195–197
28. Bishop CM (1994) Neural networks and their applications. Rev Sci Instrum 65(6):1803–1832
29. LeCun Y, Bengio Y, Hinton G (2015) Deep learning. Nature 521(7553):436–444
30. Alzubi J, Nayyar A, Kumar A (ed) (2018) Machine learning from theory to algorithms: an overview. J Phys: Confer Ser. IOP Publishing
31. Shoeibi A, Khodatars M, Jafari M, Moridian P, Rezaei M, Alizadehsani R et al (2021) Applications of deep learning techniques for automated multiple sclerosis detection using magnetic resonance imaging: a review. Comput Biol Med 136:104697
32. Brosch T, Tang LY, Yoo Y, Li DK, Traboulsee A, Tam R (2016) Deep 3D convolutional encoder networks with shortcuts for multiscale feature integration applied to multiple sclerosis lesion segmentation. IEEE Trans Med Imaging 35(5):1229–1239
33. Bot JC, Barkhof F, Polman C, à Nijeholt GL, De Groot V, Bergers E et al (2004) Spinal cord abnormalities in recently diagnosed MS patients: added value of spinal MRI examination. Neurology 62(2):226–233
34. Thompson AJ, Banwell BL, Barkhof F, Carroll WM, Coetzee T, Comi G et al (2018) Diagnosis of multiple sclerosis: 2017 revisions of the McDonald criteria. Lancet Neurol 17(2):162–173
35. Xu J, Xue K, Zhang K (2019) Current status and future trends of clinical diagnoses via image-based deep learning. Theranostics. 9(25):7556
36. Pretorius P, Quaghebeur G (2003) The role of MRI in the diagnosis of MS. Clin Radiol 58(6):434–448
37. Avanzo M, Porzio M, Lorenzon L, Milan L, Sghedoni R, Russo G et al (2021) Artificial intelligence applications in medical imaging: a review of the medical physics research in Italy. Physica Med 83:221–241
38. Alloghani M, Al-Jumeily D, Aljaaf AJ, Khalaf M, Mustafina J, Tan SY (eds) (2019) The application of artificial intelligence technology in healthcare: a systematic review. In: Applied computing to support industry: innovation and technology: first international conference, ACRIT 2019, Ramadi, Iraq, September 15–16, 2019, Revised Selected Papers; 2020: Springer
39. Vrenken H, Jenkinson M, Pham DL, Guttmann CRG, Pareto D, Paardekooper M et al (2021) Opportunities for understanding MS mechanisms and progression with MRI using large-scale data sharing and artificial intelligence. Neurology 97(21):989–999
40. Aslam N, Khan IU, Bashamakh A, Alghool FA, Aboulnour M, Alsuwayan NM et al (2022) Multiple sclerosis diagnosis using machine learning and deep learning: challenges and opportunities. Sensors 22(20):7856
41. Willemink MJ, Koszek WA, Hardell C, Wu J, Fleischmann D, Harvey H et al (2020) Preparing medical imaging data for machine learning. Radiology 295(1):4–15
42. Dankwa-Mullan I, Weeraratne D (2022) Artificial intelligence and machine learning technologies in cancer care: addressing disparities, bias, and data diversity. Cancer Discov 12(6):1423–1427
43. Ranschaert ER, Morozov S, Algra PR (2019) Artificial intelligence in medical imaging: opportunities, applications and risks. Springer
44. Myszczynska MA, Ojamies PN, Lacoste AM, Neil D, Saffari A, Mead R et al (2020) Applications of machine learning to diagnosis and treatment of neurodegenerative diseases. Nat Rev Neurol 16(8):440–456
45. Shaikh F, Dehmeshki J, Bisdas S, Roettger-Dupont D, Kubassova O, Aziz M et al (2021) Artificial intelligence-based clinical decision support systems using advanced medical imaging and radiomics. Curr Probl Diagn Radiol 50(2):262–267
46. McKinley R, Wepfer R, Aschwanden F, Grunder L, Muri R, Rummel C et al (2021) Simultaneous lesion and brain segmentation in multiple sclerosis using deep neural networks. Sci Rep 11(1):1087

47. McKinley R, Meier R, Wiest R (eds) Ensembles of densely-connected CNNs with label-uncertainty for brain tumor segmentation. In: Brainlesion: glioma, multiple sclerosis, stroke and traumatic brain injuries: 4th international workshop, BrainLes 2018, Held in Conjunction with MICCAI 2018, Granada, Spain, September 16, 2018, Revised Selected Papers, Part II 4; 2019. Springer
48. Eshaghi A, Young AL, Wijeratne PA, Prados F, Arnold DL, Narayanan S et al (2021) Identifying multiple sclerosis subtypes using unsupervised machine learning and MRI data. Nat Commun 12(1):2078
49. Pemberton HG, Zaki LAM, Goodkin O, Das RK, Steketee RME, Barkhof F et al (2021) Technical and clinical validation of commercial automated volumetric MRI tools for dementia diagnosis—a systematic review. Neuroradiology 63(11):1773–1789
50. Mendelsohn Z, Pemberton HG, Gray J, Goodkin O, Carrasco FP, Scheel M et al (2023) Commercial volumetric MRI reporting tools in multiple sclerosis: a systematic review of the evidence. Neuroradiology 65(1):5–24
51. Mande SS, Bose C, Kaur H (2022) System and method for risk assessment of multiple sclerosis. Google Patents
52. Sati P, Patil SG, Reich D (2022) Automatic identification of subjects at risk of multiple sclerosis. Google Patents
53. Keller A, Meese E, Borries A, Staehler PF, Beier M (2015) miRNA fingerprint in the diagnosis of multiple sclerosis. Google Patents
54. Schaevitz L, Ford DJ (2019) Method of predicting severity of multiple sclerosis. Google Patents

Diagnosis and Analysis of Multiple Sclerosis Disease Using Artificial Intelligence

Shafaque Aziz, Mohammad Amjad, Faiz Akram, Neha Sami, and Azra Parveen

Abstract Multiple sclerosis (MS) is a chronic acquired idiopathic, autoimmune inflammatory demyelinating disorder of the central nervous system (CNS) that results in disruption of myelin sheath due to environmental and genetic factors. Demyelination and inflammation occur at the early stages of plaque formation which progresses to axonal damage and neuronal loss in the later stages of the disease. Despite having a typical progression there are no specific markers that can help in its easy and early diagnosis. Consequently, MS diagnosis primarily depends on the medical history of the patient, neurological examination including MRI scan, evoked potential test, Lumbar puncture, and some blood. However, it still takes some years to make a correct diagnosis since the condition worsens gradually. Moreover, the last decade has seen a significant rise in MS. However, advances in the applications of information technology and their intertwining with the medical domain have accounted for a considerable amount of data from normal and diseased individuals alike. More recently, artificial intelligence (AI) techniques in MS research have increased interest and provide means to facilitate its early diagnosis and better prognosis. The traditional methods, on the contrary, have relatively lower values of performance measures that reduce the effectiveness of the method. The AI approaches can make efficient utilization of observational data for early identification and prediction of the disease

S. Aziz (✉) · M. Amjad · F. Akram
Faculty of Engineering and Technology, Department of Computer Engineering, Jamia Millia Islamia, A Central University, New Delhi 110025, India
e-mail: shafaque.phd@gmail.com

M. Amjad
e-mail: mamjad@jmi.ac.in

F. Akram
e-mail: syedfaiz.phd@gmail.com

N. Sami
Department of Biosciences, A Central University, Jamia Millia Islamia, New Delhi 110025, India
e-mail: nsami.mail@gmail.com

A. Parveen
Postdoctoral Research Fellow, IIIS Delhi, New Delhi, India
e-mail: parveenazra999@gmail.com

K. Raza and S. Singh (eds.), *Artificial Intelligence and Autoimmune Diseases*, Studies in Computational Intelligence 1133, https://doi.org/10.1007/978-981-99-9029-0_7

progression. In this paper, we have discussed the different ways through which AI techniques can help in the prognosis and early diagnosis of MS and the associated challenges of AI methods in MS research.

Keywords Multiple sclerosis · Artificial intelligence · Machine learning · Deep learning · Autoimmune disease · MS diagnosis · MS prognosis

1 Introduction

Multiple sclerosis (MS) is an acquired dreadful autoimmune disease constrained to the central nervous system (CNS), exempting the peripheral nervous system (PNS). The disease induces an unusual CNS-directed immune response and inflammation that causes demyelination at the initial stages; nerve damage and axon loss in the later stages [1–3]. The major symptoms include tremors, acute fatigue, visual difficulties, slurred speech, and balance and coordination loss [4]. As these symptoms affect the complete body, the diagnosis of MS gets difficult. Thus, there is a dire need for advanced tools and programs to detect its occurrence in the initial stages to prevent the worsening condition.

MS has symptoms that are very similar to other diseases, thus over time the diagnosis methods for MS have evolved over time [5]. Cerebrospinal fluids (CSF) are the basis of the evaluation of the progression of the disease and show immunological disorder enhancing with time. The detection based on CSF is a global standard for diagnosing MS. But, this method of clinical diagnosis is time-consuming and is based on the subjective judgments of operator interpretations. Additionally, this method does not detail the information on overlapping symptoms of MS with other diseases. There is no specific laboratory method to detect MS but a combination of various methods like CSF, blood tests, and MRI scans [6]. Furthermore, the detection is based on the physical conditions of the patient and assessing their medical history [7]. In recent times, a method named *McDonald diagnostic* criteria is preferred for diagnosis which uses clinical observations as well as imaging techniques like MRI for detection of MS [8]. Based on our review, MRI scans are considered one of the most appropriate diagnosis tools for predicting and understanding the course of the disease [9]. MRI has revolutionized the approach toward early detection, prognostication, and medication of the disease [10]. However, manual diagnosis using MRI scans is often tedious and prone to human errors. Thus, there is a need for better diagnostic methodology for early diagnosis of the disease and hence reduce the scalability of the worsening condition.

Recent advancements in computer-aided tools facilitated early diagnosis and better prognosis of many diseases including MS. AI is a digital system based on human intelligence that has contributed prominently to the detection and diagnosis of various neurological diseases [11]. The enhanced applications of AI have given opportunities for classification, early prediction, and identification of MS. Importantly, the AI-based tools also help in the prediction of the course of the MS disease.

This helps in determining the possible worsened condition of the patients and assists in medication for decelerating the associated symptoms of the disease [12]. Additionally, the datasets generated from AI are much more reliable, unproblematic, and time-efficient compared to traditional manual methods [13]. Therefore, AI provides a platform that can be used for developing an automated framework for early prediction, classification, and progression of MS disease utilizing ML and DL techniques [14, 15].

ML is a subclass of AI which focuses on analyzing data without being programmed explicitly while; DL is a subclass of ML which trains itself on the basis of neural networks utilizing enormous amounts of data [8]. Also, ML learns on the basis of numerous existing features of the dataset, i.e., hand-crafted features while DL expands to independent learning of features and decisive fine-tuning as per input dataset [13]. ML/DL algorithms can be supervised, unsupervised, or even semi-supervised [16]. In this paper, we have discussed various ML and DL techniques used in the automated prediction of MS. We have also discussed various AI methods to determine the progression of the disease along with the potential challenges, advantages, and disadvantages of both the subclasses of AI. The organization of the paper is as follows: Sect. 2 discusses MS as a global menace, its causes, symptoms, and pathogenesis. Section 3 describes the various types of MS. Diagnostic workup of a patient for MS is briefed in Sect. 4. Section 5 describes the various AI approaches for the diagnosis of MS followed by the associated challenges in automated diagnosis in Sect. 6. And finally, the conclusion in Sect. 7.

2 Multiple Sclerosis as a Global Menace

MS is a global problem, and its prevalence is on the rise. Alterations in the environment and day-to-day habits modulate the disease occurrence rate [17]. The occurrence of MS is linked to latitude as well, called the "*Latitude effect.*" It has been observed that it is more common in polar areas, i.e., areas away from the equator since they receive less sunlight and people are deficient in Vitamin D [18, 19]. This also explains the reason behind its high occurrence in North America, Western Europe, and Australia (>100 cases per 100,000 population), and lowest in countries centered on the equator (<30 cases per 100,000 population) [20, 21]. *National Multiple Sclerosis Society* has assessed that approximately 2.8 million people or more are suffering from MS and about 300 people get diagnosed with it every day globally [22]. Recently, it has been predicted that every five minutes, an individual gets diagnosed with MS [23]. With the advancement in technology, more cases of MS are now being diagnosed throughout India as well with a roughly estimated prevalence of 5–10 per 100,000 individuals [24]. MS threatens people of all ages but generally, individuals between the ages of 20–50 years are most affected. It shows gender skew as well with women being more prone and having three times more risk of developing MS and thus exhibiting a higher susceptibility than men [25, 26].

According to 2017 data, 74% of individuals with MS are female and 26% are male [27].

2.1 Causes of MS

The specific cause of MS is unclear, but scientists have developed numerous theories related to factors that may lead to MS, including environmental, genetic, immune factors, and infection-related [27, 28]. The environmental factors include exposure to UV radiation and Vitamin D deficiency (increased risk at levels <100 nmol/L). Many studies have reported that living in areas farther from the equator leads to reduced sunlight exposure and vitamin D levels that increase the probability of MS [29–31]. Habits like smoking and eating disorders causing obesity also increase the chances of MS [25, 32]. When it comes to genetic factors it has been observed that individuals having a family history of MS are imperiled to developing the condition. Further, the existence of factors such as Major Histocompatibility Complex (MHC) HLA-DRB1 locus also increases the possibility of developing MS [33, 34]. Alterations in the immune system make the myelin fibers vulnerable and individuals prone to MS [35–37]. Recently, it has been observed that a virus or bacteria like herpes simplex viruses and Epstein-Barr may also elicit MS [25, 32].

2.2 Symptoms of MS

It varies from individual to individual and changes over the course of the disease depending on the affected nerve fibers' location. The severity and localization of MS injuries within the spinal cord and brain are random thus; it adversely affects various parts of the body in variable amounts. It has been found that individuals who are severely affected by MS become unable to walk independently or ambulate completely while some can experience long remission periods without showing any new symptoms. Subsequently, MS is said to be associated with a wide range of symptoms and multimorbidity that impact the daily activities of people and their quality of life. The common symptoms include bowel, bladder, cognitive, and sexual dysfunction. Other important symptoms include pain, spasticity, fatigue, and depression [27, 38–40]. Because no two patients with MS are alike, symptomatic problems tend to vary tremendously.

2.3 Pathogenesis of MS

MS pathogenesis is assorted and encompasses inflammatory processes, and environmental, and genetic factors, see Fig. 1. Its pathogenesis usually includes two

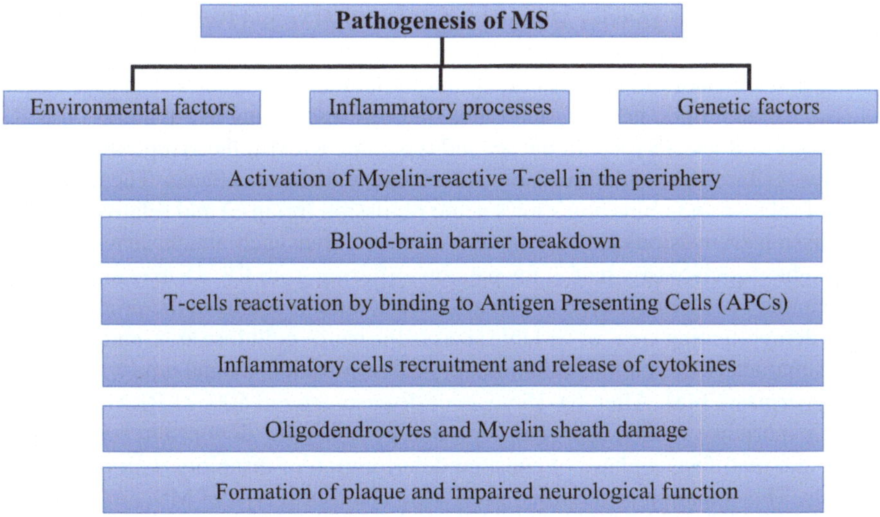

Fig. 1 Inflammatory processes, environmental, and genetic factors in MS pathogenesis

main mechanisms, i.e., inflammatory demyelination and neurodegeneration [41, 42]. Other significant hallmarks are remyelination, inflammation, reactive gliosis, and axonal loss [33, 43]. These can happen diffusely or focally, primarily affecting the white matter but also involve grey matter and nuclei of the deep brainstem [44]. The characteristic MS plaque is found around the central vein, however, the type of clinical manifestations that will develop is determined by the lesion location [43]. The progression of the diseases is normally measured by the short-term progression of disability, magnetic resonance imaging (MRI) activity, and relapses. Relapse is defined as new or deteriorating neurologic symptoms like sensory disturbances, weakness, and gait impairment that persist for 24 h or much longer in the absence of fever or infection to eliminate "pseudo relapses" [45–47]. According to the incidence and prognosis of MS, it exhibits two rare clinical types, i.e., malignant and benign MS, that overlap with the above clinical types. In the former type, patients exhibit a sudden disease onset, which progresses rapidly ensuing neurological deterioration that results in disability or sometimes death [48]. However, in benign MS, the number of relapses decreases within 10–15 years of disease onset, but the nervous system still functions well.

3 Types of MS

According to the characteristics of the clinical course, MS can be divided into five different clinical phenotypes, i.e., *Clinical isolated syndrome (CIS)*, *Relapsing-Remitting Multiple Sclerosis (RRMS)*, *Secondary Progressive Multiple Sclerosis*

(SPMS), *Primary Progressive Multiple Sclerosis (PPMS)*, and *Progressive Relapsing Multiple Sclerosis (PRMS)* [48–51].

The first attack of MS involves the spinal cord, brainstem syndrome, and/or hemispheric, isolated optic neuritis, and other findings resembling MS plaques on MRI are categorized as CIS [50]. In the second type, i.e., RRMS, the symptoms develop in relapses (flare-ups) with remission (full recovery) between attacks. The remission cycle of relapse and remission shows acute remission (relapse) and relatively stable intermission (remission) and the patient recovers after each attack, leaving no or only slight sequel. Nearly half of the patients suffering from RRMS may also exhibit the secondary progressive type of MS after some time. It results in the production of lumpy demyelinating areas of variable sizes in the neuro-cellulose area, and its pathological characteristics include inflammatory cell infiltration, axonal injury, and astrocyte hyperplasia [48]. After 10–15 years of disease, around 50% of RRMS patients do not experience relapse and remission and demonstrate slow progressive aggravation that manifests a phase of constant deterioration of disability with or without seizures. This situation is classified as SPMS. The fourth type of MS, i.e., PPMS is rare (approximately 10% of MS) and starts at a relatively older age a stable weakening without relapse or remission. The disease exhibits a course duration of a year or more which progresses slowly displaying only short-term, insignificant symptom improvement with no remission or recurrence and exhibiting reduced response to treatment. Similarly, PRMS is also clinically rare and exhibits continuing aggravation and development, random recurrence, and constant progression between two relapses [49].

4 Diagnosis of MS: Need of AI

Despite these distinctions in the symptoms, all the clinical forms of MS imitate the same underlying disease process but the course or progression of MS varies from person to person. In the literature, there are no markers specific to the diagnosis of MS and it mainly depends on the neurological examination and medical history of the patient [3, 52]. Thus, the diagnostic criteria for MS depend on factors including the presentation of symptoms, numerous lesions on MRI, and evidence of CNS damage [53]. Another predicament is that the clinical and imaging findings that are observed in MS, can also be imitated by other infectious, genetic, neo-plastic, metabolic, vascular, and other idiopathic inflammatory demyelinating disorders (IIDD) that cause diagnostic difficulty [54]. Therefore, identifying MS-related symptoms and determining the final diagnosis is vital for the correct treatment choice and long-term disability prevention.

It is known that there is no specific laboratory test for the diagnosis of the disease [6]. Therefore, the existing 2017 McDonald's MS diagnostic criteria envisage laboratory findings, imaging, and clinical assessment [55]. The main paraclinical test for MS diagnosis is MRI with an intravenous contrast agent having gadolinium which can present the nature of the lesions for differential diagnosis, i.e., inflammatory and demyelinating characteristics, as well as the distribution of the lesions within the CNS [56, 57]. Another important analysis in the MS diagnosis is lumbar puncture CSF examination, microbiological tests (cell count, ELISA tests), basic CSF biochemistry (albumin, glucose, IgG, protein, and lactate levels), and screening for malignant cells. Apart from these, electrophysiological tests (somatosensory evoked potentials (SEP) and visual evoked potentials (VEP)) can also be done [58–60]. All the tests and investigations included in the diagnostic workup of a patient with suspected MS have been mentioned in Table 1.

A reliable and detailed diagnosis of MS is critical for facilitating early interventions for MS, as disease-modifying drugs help in managing symptoms and preventing the progression of the disease [61].

Due to the above-discussed shortcomings of the existing methodologies; we need a sophisticated and fast diagnosis methodology. Moreover, increasing knowledge and expansion of the availability of advanced MRI techniques require more and more

Table 1 Diagnostic workup of a patient with suspected MS

Type of tests		Example
Primary	Blood tests	Viral serology (anti-HCV, anti-Hbs, anti-HIV, HbsAg), electrolyte levels, Lipid panel, Thyroid function tests, Hemogram, Renal and liver function tests, CRP, B12, Vitamin Dandfolate
	MRI	Cranial, cervical and thoracal
	CSF analyses	CSF protein and lactate, CSF and serum albumin, CSFIgG and IgG index, Concurrent blood glucose, CSF OCB analysis with IEF electrophoresis
Secondary tests	Evoked potentials Optic coherence tomography Urodynamic testing Cognitive testing	
For differential diagnosis	Biochemical tests	GFR evaluation, 24-h urine analysis etc
	Specific tests for infectious aetiologies	Antibodies for Lyme disease and Brucellosis, Quantiferonand PPD tests for tuberculosis
	Angiography	Cerebral, fluorescein, MRA
	Biopsy	Skin, brain and/or leptomeninx, lymph node, peripheral nerve, other
	Eye examination	Evaluation of retina for metabolic disorders, Evaluation of uvea for sarcoidosis, and Behçet's disease
	Hearing tests	For Susac
	Electrophysiology	
	Chest X-ray	
	Cardiac examination	Echocardiography
Other tests	Schirmer test Salivary gland syntigraphy	

time, resources, and expertise, which conflicts with the clinical applications of these tools.

5 Artificial Intelligence Techniques in Multiple Sclerosis

The approaches of techniques in AI are either top-down or bottom-up. The top-down AI algorithms or symbolic AI algorithms seek to mimic human intelligence but are independent of the structure of the human brain and use processed symbols for replication. On the contrary, bottom-up AI approaches are based on connections of systems with data. Bottom-up approaches are also referred to as *connectionist* as they create basic elements and allow those basic elements to communicate with data. The major goal of any AI system in MS is to automate early detection of the disease and determine the progression of the disease. Additionally, automation using AI helps to differentiate various other diseases from MS and provides proper monitoring, treatment, and medication for the illness. Any AI automation and intelligent system is highly dependent on the dataset of the problem. Researchers have primarily focussed on bottom-up AI approaches mainly based on conventional ML and DL techniques [13]. A basic block diagram of the steps in the automation of the diagnosis of MS using AI is shown in Fig. 2. First, the collected dataset or publicly available datasets are given to the intelligent MS diagnostic system. Then few processing algorithms are applied to standardise the data and enhance their capability. Finally, a robust and precise ML or DL architecture is designed for automation in the diagnosis of MS.

The dataset for diagnosis of MS consists of multiple sources such as MRIs, Optical coherence tomography (OCT) data, blood biomarkers, and clinical data. There are various publicly available datasets such as MICCAI 2008 [62], eHealth Lab [63], Private + eHealth Lab [64], Whole Brain Atlas image database [65], LabIT [66], University Medical Centre Ljubljana (UMCL) [67], etc. The modalities of various datasets are heterogeneous in nature and consist of noises, obliqueness, registration issues, standardization, and segmentation. Thus, we need low-level and high-level preprocessing methods to deal with different factors affecting our results [68].

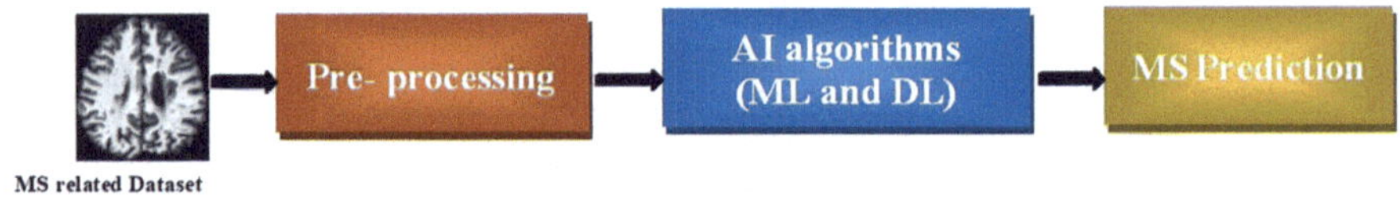

Fig. 2 Block diagram of an automated AI system for MS detection

5.1 Machine Learning in Multiple Sclerosis

ML techniques comprise various algorithms which work on a trial-and-error basis. ML is a conventional method using specific data for feature extraction. Feature engineering provides a base for creating predictive models by selecting the appropriate features. Each model uses sample data to train them and generate appropriate features for prediction and classification. ML algorithms can be supervised or unsupervised [69, 70]. Supervised ML algorithms have defined output labels based on past information and help map input values to output values. The algorithms based on supervised ML techniques are mainly used for classification and regression. On the contrary, in unsupervised learning the output labels are missing. They are trained on an unlabelled dataset. Unsupervised ML algorithms are mainly focused on clustering and association. Supervised algorithms include classification and regression algorithms while unsupervised algorithms include clustering and dimensionality reduction algorithms.

In various medical implications of MS, both supervised and unsupervised leanings provide a crucial basis for diagnosis and medical treatments at various stages of MS. In MS, ML influences the classification aspect of the disease based on MRI images and points out the symptoms of the continuous evolution of the disease. The popular ML classification algorithms classify a person as healthy or an MS patient. The Regression algorithms help to calculate the speed of gait for any wearable device used in the prediction of MS. A few popular supervised ML algorithms used for the classification, prediction, and diagnosis of MS are Support Vector Machine (SVM) [71–73], Random Forest (RF) [74–76], K-Nearest Neighbour (K-NN) [77], and Logistic Regression [78, 79]. Clustering ML algorithms facilitate the recognition of MRI Phenotypes in MS patients. Association rules-based ML algorithm simplifies DNA comparison among genetically affected patients of MS. Few popular unsupervised ML algorithms [71] preferring medical assistance are K-Means [80], Fuzzy C-Means [5], and Apriori algorithm [81]. The role of various supervised and unsupervised machine learning algorithms used in the diagnosis and prognosis of MS are described below.

Linear and Logistic Regression

Linear and Logistic regression are supervised machine learning algorithms used to determine the relationship among dependent variables and independent variables [82] The predictors are based on independent variables and the correlation among these variables must not be too high. In MS, the regression algorithm helps in the prediction of disease and most importantly, it supports wearable devices for better prediction for automated diagnosis of MS [79].

Support Vector Machine

SVM is a binary classifier that calculates the distance of hyperplanes based on data points and draws a line to segregate the data into N-dimensional space. The final classification is based on optimal distance among hyperplanes and data points or support vectors. SVMs are also extended to be used in regression [83]. They can

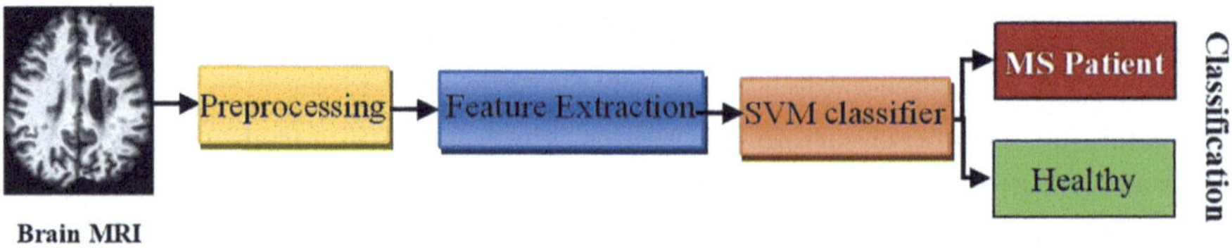

Fig. 3 Diagnosis of MS patients using SVM classifier (supervised learning)

be used for nonlinear classifier problems using kernels and supports to determine misclassified points. Although SVM is a highly complex algorithm it works well with less data [84]. SVM is one of the most popular ML algorithms used in the classification and automatic diagnosis of MS [71, 72]. In MS, SVM has also been used in the prediction of prognosis of disease [73] and differentiating disease from other diseases with similar symptoms [85]. The automatic diagnosis of MS with the help of SVM is illustrated in Fig. 3.

K-Nearest Neighbors

K-NN is a supervised ML algorithm which calculates nearest neighbors among data points and classifies them on the basis of calculated minimum distance. Thus, K-NN comprises two steps: Calculating distance metrics among data points and then classifying data into labeled classes by finding nearest neighbors [86]. K-NN is quite helpful in the automatic diagnosis and prognosis of MS [77].

Ensemble Algorithms

Ensemble algorithms are the combination of multiple ML algorithms to enhance the performance of existing architecture [87]. Ensemble learning algorithms are based on deciding rules to determine the performance of algorithms. Ensemble methods can be divided into Bagging and Boosting algorithms. Random Forest is the most popular bagging algorithm used for classification [87]. In Bagging, a subset is extracted from the initial dataset given to various models and finally average of the results obtained from those models is done. Random Forest combines multiple Decision tree (DT) rules and aggregates the final output. The other group of ensemble methods is boosting which combines weak classifiers to make them strong and incrementally increases the performance capability of classifiers. AdaBoost [88, 89], XgBoost [90], CatBoost [91], etc., are some popular boosting algorithms. Figure 4 depicts a bagging method using a random forest algorithm required in the automatic diagnosis of MS.

Apart from this, there are many ML algorithms like Naive Bayes [92], Decision tree [93], LDA [85], etc., assisting in clinical diagnosis and prognosis of MS. Some of the ML algorithms used in MS diagnosis, MS prognosis, and MS classification are summarized in Table 2. The studies also show ML algorithms are used to determine the progress of the disease at various stages with the help of MRI scans. The algorithms detect lesions in the brain, and their sizes and differentiate MS from many other diseases with similar symptoms accurately.

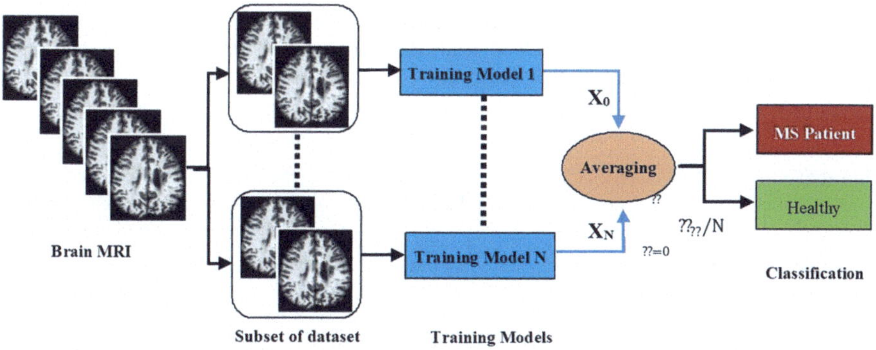

Fig. 4 Automatic classification of MS patients from healthy brain MRIs using random forest

5.2 *Deep Learning in Multiple Sclerosis*

Recently, with the increase in the usage of MRI modalities, DL algorithms have become quite supportive in clinical interpretations of MS. DL algorithms are different from conventional ML algorithms which require complex pre-processing tasks to achieve the highest accuracy. DL includes deep neural networks working intelligently to extract features for prediction, diagnosis, and medical associations [96]. DL algorithms use a large amount of MRI data and are robust to noise. Thus, DL algorithms solve the limitation of the dataset with the ability of augmentations. DL techniques skip the step of feature engineering and neural networks diligently learn from data itself. DL algorithms can be based on supervised or unsupervised learning. The most popular DL algorithm in the analysis of medical images is the Convolutional Neural Network (CNN) [97, 98]. CNN is a type of supervised learning used for the detection of MS using MRI modalities. The other popular DL algorithms are Autoencoders (AEs) [79, 99], CNN-Recurrent Neural Network (RNN) [100], and Generative Adversarial Networks (GANs) [101, 102, 121]. AEs are unsupervised DL techniques used in the diagnosis and prognosis of MS. The roles of various DL techniques used in MS are described below.

CNN

A CNN model does not require any manual feature. They have many hidden layers to extract the features from the MRI of any patient of MS. As we go deeper with layers in CNN, the higher we can extract features from the dataset [103]. CNN focuses on finding relevant features from images rather than going through the process of feature engineering as in classical ML algorithms. Although CNN has given outstanding observations and results it requires heavy computations using Graphical Processing Unit (GPU) and Tensor Processing Unit (TPU) [97]. CNNs have been used for many applications like image classification [104], image segmentation [105], and more [106–108]. The major components of CNN are convolution, pooling, batch normalization, and fully connected layers [98].

Table 2 Studies showing ML algorithms used in MS diagnosis, prognosis, and classification. *Clinically isolated syndrome (CIS) and **radiologically isolated syndrome (RIS); ***Subtype and Stage Inference (SuStaIn), Dice similarity coefficient (DSC)#, Area Under the ROC Curve (AUC)#

Author and year	Data type	ML Algorithms	Subjects	Performance matrix	Application
Guo et al. [71]	MRI	SVM and unsupervised learning	60 strokes Patients	DSC#—66.5%	Detecting brain lesions in MS patients
Fartaria et. al. [77]	MRI	K-NN	44 patients	Sensitivity of 77%	Detection of lesions as small as 0.0036 mL
Mărgineanu et al. [85]	MRI	LDA, SVM with Gaussian kernel	13 HCs and 87 MS patients	F1-score of 87%	Differentiating the disease starting points of each MS form
Melingi and Vijayalakshmi [75]	MRI	RF	–	Accuracy of 99.40%	Automatic diagnosis of MS
Eitel et al. [72]	MRI	SVM	20 Healthy Controls (HCs) and MS patients	Accuracy of 95%	Classify MS patients from HCs
Salem et al. [79]	MRI	Logistic Regression	60 patients	DSC of 0.77	Detection of new T2-w lesions in MS
Mato-Abad et al. [92]	MRI	Naïve Bayes	34 MS patients	AUC# of 76.50%	Differentiation among the earliest status of MS (CIS and RIS**)
Acquaviva et al. [88]	Clinical data	Functional trees (FT), and ADAboost FT	313 individuals: 60 HCs, 57 CIs, 108 RRMS, 26 SPMS, 35 PPMS, and 27 with other Diseases	Maximum Accuracy of 88.7%	Classify MS patients from HCs Classify CIS* patients from HCs Differentiate between PPMS and/or SPMS from RRMS
Jain et al. [93]	MRI	GLCoM + Decision tree with Logitboost	103 HCs and 190 MS patients	Accuracy of 94.17%	Classify MS patients from HCs

(continued)

Table 2 (continued)

Author and year	Data type	ML Algorithms	Subjects	Performance matrix	Application
Martynova et al. [90]	Clinical data	KNN, DT, XgBoost, Gaussian naïve Bayes, RF	101 MS patients and 25 HCs	Maximum Accuracy of 99.0%	Determining serum and CSF cytokine-based markers for MS diagnosis
Buyukturkoglu et al. [76]	MRI	RF	183 MS patients	AUC of 0.90	Prediction of changes in early MS diagnosis
Monaghan et al. [94]	MRI	PCA	122 patients with RRMS and 45 HCs	Gait variance of 79%	Classify MS patients from HCs using MS-specific model of gait
Kenney et al. [73]	OCT data	SVM	1568 MS patients and 552 HCs	AUC of 0.89	Classify MS patients from HCs using thresholds for OCT inter-eye differences (IEDs)
Pontillo et al. [95]	MRI	Unsupervised ML based on SuStaIn*** algorithm	148 HCs and 425 MS patients	Atrophy pattern is 0.806	Stratifying patients with SPMS

There are various architectures of CNN which use MRI modalities for various clinical aspects of MS. One of the most popular CNN architectures are 2D and 3D CNNs architectures for the classification of MS [106, 109]. The basic architecture of 2D CNN for diagnosis of MS can be seen in Fig. 5. U-Nets [110] and Fully Convolutional Neural Networks (FCNs) [111] are preferred for image segmentation of MS using MRI images. U-Net was designed by Ronneberger et al. [112] for segmentation of images. U-Net is divided into two parts: Encoder and Decoder. The encoder consists of multiple down-sampling and convolutional layers while the decoder has up-sampling and convolutional layers [112]. The main advantages of U-Net are that it can work with limited available datasets and has the ability to skip connections. FCNs are the combination of fully connected and convolutional layers, as proposed by Shelhamer et al. (2017) [113]. FCN receives arbitrary-sized input to produce corresponding-sized output with learning.

Autoencoders

Autoencoder is a type of DL network, originally given by LeCun et al. (1987) [114]. An autoencoder is divided into two parts: An Encoder and a Decoder [97]. Both

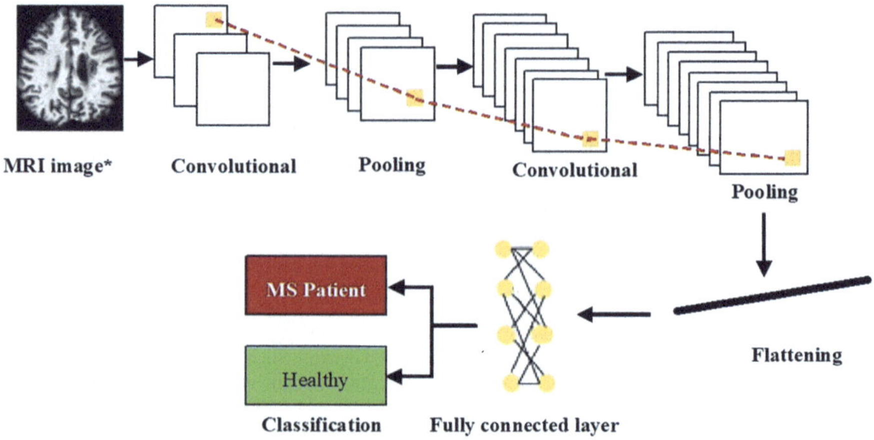

Fig. 5 Automatic diagnosis of MS using 2D-CNN

Encoders and Decoders are implemented using neural networks and find low dimensional data of a high dimensional dataset. An encoder compresses high dimensional data into low dimension while a decoder reconstructs the original data. A block diagram of autoencoders used in the diagnosis of MS can be seen in Fig. 6.

CNN-RNN

CNN-RNN is a hybrid DL architecture combining networks of CNN and RNN in the diagnosis and prognosis of MS. The design of this hybrid architecture paved the path for AI professionals to work with temporal and spatial feature sets of data. CNN has the capability to learn spatial features while RNN has expertise in the temporal study of feature sets. In this network, the input set is fed to CNN and after passing through various convolutional and pooling layers, the output feature maps are fed to RNN. Finally, RNN succors the network for image classification with greater accuracy [68, 100]. Figure 7 shows the image classification of MS using hybrid CNN-RNN architecture.

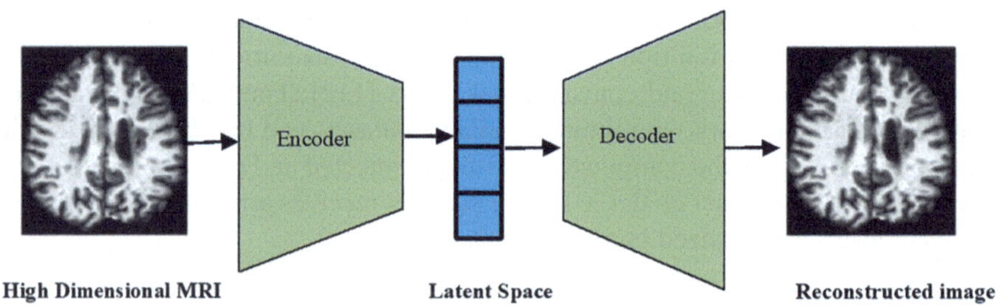

Fig. 6 Autoencoders used for diagnosis of MS

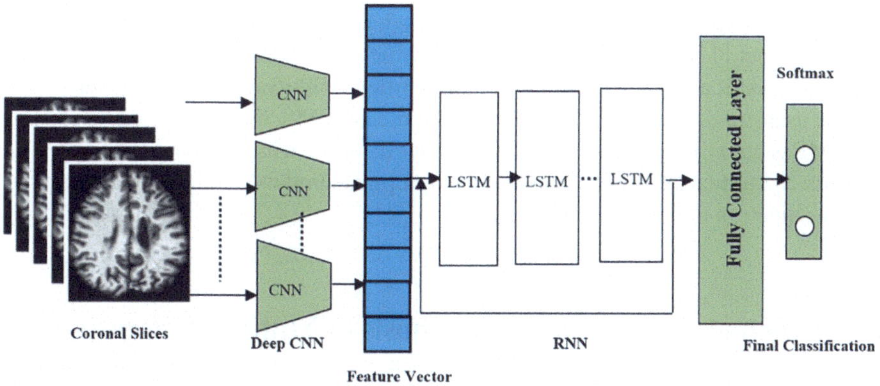

Fig. 7 Automated MS classification using CNN-RNN hybrid architecture

General Adversarial Networks

GANs are novel architecture of DL proposed by Ian Goodfellow [101]. GANs act as a generative model and comprise of two neural networks called Generator G and Discriminator D. Generator G estimates the probability distribution of original data and generates similar data. The role of Discriminator D includes likelihood estimation and distinguishing between artificial and original sets of data. Thus, in this architecture generator generates images to mislead the discriminator while the discriminator identifies the most similar samples [102]. Figure 8 displays the GAN used for the automated detection of MS.

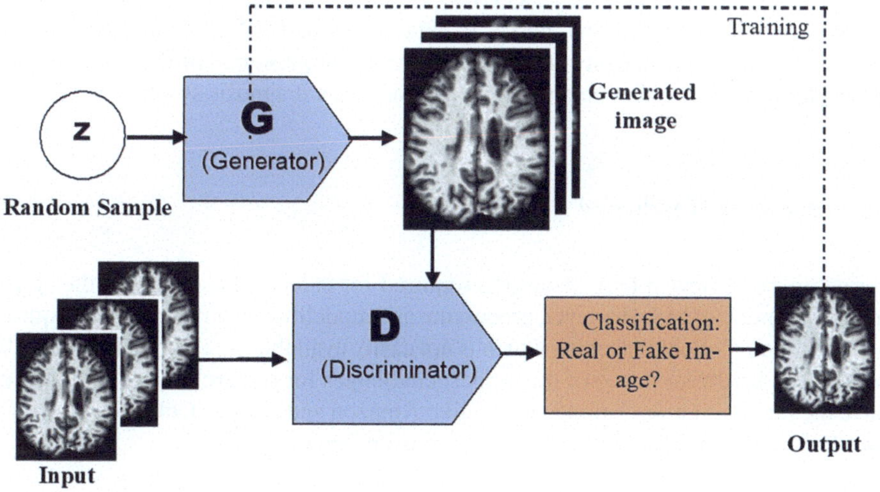

Fig. 8 Automatic diagnosis of MS using GAN

There are many variants of deep learning models like Gated Recurrent Unit (GRU) [115], CVSnet [116], DeepScan [117], etc., which are used in diagnosis, segmentation, and classification of MS using MRI modalities. Table 3 summarizes different DL models used for extracting lesion points, diagnosis of MS at an early stage, subsampling MRIs, and differentiating MS from other diseases with similar symptoms. The majority of studies depict CNN as the most popular model on MRI modalities used for classification and segmentation.

6 Challenges in Automated Diagnosis of Multiple Sclerosis

6.1 *Unavailability of Dataset*

A huge amount of data is regularly required for better accuracy, precision, and sensitivity in automated diagnosis of MS. But the accessibility to large datasets is limited and most of the studies used smaller datasets. The usage of smaller datasets suggests the results obtained are not reliable for real-world predictions. Also, there are various real-world scenarios which consist of many unavoidable noises such as "*patients visit multiple doctors and do not maintain any record*". These noises cannot be obtained while preparing the dataset reducing the precision of the model. As per the studies in Tables 2 and 3, we can also find that the majority of the researchers have focussed on MRIs in the diagnosis and analysis of MS. However, the analysis of MS requires regular monitoring and is mainly dependent on functional MRIs (fMRIs). fMRIs are used to record metabolic activities with time. The other major problem is the unavailability of these fMRI datasets [68]. Based on the studies, better information on cognitive, motor, and visual nerves is obtained using fMRIs for automated diagnosis, prognosis, and analysis of MS [120]. Thus, a large source of fMRI datasets is quite important for researchers to develop an accurate diagnosis system for MS.

6.2 *Lack of Hardware Aspect*

Based on the review, a large dataset is required for enhanced accuracy in the automated diagnosis of MS. However, processing and modelling on larger datasets require a higher computational machine which is not easily available to researchers. The lack of required hardware is one of the biggest challenges for researchers. Although, we have the facility of many online servers like Amazon and Google Colab to solve this problem, however, these servers are risks to users' privacy [68].

Table 3 Studies showing DL algorithms used in MS. Artificial Neural Network (ANN)*, Multi-dimensional gated recurrent units (MD-GRU) **. Gray matter (GM)***, White matter (WM)****, and Cerebrospinal fluid (CSF)*****. Peak signal-to-noise ratio (PSNR)$^{\#}$, Dice similarity coefficient (DSC)

Author and year	Data type	DNN	Subject	Performance matrix	Application
Garcia-Martin et al. [108]	OCT data	ANN*	106 MS patients, 115 HCs	–	Compare axonal loss in ganglion cells in the eyes of patients with MS versus HCs
Birenbaum and Greenspan [105]	MRI	CNN	19 MS patients	DSC of 62.7	Longitudinal Lesion Segmentation
Andermatt et al. [115]	MRI	MD-GRU**	20 MS patients	DSC of 62.85	Automated lesion segmentation in MS
Zhang et al. [102]	MRI	MS-GAN	69 MS patients	DSC of 67.2	Localize MS lesions in MRIs
Siar and Teshnehlab [106]	MRI	2D-CNN	320 MS patients, 791 HCs	Accuracy-96.88%	Diagnose and differentiae brain tumour and MS
Yoo et al. [109]	MRI	3D-CNN	140 MS patients	Accuracy 75%	Extraction of latent features of MS lesion and predicting prognosis
Eitel et al. [72]	MRI	2D-CNN	76 MS patients, 71 HCs	Accuracy 80.92%	Harnessing Spatial MRI Normalization
Salem et al. [79]	MRI	Encoder-Decoder U-NET	65 MS patients, 15 HCs	DSC of 63	Multiple Sclerosis Lesion Synthesis in MRIs
Vatian et al. [100]	MRI and textual clinical records	CNN and RNN	19 patients	Accuracy 87.5%	Diagnosis of MS
Sujit et al. [118]	MRI	Ensemble DL model	1112 Subjects, 110 MS patients	AUC of 0.90	Automatically Evaluate the Quality of Multicentre Structural Brain MRIs

(continued)

Table 3 (continued)

Author and year	Data type	DNN	Subject	Performance matrix	Application
Narayana et al. [110]	MRI	Multiclass U-Net	1008 MS patients	GM***-DSC of 94, WM****-DSC of 94, CSF*****-DSC of 96, Lesion-DSC of 86	Brain MRI segmentation in MS
Gabr et al. [111]	MRI	FCNN	1008 MS patients	WM-DSC of 95, GM-DSC of 96, CSF-DSC of 99, T2 Lesions DSC of 82	Automatically segment MS brain tissues
Shaul et al. [119]	MRI	GAN	80 MS patients	PSNR# of 28.26	Subsampling of Brain MRI for accelerating MRI acquisition
Vogelsanger and Federau [104]	MRI	Introspective Variational Autoencoder (intro-VAE or IVAE)	616 MS patients	Precision 92	Classify multiple sclerosis, leukoencephalopathy and healthy patients in the latent space of network
López-Dorado et al. [107]	OCT data	CNN	48 MS patients, 48 HCs	Accuracy 100%	Diagnosis of MS in its initial stages

6.3 Unreliability on Models

We have seen many studies showing ML and DL algorithms as very successful techniques for an automated diagnosing system of MS. The results of these models are mainly dependent on the input dataset. Also, DL and ML algorithms lack internal interpretation and working of the model which can be a risk to the accuracy of the automated system [8]. Therefore, researchers are suggested to understand, interpret, and explain the algorithms well.

7 Conclusion

MS is a chronic neural disease which requires early diagnosis, regular monitoring, and on-time treatment. It is a global menace that directly affects the brain, optic nerves, and spinal cord. The diagnosis, prognosis, and assessment of the disease can be found through MRI modalities. The precision of the diagnosed MS is crucial as there are multiple causes of the disease. Additionally, some of the symptoms of MS are very similar and somewhat overlapping to the symptoms of other neurological diseases. This makes its clinical diagnosis all the more difficult. MS has five different clinical phenotypes varying from person to person. This further complicates the diagnosis of the disease. Neurological examination and medical history of the patient are the prominent determining factors that facilitate the diagnosis of MS. The traditional diagnostic workup of a patient is time-consuming, thus in our work, we have explored the prospects of AI in the early diagnosis of MS.

Our work intends to provide a comprehensive overview of the MS disease and the applications of AI in its analysis, clinical diagnosis, and prognosis that will facilitate in providing proper monitoring, treatment, and medication to the patient. Different supervised and unsupervised ML algorithms that are used in the diagnosis of MS are discussed. Additionally, various significant DL algorithms are discussed that facilitate the diagnosis of MS. There are also various challenges associated with the automated diagnosis of MS, e.g., unavailability of relevant dataset, high computational capacity for data processing, etc., that hinder the implementation.

References

1. Charcot M (1868) Histologie de la sclerose en plaque. Gaz Hosp 41:554–556
2. Kalaria R, Ferrer I, Love S, Perry A, Ironside J (2015) Greenfield's neuropathology
3. Lucchinetti C, Brück W, Parisi J, Scheithauer B, Rodriguez M, Lassmann H (2000) Heterogeneity of multiple sclerosis lesions: implications for the pathogenesis of demyelination. Ann Neurol: Off J Am Neurol Assoc Child Neurol Soc 47(6):707–717. https://doi.org/10.1002/1531-8249(200006)47:6%3c707::AID-ANA3%3e3.0.CO;2-Q
4. Dendrou CA, Fugger L, Friese MA (2015) Immunopathology of multiple sclerosis. Nat Rev Immunol 15(9):545–558. https://doi.org/10.1038/nri3871
5. Arani LA, Hosseini A, Asadi F, Masoud SA, Nazemi E (2018) Intelligent computer systems for multiple sclerosis diagnosis: a systematic review of reasoning techniques and methods. Acta Inform Med 26(4). https://doi.org/10.5455/aim.2018.26.258-264
6. Fangerau T, Schimrigk S, Haupts M, Kaeder M, Ahle G, Brune N, Klinkenberg K, Kotterba S, Möhring M, Sindern E (2004) Diagnosis of multiple sclerosis: comparison of the poser criteria and the new McDonald criteria. Acta Neurol Scand 109(6):385–389. https://doi.org/10.1111/j.1600-0404.2004.00246.x
7. Ghadirian P, Dadgostar B, Azani R, Maisonneuve P (2001) A case-control study of the association between socio-demographic, lifestyle and medical history factors and multiple sclerosis. Can J Public Health 92(4):281–285. https://doi.org/10.1007/bf03404961
8. Aslam N, Khan IU, Bashamakh A, Alghool FA, Aboulnour M, Alsuwayan NM, Alturaif RK, Brahimi S, Aljameel SS, Ghamdi K, et al (2022) Multiple sclerosis diagnosis using machine learning and deep learning: challenges and opportunities. Sensors 22(20). https://doi.org/10.3390/s22207856
9. Wildner P, Stasiołek M, Matysiak M (2020) Differential diagnosis of multiple sclerosis and other inflammatory CNS diseases. Mult Scler Relat Disord 37. https://doi.org/10.1016/j.msard.2019.101452
10. Wattjes MP, Ciccarelli O, Reich DS, Banwell B, de Stefano N, Enzinger C, Fazekas F, Filippi M, Frederiksen J, Gasperini C, Hacohen Y, Kappos L, Li DKB, Mankad K, Montalban X,

Newsome SD, Oh J, Palace J, Rocca MA, Tintore M (2021) 2021 MAGNIMS–CMSC–NAIMS consensus recommendations on the use of MRI in patients with multiple sclerosis. Lancet Neurol 20(8):653–670. https://doi.org/10.1016/S1474-4422(21)00095-8

11. Qazi S, Raza K, Iqbal N (2021) 5 Artificial intelligence in medicine (AIM): machine learning in cancer diagnosis, prognosis and therapy. In: Gupta D, U Kose, Le Nguyen B, Bhattacharyya S (eds) Artificial intelligence for data-driven medical diagnosis. De Gruyter, Berlin, Boston, pp 103–126. https://doi.org/10.1515/9783110668322-005
12. Montolío A, Martín-Gallego A, Cegoñino J, Orduna E, Vilades E, Garcia-Martin E, Del Palomar AP (2021) Machine learning in diagnosis and disability prediction of multiple sclerosis using optical coherence tomography. Comput Biol Med 133:104416. https://doi.org/10.1016/j.compbiomed.2021.104416
13. Afzal HMR, Luo S, Ramadan S, Lechner-Scott J (2022) The emerging role of artificial intelligence in multiple sclerosis imaging. Mult Scler J 28(6):849–858. https://doi.org/10.1177/1352458520966298
14. Qazi W, Qazi S, Iqbal N, Raza K (2023) The scope and applications of nature-inspired computing in bioinformatics. In: Raza K (ed) Nature-inspired intelligent computing techniques in bioinformatics. Studies in computational intelligence, vol 1066. Springer, Singapore. https://doi.org/10.1007/978-981-19-6379-7_1
15. Bonacchi R, Filippi M, Rocca MA (2022) Role of artificial intelligence in MS clinical practice. NeuroImage: Clin 35:103065. https://doi.org/10.1016/j.nicl.2022.103065
16. Raza K, Singh NK (2021) A tour of unsupervised deep learning for medical image analysis. Curr Med Imaging 17(9):1059–1077. https://doi.org/10.2174/1573405617666210127154257
17. Wiendl H, Gold R, Berger T, Derfuss T, Linker R, Mäurer M, Aktas O, Baum K, Berghoff M, Bittner S, die Multiple Sklerose Therapie Konsensus Gruppe (MSTKG) (2021) Multiple sclerosis treatment consensus group (MSTCG): position paper on disease-modifying treatment of multiple sclerosis 2021 (white paper). Der Nervenarzt 92:773–801.https://doi.org/10.1007/s00115-021-01157-2
18. Simpson S, Wang W, Otahal P, Blizzard L, van der Mei IA, Taylor BV (2019) Latitude continues to be significantly associated with the prevalence of multiple sclerosis: an updated meta-analysis. J Neurol Neurosurg Psychiatry 90(11):1193–1200. https://doi.org/10.1136/jnnp-2018-320189
19. Tao C, Simpson S, van der Mei I, Blizzard L, Havrdova E, Horakova D, Shaygannejad V, Lugaresi A, Izquierdo G, Trojano M, Duquette P, Taylor BV (2016) Higher latitude is significantly associated with an earlier age of disease onset in multiple sclerosis. J Neurol Neurosurg Psychiatry 87(12):1343–1349. https://doi.org/10.1136/jnnp-2016-314013
20. Campbell JA, Simpson S Jr, Ahmad H, Taylor BV, van der Mei I, Palmer AJ (2020) Change in multiple sclerosis prevalence over time in Australia 2010–2017 utilising disease-modifying therapy prescription data. Mult Scler J 26(11):1315–1328. https://doi.org/10.1177/1352458519861270
21. Qian Z, Li Y, Guan Z, Guo P, Zheng K, Du Y, Yin S, Chen B, Wang H, Jiang J, Qiu K, Zhang M (2023) Global, regional, and national burden of multiple sclerosis from 1990 to 2019: findings of global burden of disease study 2019. Front Public Health 11:220. https://doi.org/10.3389/fpubh.2023.1073278
22. Walton C, King R, Rechtman L, Kaye W, Leray E, Marrie RA, Robertson N, La Rocca N, Uitdehaag B, van der Mei I, Baneke P (2020) Rising prevalence of multiple sclerosis worldwide: Insights from the Atlas of MS. Mult Scler J 26(14):1816–1821. https://doi.org/10.1177/1352458520970841
23. Atlas of MS (2021) Atlas-3rd edn-Epidemiology-report-EN-updated-30-9-20.pdf (msif.org)
24. Singhal BS, Advani H (2015) Multiple sclerosis in India: an overview. Ann Indian Acad Neurol 18(Suppl 1):S2. https://doi.org/10.4103/0972-2327.164812
25. Dobson R, Giovannoni G (2019) Multiple sclerosis-a review. Eur J Neurol 26(1):27–40. https://doi.org/10.1111/ene.13819
26. Hauser SL, Cree BA (2020) Treatment of multiple sclerosis: a review. Am J Med 133(12):1380–1390. https://doi.org/10.1016/j.amjmed.2020.05.049

27. Doshi A, Chataway J (2017) Multiple sclerosis, a treatable disease. Clin Med 17(6):530. https://doi.org/10.7861/clinmedicine.16-6-s53
28. Koriem KMM (2016) Multiple sclerosis: new insights and trends. Asian Pac J Trop Biomed 6(5):429–440. https://doi.org/10.1016/j.apjtb.2016.03.009
29. Loma I, Heyman R (2011) Multiple sclerosis: pathogenesis and treatment. Curr Neuropharmacol 9(3):409–416. https://doi.org/10.2174/157015911796557911
30. Belbasis L, Bellou V, Evangelou E, Ioannidis JP, Tzoulaki I (2015) Environmental risk factors and multiple sclerosis: an umbrella review of systematic reviews and meta-analyses. Lancet Neurology 14(3):263–273. https://doi.org/10.1016/S1474-4422(14)70267-4
31. Zarghami A, Li Y, Claflin SB, van der Mei I, Taylor BV (2021) Role of environmental factors in multiple sclerosis. Expert Rev Neurother 21(12):1389–1408. https://doi.org/10.1080/14737175.2021.1978843
32. Teymoori-Rad M, Sahraian MA, Mokhtariazad T, Nejati A, Mozdabadi RSK, Amiri MM, Shokri F, Marashi SM (2021) Illuminating the in vitro effects of Epstein-Barr virus and vitamin D on immune response in multiple sclerosis patients. J Neurovirol 27:260–271. https://doi.org/10.1007/s13365-021-00951-7
33. Baecher-Allan C, Kaskow BJ, Weiner HL (2018) Multiple sclerosis: mechanisms and immunotherapy. Neuron 97(4):742–768. https://doi.org/10.1016/j.neuron.2018.01.021
34. Howard J, Trevick S, Younger DS (2016) Epidemiology of multiple sclerosis. Neurol Clin 34(4):919–939. https://doi.org/10.1016/j.ncl.2016.06.016
35. Cencioni MT, Mattoscio M, Magliozzi R, Bar-Or A, Muraro PA (2021) B cells in multiple sclerosis—from targeted depletion to immune reconstitution therapies. Nat Rev Neurol 17(7):399–414. https://doi.org/10.1038/s41582-021-00498-5
36. Comi G, Bar-Or A, Lassmann H, Uccelli A, Hartung HP, Montalban X, Sørensen PS, Hohlfeld R, Hauser SL (2021) Expert panel of the 27th annual meeting of the european charcot foundation: role of B cells in multiple sclerosis and related disorders. Ann Neurol 89(1):13–23https://doi.org/10.1002/ana.25927
37. Guerrero BL, Sicotte NL (2020) Microglia in multiple sclerosis: friend or foe? Front Immunol 11:374. https://doi.org/10.3389/fimmu.2020.00374
38. de Sa JCC, Airas L, Bartholome E, Grigoriadis N, Mattle H, Oreja-Guevara C, O'Riordan J, Sellebjerg F, Stankoff B, Vass K, Kieseier BC (2011) Symptomatic therapy in multiple sclerosis: a review for a multimodal approach in clinical practice. Ther Adv Neurol Disord 4(3):139–168. https://doi.org/10.1177/1756285611403646
39. Bainbridge J, Miravalle A, Wong P (2017) Multiple sclerosis. In: DiPiro J, Talbert R, Yee G, Matzke G, Wells B, Posey L (eds) Pharmacotherapy: a pathophysiological approach, 10th edn. McGraw-Hill Education, New York, NY, pp 815–836
40. Goldman MD, Cohen JA, Fox RJ, Bethoux FA (2006) Multiple sclerosis: treating symptoms, and other general medical issues. Clevel Clin J Med 73(2):177–186. https://doi.org/10.3949/ccjm.73.2.177
41. Brück W, Stadelmann C (2003) Inflammation and degeneration in multiple sclerosis. Neurol Sci 24:s265–s267. https://doi.org/10.1007/s10072-003-0170-7
42. Meltzer EI, Costello FE, Frohman EM, Frohman TC (2018) New ways of "seeing" the mechanistic heterogeneity of multiple sclerosis plaque pathogenesis. J Neuroophthalmol 38(1):91–100. https://doi.org/10.1097/WNO.0000000000000633
43. Kamm CP, Uitdehaag BM, Polman CH (2014) Multiple sclerosis: current knowledge and future outlook. Eur Neurol 72(3–4):132–141. https://doi.org/10.1159/000360528
44. Ghasemi N, Razavi S, Nikzad E (2017) Multiple sclerosis: pathogenesis, symptoms, diagnoses and cell-based therapy. Cell J (Yakhteh) 19(1):1–10. https://doi.org/10.22074/cellj.2016.4867
45. Kalincik T, Buzzard K, Jokubaitis V, Trojano M, Duquette P, Izquierdo G, Girard M, Lugaresi A, Grammond P, Grand'Maison F, Oreja-Guevara C, MS Base Study Group (2014) Risk of relapse phenotype recurrence in multiple sclerosis. Mult Scler J 20(11):1511–1522. https://doi.org/10.1177/1352458514528
46. Repovic P, Lublin FD (2011) Treatment of multiple sclerosis exacerbations. Neurol Clin 29(2):389–400. https://doi.org/10.1016/j.ncl.2010.12.012

47. Vollmer T (2007) The natural history of relapses in multiple sclerosis. J Neurol Sci 256:S5–S13. https://doi.org/10.1016/j.jns.2007.01.065
48. Wei W, Ma D, Li L, Zhang L (2021) Progress in the application of drugs for the treatment of multiple sclerosis. Front Pharmacol 12:724718. https://doi.org/10.3389/fphar.2021.724718
49. Lublin FD, Reingold SC, Cohen JA, Cutter GR, Sørensen PS, Thompson AJ, Wolinsky JS, Balcer LJ, Banwell B, Barkhof F, Bebo B, Polman CH (2014) Defining the clinical course of multiple sclerosis: the 2013 revisions. Neurology 83(3):278–286. https://doi.org/10.1212/WNL.0000000000000560
50. Miller D, Barkhof F, Montalban X, Thompson A, Filippi M (2005) Clinically isolated syndromes suggestive of multiple sclerosis, part I: natural history, pathogenesis, diagnosis, and prognosis. Lancet Neurology 4(5):281–288. https://doi.org/10.1016/S1474-4422(05)70071-5
51. Sand IBK, Lublin FD (2013) Diagnosis and differential diagnosis of multiple sclerosis. CONTINUUM: Lifelong Learn Neurol 19(4):922–943. https://doi.org/10.1212/01.CON.0000433290.15468.21
52. Sobel RA (2015) Greenfield's neuropathology, vol 2 Set
53. McDonald WI, Compston A, Edan G, Goodkin D, Hartung HP, Lublin FD, McFarland HF, Paty DW, Polman CH, Reingold SC, Sandberg-Wollheim M, Wolinsky JS (2001) Recommended diagnostic criteria for multiple sclerosis: guidelines from the International Panel on the diagnosis of multiple sclerosis. Ann Neurol: Off J Am Neurol Assoc Child Neurol Soc 50(1):121–127. https://doi.org/10.1002/ana.1032
54. Miller DH, Weinshenker BG, Filippi M, Banwell BL, Cohen JA, Freedman MS, Galetta SL, Hutchinson M, Johnson RT, Kappos L, Kira J, Polman CH (2008) Differential diagnosis of suspected multiple sclerosis: a consensus approach. Mult Scler J 14(9):1157–1174. https://doi.org/10.1177/1352458508096878
55. Thompson AJ, Banwell BL, Barkhof F, Carroll WM, Coetzee T, Comi G, Correale J, Fazekas F, Filippi M, Freedman MS, Fujihara K, Cohen JA (2018) Diagnosis of multiple sclerosis: 2017 revisions of the McDonald criteria. Lancet Neurology 17(2):162–173. https://doi.org/10.1016/S1474-4422(17)30470-2
56. Kuhlmann T, Lassmann H, Brück W (2008) Diagnosis of inflammatory demyelination in biopsy specimens: a practical approach. Acta Neuropathol 115:275–287. https://doi.org/10.1007/s00401-007-0320-8
57. Ömerhoca S, Akkaş SY, İçen NK (2018) Multiple sclerosis: diagnosis and differential diagnosis. Arch Neuropsychiatry 55(Suppl 1):S1. https://doi.org/10.29399/npa.23418
58. Hegen H, Teunissen CE, Sellebjerg F, Tumani H, Deisenhammer F (2015) Guidelines on cerebrospinal fluid analysis. Cerebrospinal Fluid Clin Neurol 407–428
59. Tumani H, Petereit HF, Gerritzen A, Gross CC, Huss A, Isenmann S, Jesse S, Khalil M, Lewczuk P, Lewerenz J, Zimmermann T (2020) S1 guidelines "lumbar puncture and cerebrospinal fluid analysis" (abridged and translated version). Neurol Res Pract 2:1–28. https://doi.org/10.1186/s42466-020-0051-z
60. Zheng Y, Cai MT, Yang F, Zhou JP, Fang W, Shen CH, Zhang YX, Ding MP (2020) IgG index revisited: diagnostic utility and prognostic value in multiple sclerosis. Front Immunol 11:1799. https://doi.org/10.3389/fimmu.2020.01799
61. Murray TJ (2006) Diagnosis and treatment of multiple sclerosis. BMJ 332(7540):525–527. https://doi.org/10.1136/bmj.332.7540.525
62. Styner M, Lee J, Chin B, Chin M, Commowick O, Tran H, Warfield S (2008) 3D segmentation in the clinic: a grand challenge II: MS lesion segmentation. MIDAS journal 2008:1–6
63. Alijamaat A, NikravanShalmani A, Bayat P (2021) Multiple sclerosis identification in brain MRI images using wavelet convolutional neural networks. Int J Imaging Syst Technol 31(2):778–785. https://doi.org/10.1002/ima.22492
64. E-Health Lab Dataset. http://www.medinfo.cs.ucy.ac.cy/index.php/facilities/32-software/218-datasets
65. Iswisi AF, Karan O, Rahebi J (2021) Diagnosis of multiple sclerosis disease in brain magnetic resonance imaging based on the Harris hawks optimization algorithm. Biomed Res Int 2021. https://doi.org/10.1155/2021/3248834

66. Acar ZY, Başçiftçi F, Ekmekci AH (2022) A Convolutional Neural Network model for identifying multiple sclerosis on brain FLAIR MRI. Sustain Comput: Inform Syst 35:100706. https://doi.org/10.1016/j.suscom.2022.100706
67. Shmueli OZ, Solomon C, Ben-Eliezer N, Greenspan H (2022) Deep learning based multiple sclerosis lesion detection utilizing synthetic data generation and soft attention mechanism. In: Medical imaging 2022: computer-aided diagnosis, vol 12033. SPIE, pp 191–199. https://doi.org/10.1117/12.2613283
68. Shoeibi A, Khodatars M, Jafari M, Moridian P, Rezaei M, Alizadehsani R, Khozeimeh F, Gorriz JM, Heras J, Panahiazar M, Nahavandi S, Acharya UR (2021) Applications of deep learning techniques for automated multiple sclerosis detection using magnetic resonance imaging: a review. Comput Biol Med 136. https://doi.org/10.1016/j.compbiomed.2021.104697
69. Lundervold AS, Lundervold A (2019) An overview of deep learning in medical imaging focusing on MRI. Zeitschrift fur Medizinische Phys. 29(2):102–127. https://doi.org/10.1016/j.zemedi.2018.11.002
70. Moazami F, Lefevre-Utile A, Papaloukas C, Soumelis V (2021) Machine learning approaches in study of multiple sclerosis disease through magnetic resonance images. Front Immunol 12:700582. https://doi.org/10.3389/fimmu.2021.700582
71. Guo D, Fridriksson J, Fillmore P, Rorden C, Yu H, Zheng K, Wang S (2015) Automated lesion detection on MRI scans using combined unsupervised and supervised methods. BMC Med Imaging 15(1):1–21. https://doi.org/10.1186/s12880-015-0092-x
72. Eitel F, Soehler E, Bellmann-Strobl J, Brandt AU, Ruprecht K, Giess RM, Kuchling J, Asseyer S, Weygandt M, Haynes JD, Scheel M, Paul F, Ritter K (2019) Uncovering convolutional neural network decisions for diagnosing multiple sclerosis on conventional MRI using layer-wise relevance propagation. NeuroImage: Clin 24. https://doi.org/10.1016/j.nicl.2019.102003.
73. Kenney RC, Liu M, Hasanaj L, Joseph B, Al-Hassan AA, Balk LJ, Balcer LJ (2022) The role of optical coherence tomography criteria and machine learning in multiple sclerosis and optic neuritis diagnosis. Neurology 99(11):e1100–e1112. https://doi.org/10.1212/WNL.0000000000200883
74. Breiman L (2001) Random forests. Mach Learn 45:5–32. https://doi.org/10.1023/A:1010933404324
75. Melingi SB, Vijayalakshmi V (2018) A hybrid approach for sub-acute ischemic stroke lesion segmentation using random decision forest and gravitational search algorithm. Curr Med Imaging Former Curr Med Imaging Rev 15(2):170–183. https://doi.org/10.2174/1573405614666180209150338
76. Buyukturkoglu K, Zeng D, Bharadwaj S, Tozlu C, Mormina E, Igwe KC, Lee S, Habeck C, Brickman AM, Riley CS, de Jager PL, Sumowski JF, Leavitt VM (2021) Classifying multiple sclerosis patients on the basis of SDMT performance using machine learning. Mult Scler J 27(1):107–116. https://doi.org/10.1177/1352458520958362
77. Fartaria MJ, Bonnier G, Roche A, Kober T, Meuli R, Rotzinger D, Frackowiak R, Schluep M, du Pasquier R, Thiran JP, Krueger G, Bach Cuadra M, Granziera C (2016) Automated detection of white matter and cortical lesions in early stages of multiple sclerosis. J Magn Reson Imaging 43(6):1445–1454. https://doi.org/10.1002/jmri.25095
78. Wang QQ, Yu SC, Qi X, Hu YH, Zheng WJ, Shi JX, Yao HY (2019) Overview of logistic regression model analysis and application. Zhonghua yu fang yi xue za zhi [Chin J Prev Med] 53(9):955–960. https://doi.org/10.3760/cma.j.issn.0253-9624.2019.09.018
79. Salem M, Valverde S, Cabezas M, Pareto D, Oliver A, Salvi J, Rovira A, Llado X (2019) Multiple sclerosis lesion synthesis in MRI using an encoder-decoder U-NET. IEEE Access 7. https://doi.org/10.1109/ACCESS.2019.2900198
80. Krishna K, Murty MN (1999) Genetic K-means algorithm. IEEE Trans Syst, Man, Cybern, Part B (Cybernetics) 29(3):433–439. https://doi.org/10.1109/3477.764879
81. Khayati R, Vafadust M, Towhidkhah F, Nabavi M (2008) Fully automatic segmentation of multiple sclerosis lesions in brain MR FLAIR images using adaptive mixtures method and

Markov random field model. Comput Biol Med 38(3):379–390. https://doi.org/10.1016/j.compbiomed.2007.12.005
82. Mata J (2011) Interpretation of concrete dam behaviour with artificial neural network and multiple linear regression models. Eng Struct 33(3):903–910. https://doi.org/10.1016/j.engstruct.2010.12.011
83. Drucker H, Burges CJ, Kaufman L, Smola A, Vapnik V (1996) Support vector regression machines. Adv Neural Inf Process Syst 9:155–161
84. Chang CC, Lin CJ (2011) LIBSVM: a Library for support vector machines. ACM Trans Intell Syst Technol 2(3):1–27. https://doi.org/10.1145/1961189.1961199
85. Ion-Margineanu A, Kocevar G, Stamile C, Sima DM, Durand-Dubief F, van Huffel S, Sappey-Marinier D (2017) Machine learning approach for classifying multiple sclerosis courses by combining clinical data with lesion loads and magnetic resonance metabolic features. Front Neurosci 11:398. https://doi.org/10.3389/fnins.2017.00398
86. Cunningham P, Delany SJ (2021) K-Nearest neighbour classifiers-A tutorial. ACM Comput Surv 54(6):1–17. https://doi.org/10.1145/3459665
87. Qi Y (2012) Random forest for bioinformatics. in ensemble machine learning. Springer, Berlin/Heidelberg, Germany, pp 307–323.https://doi.org/10.1007/978-1-4419-9326-7_11
88. Acquaviva M, Menon R, Di Dario M, Dalla Costa G, Romeo M, Sangalli F, Farina C (2020) Inferring multiple sclerosis stages from the blood transcriptome via machine learning. Cell Rep Med 1(4):100053. https://doi.org/10.1016/j.xcrm.2020.100053
89. Afreen N, Patel R, Ahmed M, Sameer M (2021) A novel machine learning approach using boosting algorithm for liver disease classification. In: 2021 5th international conference on information systems and computer networks (ISCON). IEEE, pp 1–5. https://doi.org/10.1109/ISCON52037.2021.9702488
90. Martynova E, Goyal M, Johri S, Kumar V, Khaibullin T, Rizvanov AA, Baranwal M (2020) Serum and cerebrospinal fluid cytokine biomarkers for diagnosis of multiple sclerosis. Mediat Inflamm 2020. https://doi.org/10.1155/2020/2727042
91. Schapire RE (2013) Explaining adaboost. In: Empirical inference. Springer, Berlin/Heidelberg, Germany, pp 37–52.https://doi.org/10.1007/978-3-642-41136-6_5
92. Mato-Abad V, Labiano-Fontcuberta A, Rodríguez-Yáñez S, García-Vázquez R, Munteanu CR, Andrade-Garda J, Domingo-Santos A, Galán Sánchez-Seco V, Aladro Y, Martínez-Ginés ML, Ayuso L, Benito-León J (2019) Classification of radiologically isolated syndrome and clinically isolated syndrome with machine-learning techniques. Eur J Neurol 26(7):1000–1005. https://doi.org/10.1111/ene.13923
93. Jain S, Rajpal N, Yadav J (2020) Multiple sclerosis identification based on ensemble machine learning technique. SSRN Electron J. https://doi.org/10.2139/ssrn.3734806
94. Monaghan AS, Huisinga JM, Peterson DS (2021) The application of principal component analysis to characterize gait and its association with falls in multiple sclerosis. Sci Rep 11(1):12811. https://doi.org/10.1038/s41598-021-92353-2
95. Pontillo G, Penna S, Cocozza S, Quarantelli M, Gravina M, Lanzillo R, Marrone S, Costabile T, Inglese M, Morra VB, Riccio D, Elefante A, Petracca M, Sansone C, Brunetti A (2022) Stratification of multiple sclerosis patients using unsupervised machine learning: a single-visit MRI-driven approach. Eur Radiol 32(8):5382–5391. https://doi.org/10.1007/s00330-022-08610-z
96. Zhang L, Wang M, Liu M, Zhang D (2020) A survey on deep learning for neuroimaging-based brain disorder analysis. Front Neurosci 14. https://doi.org/10.3389/fnins.2020.00779
97. Wani MA, Bhat FA, Afzal S, Khan AI (2020) Advances in deep learning. Springer
98. Goodfellow I, Bengio Y, Courville A (2016) Deep learning. MIT Press
99. Gulli A, Pal S (2017) Deep learning with Keras. Packt Publishing Ltd
100. Vatian A, Gusarova N, Dobrenko N, Klochkov A, Nigmatullin N, Lobantsev A, Shalyto A (2019) Fusing of medical images and reports in diagnostics of brain diseases. In: Proceedings of the 2019 the international conference on pattern recognition and artificial intelligence, pp 102–108. https://doi.org/10.1145/3357777.3357793

101. Goodfellow IJ, Pouget-Abadie J, Mirza M, Xu B, Warde-Farley D, Ozair S, Courville A, Bengio Y (2014) Generative adversarial nets. Adv Neural Inf Process Syst 3(January). https://doi.org/10.1007/978-3-658-40442-0_9
102. Zhang C, Song Y, Liu S, Lill S, Wang C, Tang Z, You Y, Gao Y, Klistorner A, Barnett M, Cai W (2019) MS-GAN: GAN-based semantic segmentation of multiple sclerosis lesions in brain magnetic resonance imaging. In: 2018 international conference on digital image computing: techniques and applications, DICTA 2018. https://doi.org/10.1109/DICTA.2018.8615771
103. Singh NK, Raza K (2022) Progress in deep learning-based dental and maxillofacial image analysis: a systematic review. Expert Syst Appl 199:116968. https://doi.org/10.1016/j.eswa.2022.116968
104. Vogelsanger C, Federau C (2021) Latent space analysis of vae and intro-vae applied to 3-dimensional mr brain volumes of multiple sclerosis, leukoencephalopathy, and healthy patients. arXiv:2101.06772
105. Birenbaum A, Greenspan H (2017) Multi-view longitudinal CNN for multiple sclerosis lesion segmentation. Eng Appl Artif Intell 65:111–118. https://doi.org/10.1016/j.engappai.2017.06.006
106. Siar H, Teshnehlab M (2019) Diagnosing and classification tumors and MS simultaneous of magnetic resonance images using convolution neural network∗. In: 2019 7th Iranian joint congress on fuzzy and intelligent systems, CFIS 2019, pp 1–4.https://doi.org/10.1109/CFIS.2019.8692148
107. López-Dorado A, Ortiz M, Satue M, Rodrigo MJ, Barea R, Sánchez-Morla EM, Garcia-Martin E (2022) Early diagnosis of multiple sclerosis using swept-source optical coherence tomography and convolutional neural networks trained with data augmentation. Sensors 22(1):167. https://doi.org/10.3390/s22010167
108. Garcia-Martin E, Pablo LE, Herrero R, Ara JR, Martin J, Larrosa JM, Fernandez J (2013) Neural networks to identify multiple sclerosis with optical coherence tomography. Acta Ophthalmol 91(8):e628-634. https://doi.org/10.1111/aos.12156
109. Yoo Y, Tang LYW, Li DKB, Metz L, Kolind S, Traboulsee AL, Tam RC (2019) Deep learning of brain lesion patterns and user-defined clinical and MRI features for predicting conversion to multiple sclerosis from clinically isolated syndrome. Comput Methods Biomech Biomed Eng: Imaging Vis 7(3):250–259. https://doi.org/10.1080/21681163.2017.1356750
110. Narayana PA, Coronado I, Sujit SJ, Wolinsky JS, Lublin FD, Gabr RE (2020) Deep-learning-based neural tissue segmentation of mri in multiple sclerosis: effect of training set size. J Magn Reson Imaging 51(5):1487–1496. https://doi.org/10.1002/jmri.26959
111. Gabr RE, Coronado I, Robinson M, Sujit SJ, Datta S, Sun X, Allen WJ, Lublin FD, Wolinsky JS, Narayana PA (2020) Brain and lesion segmentation in multiple sclerosis using fully convolutional neural networks: a large-scale study. Mult Scler J 26(10):1217–1226. https://doi.org/10.1177/1352458519856843
112. Ronneberger O, Fischer P, Brox T (2015) U-net: convolutional networks for biomedical image segmentation. Lecture notes in computer science (Including subseries lecture notes in artificial intelligence and lecture notes in bioinformatics), vol 9351, pp 234–241.https://doi.org/10.1007/978-3-319-24574-4_28
113. Shelhamer E, Long J, Darrell T (2017) Fully convolutional networks for semantic segmentation. IEEE Trans Pattern Anal Mach Intell 39(4):3431–3440. https://doi.org/10.1109/TPAMI.2016.2572683
114. LeCun Y (1987) PhD thesis: modeles connexionnistes de l'apprentissage (connectionist learning models)
115. Andermatt S, Pezold S, Cattin PC (2018) Automated segmentation of multiple sclerosis lesions using multi-dimensional gated recurrent units. Lecture notes in computer science (Including subseries lecture notes in artificial intelligence and lecture notes in bioinformatics), vol 10670. LNCS, pp 31–42. https://doi.org/10.1007/978-3-319-75238-9_3
116. Maggi P, Fartaria MJ, Jorge J, La Rosa F, Absinta M, Sati P, Kober T (2020) CVSnet: a machine learning approach for automated central vein sign assessment in multiple sclerosis. NMR Biomed 33(5):e4283. https://doi.org/10.1002/nbm.4283

117. McKinley R, Wepfer R, Aschwanden F, Grunder L, Muri R, Rummel C, Wiest R (2021) Simultaneous lesion and brain segmentation in multiple sclerosis using deep neural networks. Sci Rep 11(1):1087. https://doi.org/10.1038/s41598-020-79925-4
118. Sujit SJ, Coronado I, Kamali A, Narayana PA, Gabr RE (2019) Automated image quality evaluation of structural brain MRI using an ensemble of deep learning networks. J Magn Reson Imaging 50(4):1260–1267. https://doi.org/10.1002/jmri.26693
119. Shaul R, David I, Shitrit O, Riklin Raviv T (2020) Subsampled brain MRI reconstruction by generative adversarial neural networks. Med Image Anal 65:101747. https://doi.org/10.1016/j.media.2020.101747
120. Hluštík P (2015) 3. Functional MRI in the diagnosis and prognosis of multiple sclerosis. Clin Neurophysiol 126(3):e30. https://doi.org/10.1016/j.clinph.2014.10.1621799. https://doi.org/10.3389/fimmu.2020.01799
121. Singh NK, Raza K (2021) Medical image generation using generative adversarial networks: a review. In: Health informatics: a computational perspective in healthcare, studies in computational intelligence, vol 932. Springer, Berlin, pp 77–96.https://doi.org/10.1007/978-981-15-9735-0_5

Exploring Challenges and Opportunities for the Early Detection of Multiple Sclerosis Using Deep Learning

K. O. Mohammed Aarif, Afroj Alam, Pakruddin, and J. Riyazulla Rahman

Abstract MS stands as a persistent autoimmune condition impacting the central nervous system, leading to inflammation and the loss of myelin. Early and accurate diagnosis of MS is crucial for initiating timely medication and refining patient results. Deep learning, a branch of artificial intelligence, has displayed significant promise across a range of medical uses, encompassing the identification and prognosis of MS. This research aims to delve into the difficulties and prospects surrounding the application of deep learning methods to promptly detect MS. The study delves into the existing scenario of MS diagnosis and the confines of conventional approaches. It delves into the capacity of deep learning algorithms, specifically convolutional neural networks (CNNs), in scrutinizing medical imagery like magnetic resonance imaging (MRI) to pinpoint distinctive MS-related structures and characteristics that might signal the initial stages of the disease. The challenges encountered in leveraging deep learning for MS diagnosis are discussed, including the need for large annotated datasets, the interpretability of deep learning models, and the synthesis of multimodal data sources. The study also addresses concerns related to the generalizability and robustness of deep learning models when applied to diverse patient populations and imaging protocols. Furthermore, the study highlights the opportunities and advancements in deep learning approaches for MS detection, such as transfer learning, data augmentation, and ensemble methods. Additionally, this study discusses the potential clinical implications of deep learning-based MS diagnosis, including the potential for improved early intervention, personalized treatment plans, and monitoring disease progression. Overall, this research contributes to a comprehensive understanding of the challenges and opportunities in utilizing deep learning for the early detection of

K. O. Mohammed Aarif (✉)
Department of Electronics & Communication Engineering, Presidency University, Bangalore, India
e-mail: aarifko@gmail.com

Afroj Alam · Pakruddin · J. Riyazulla Rahman
Department of Computer Science Engineering, Presidency University, Bangalore, India
e-mail: alamafroj@student.iul.ac.in

J. Riyazulla Rahman
e-mail: riyaz@presidencyuniversity.in

K. Raza and S. Singh (eds.), *Artificial Intelligence and Autoimmune Diseases*, Studies in Computational Intelligence 1133, https://doi.org/10.1007/978-981-99-9029-0_8

MS. The results of this study could open doors to creating better diagnostic tools that are both precise and effective, resulting in enhanced patient outcomes and progress in the field of diagnosing and treating multiple sclerosis.

Keywords Multiple Sclerosis · Artificial Intelligence · Machine Learning · Deep Learning · Convolutional Neural Network CNN · magnetic resonance imaging MRI

1 Introduction

MS stands out as an autoimmune ailment distinguished by its persistent character and unpredictable trajectory. Its primary impact is felt within the central nervous system (CNS), spanning the brain and spinal cord. Classified as a disorder characterized by the loss of myelin, MS involves the impairment or depletion of the protective coating around nerve fibers referred to as myelin. As a result, this disruption to the myelin covering obstructs the normal transmission of electrical signals along nerves, leading to a diverse range of symptoms that exhibit considerable variation among individuals. The exact origin of multiple sclerosis remains undisclosed, although it is presumed to be shaped by a blend of genetic and environmental elements. Its occurrence is more prevalent among young adults, typically falling within the age bracket of 20 to 40 years, and women are more frequently impacted than men. The symptoms associated with MS can exhibit considerable diversity and may include fatigue, difficulty in walking, sensations of numbness or tingling in the limbs, muscle weakness, coordination-balance issues, vision problems, cognitive impairments, and emotional changes. These symptoms can come and go or worsen over time, leading to periods of relapse and remission. The diagnosis of multiple sclerosis usually involves a combination of medical history, physical examination, neurological tests, and imaging studies, such as MRI, to detect areas of demyelination in the CNS. Despite the absence of a current remedy for multiple sclerosis, individuals with MS have access to diverse treatment alternatives that help alleviate symptoms, decelerate the advancement of the disease, and enhance their quality of life. These may include disease-modifying therapies, symptomatic treatments, rehabilitation therapies, and lifestyle modifications. Research into multiple sclerosis is ongoing, and advancements in understanding the disease and developing new treatment approaches continue to offer hope for better outcomes for individuals living with this complex condition. The diagnosis and assessment of multiple sclerosis heavily rely on the pivotal role of magnetic resonance imaging (MRI). When diagnosing multiple sclerosis, MRI scans are used to visualize the brain and spinal cord and detect characteristic abnormalities. These scans can reveal the presence of multiple areas of demyelination, also known as lesions or plaques, in different parts of the CNS. These lesions appear as bright or dark spots on the MRI images. The prevalent form of MRI employed to detect multiple sclerosis is a T2-weighted MRI, adept at detecting irregularities in the brain and spinal cord's white matter. T2-weighted images can reveal both recent and

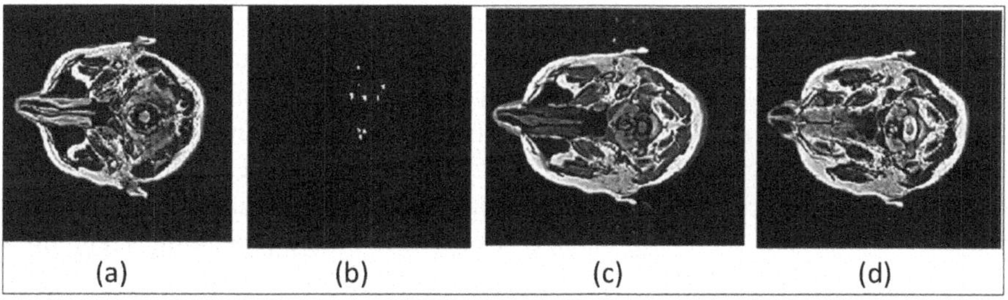

Fig. 1 Multi-sequence MRI image with consensus manual lesion segmentation. **a** Fluid-attenuated inversion recovery (FLAIR). **b** MS-lesion segmentation, **c** and **d** MRI sequences T1-weighted, T2-weighted

longstanding lesions, aiding in the identification and measurement of disease activity levels. Figure 1 shows the multi-sequence MRI image with consensus manual lesion segmentation. Another MRI technique used in multiple sclerosis diagnosis is gadolinium-enhanced MRI [1]. In this procedure, a contrast agent called gadolinium is administered intravenously to highlight active areas of inflammation and new or active lesions. Gadolinium-enhanced MRI can provide valuable information about disease activity and the effectiveness of treatment. MRI can also be used to assess the size, location, and volume of lesions, as well as to evaluate the presence of other conditions that may mimic multiple sclerosis symptoms. Additionally, MRI can help identify other features of MS, such as brain atrophy, which is the loss of brain tissue over time. Although MRI is an essential tool for diagnosing multiple sclerosis, it is not the only factor considered. Medical history, physical examination, and other diagnostic tests, such as cerebrospinal fluid analysis, are also taken into account to establish a comprehensive diagnosis.

The utilization of MRI imaging is of significant importance in the diagnosis and control of multiple sclerosis. This imaging technique offers valuable insights into the existence, site, and activity of lesions, facilitating the development of treatment strategies and enabling the monitoring of disease progression over a period of time. Image processing techniques applied to MRI data can assist in automating the detection and quantification of MS lesions, providing valuable information to clinicians [2]. One of the primary challenges in MS diagnosis is the accurate identification and segmentation of lesions from MRI scans. Manual segmentation by experts is time-consuming and subjective, making automated or semi-automated methods highly desirable.

Several image processing algorithms have been developed to address this challenge. These algorithms utilize sophisticated techniques such as thresholding, edge detection, region growth, and classification to identify and segment MS lesions from MRI images. These algorithms analyze the intensity, texture, and spatial information of the image to distinguish between normal tissue and MS lesions. By applying image processing techniques, the segmentation process can be accelerated, leading to quicker and more reliable MS lesion detection. These automated methods can assist clinicians in quantifying the lesion burden, tracking disease progression, and evaluating treatment efficacy. Additionally, image processing techniques can provide additional insights into the spatial distribution, size, and shape characteristics of MS lesions. Furthermore, image processing can aid in the analysis of MRI features beyond lesion detection. It can be utilized for the assessment of brain atrophy, which is a critical aspect of MS progression. By extracting quantitative measures of brain volume and analyzing changes over time, image processing techniques can provide valuable information about the neurodegenerative aspects of MS [3]. The integration of image processing techniques with MRI in MS diagnosis holds the promise of enhancing the precision, speed, and impartiality of identifying and describing lesions. It allows for standardized and reproducible analyses, reducing inter-observer variability and enhancing the reliability of MS diagnosis and monitoring. While image processing techniques have shown promise in MS diagnosis, they are still evolving. Ongoing research focuses on refining existing algorithms, developing machine learning approaches, and exploring advanced imaging modalities to improve the sensitivity and specificity of lesion detection. The application of image processing techniques to MRI data in multiple sclerosis diagnosis offers great potential in enhancing lesion detection, segmentation, and quantitative analysis [4]. These advancements contribute to more accurate and efficient diagnosis, monitoring disease progression, and evaluating treatment response, ultimately improving patient care in the management of multiple sclerosis.

Machine learning methods have become valuable assets in identifying and diagnosing MS. These techniques leverage the power of algorithms and data analysis to identify patterns and make predictions based on large datasets. In the context of MS, machine learning algorithms can aid in the early detection of the disease, improve accuracy in distinguishing MS from other conditions, and assist in predicting disease progression. One area where machine learning has shown promise is in the classification of MS lesions in MRI scans. By training algorithms on a large dataset of annotated MRI images, machine learning models can learn to differentiate between MS lesions and normal brain tissue [5]. These models can then be applied to new MRI scans to automatically detect and segment MS lesions, providing valuable information for diagnosis and monitoring. Additionally, these algorithms can be employed to analyze different characteristics derived from MRI scans, including lesion volume, shape, and spatial distribution. By combining multiple imaging biomarkers, these algorithms can develop predictive models to estimate disease progression, prognosis, and treatment response [6]. This information can aid clinicians in making informed decisions about patient management and selecting appropriate therapies. In addition to MRI data, machine learning algorithms can incorporate clinical and demographic information to enhance MS detection and diagnosis. By integrating data such as patient age, gender, medical history, and symptoms, machine learning models can learn complex patterns and develop diagnostic algorithms that improve accuracy and reduce false positives/negatives. Moreover, machine learning techniques have been extended to other data sources, such as genomic data, analysis of cerebrospinal fluid, and neurophysiological measurements, with the goal of identifying biomarkers linked to MS [7]. These biomarkers can provide insights into disease mechanisms, improve understanding of MS subtypes, and aid in personalized treatment strategies.

It is important to note that machine learning algorithms in MS detection and diagnosis are not meant to replace clinical expertise but rather complement and support healthcare professionals. The algorithms serve as decision support tools, assisting clinicians in interpreting complex data and making informed decisions. there are hurdles to confront in the realm of machine learning for multiple sclerosis detection. The availability of expansive, varied, and meticulously annotated datasets is essential for effectively training precise models. Ensuring the robustness, interpretability, and generalizability of machine learning models remains an ongoing area of research.

Machine learning techniques offer significant potential in the detection and diagnosis of multiple sclerosis. These algorithms can leverage various data sources, including MRI scans, clinical information, and biomarkers, to improve accuracy, efficiency, and personalized care. Continued research and development in machine learning for MS hold promise for advancing early detection, individualized treatment approaches, and ultimately improving patient outcomes in the management of multiple sclerosis. Deep learning, which falls under the umbrella of machine learning, has demonstrated significant potential in detecting and diagnosing MS. Leveraging their capacity to autonomously acquire hierarchical representations from intricate data, deep learning algorithms can proficiently examine medical images like MRI scans. This aids in the identification and characterization of MS lesions. An area where deep learning is applied in MS detection involves the automated segmentation of MS lesions in MRI scans. Convolutional neural networks (CNNs), a widely utilized deep learning framework, have exhibited remarkable effectiveness in accomplishing this task with high accuracy. By training on large datasets of annotated MRI scans, CNNs can learn to recognize and segment MS lesions with high accuracy and efficiency. This automated lesion segmentation can assist clinicians in quantifying lesion burden, monitoring disease progression, and evaluating treatment response.

Deep learning algorithms can also leverage the rich information contained within MRI images to classify and differentiate MS from other conditions. By training on large datasets of MRI scans from individuals with and without MS, deep learning models can learn to extract discriminative features and classify new cases accurately. This can aid in the early detection and accurate diagnosis of MS, reducing delays in treatment initiation and improving patient outcomes. Furthermore, deep learning techniques can incorporate multimodal data sources to enhance MS detection and diagnosis. By combining MRI scans with clinical information, genetic data, and other biomarkers, deep learning models can leverage complementary information to improve diagnostic accuracy and provide personalized predictions regarding disease progression and treatment response. Here's a brief introduction to various deep learning techniques:

Feedforward Neural Networks (FNNs): These are the foundational blocks of deep learning. Feedforward neural networks (FNNs) comprise an initial layer for input, one or more intermediary layers, and a concluding output layer. They're used for tasks like image classification, regression, and basic pattern recognition.

Convolutional Neural Networks (CNNs): Convolutional Neural Networks (CNNs) are specifically crafted for handling data arranged in a grid-like fashion, like images or video frames. They employ convolutional layers to autonomously acquire layered features, rendering them remarkably proficient in endeavors such as recognizing images, identifying objects, and producing images [8].

Recurrent Neural Networks (RNNs): RNNs are used for sequential data and have connections that loop back on themselves, allowing information to persist. They're suitable for tasks like natural language processing, time series analysis, and speech recognition.

Long Short-Term Memory (LSTM) Networks: LSTMs are a specialized type of RNN that can capture long-range dependencies in sequences. They mitigate the vanishing gradient problem and are widely used for tasks requiring memory, like language translation and sentiment analysis.

Gated Recurrent Units (GRUs): GRUs are similar to LSTMs but have a simplified structure. They're efficient and effective for many sequence-based tasks, striking a balance between complexity and performance.

Autoencoders: Autoencoders are used for unsupervised learning and dimensionality reduction. These encompass an encoder to condense data into an underlying representation and a decoder to restore the initial data. Variational Autoencoders (VAEs) and Generative Adversarial Networks (GANs) are well-recognized expansions of this concept.

Generative Adversarial Networks (GANs): GANs consist of a generator and a discriminator that play a game. The generator creates data samples to try and fool the discriminator, which in turn learns to distinguish real from generated data. GANs are used for tasks like image generation, style transfer, and data augmentation [9].

Transformers: Transformers revolutionized NLP by allowing models to capture context from entire sequences simultaneously. The self-attention mechanism enables bidirectional processing, making them highly effective for tasks like machine translation (e.g., the famous model "BERT") and text generation.

Attention Mechanisms: Attention mechanisms enhance neural networks' ability to focus on specific parts of the input, often used in conjunction with RNNs and Transformers. They have applications in machine translation, image captioning, and summarization.

Transfer Learning: Transfer learning entails initially training a model on an extensive dataset for a specific task, followed by refining its performance on a smaller dataset geared toward a related task. Pretrained models like VGG, ResNet, and GPT have demonstrated remarkable success in various domains.

Self-Supervised Learning: This approach leverages the inherent structure in data to create supervisory signals. For instance, predicting masked words in a sentence can lead to representations useful for downstream tasks without needing explicit annotations.

These techniques are just a glimpse into the diverse landscape of deep learning, which continues to evolve rapidly and find applications across a wide range of domains.

Deep learning has also been applied to other aspects of MS research, such as predicting disease prognosis and treatment response. By analyzing longitudinal data from individuals with MS, deep learning models can learn patterns and predict future outcomes, helping clinicians make informed decisions about patient management and treatment strategies. However, it is important to note that deep learning algorithms are data-driven and require large, diverse, and well-curated datasets for training. The availability and quality of such datasets pose challenges in the application of deep learning to MS detection. Additionally, the comprehensibility of deep learning models continues to be a subject of ongoing study, given that their decision-making procedures can be intricate and less straightforward when contrasted with conventional machine learning techniques. The deep learning algorithms can automate lesion segmentation, aid in accurate classification, and leverage multimodal data for enhanced diagnostic accuracy and personalized predictions. Continued research and collaboration between deep learning experts and healthcare professionals are essential to harness the full potential of deep learning in improving MS diagnosis and patient care. Figure 2 describes the AI methodologies utilized in MS detection. In this chapter, a thorough comprehension of the difficulties related to the early identification of MS using conventional diagnostic approaches is presented. Furthermore, the chapter investigates the potential of deep learning techniques, specifically deep neural networks, to enhance the precision and effectiveness of MS detection. This chapter also discusses the specific challenges faced in utilizing deep learning for MS detection and highlights the opportunities and advancements in deep learning approaches for early MS detection, including transfer learning, data augmentation, and ensemble methods. The rest of the section is organized as follows: Sect. 2 presents the Deep Learning

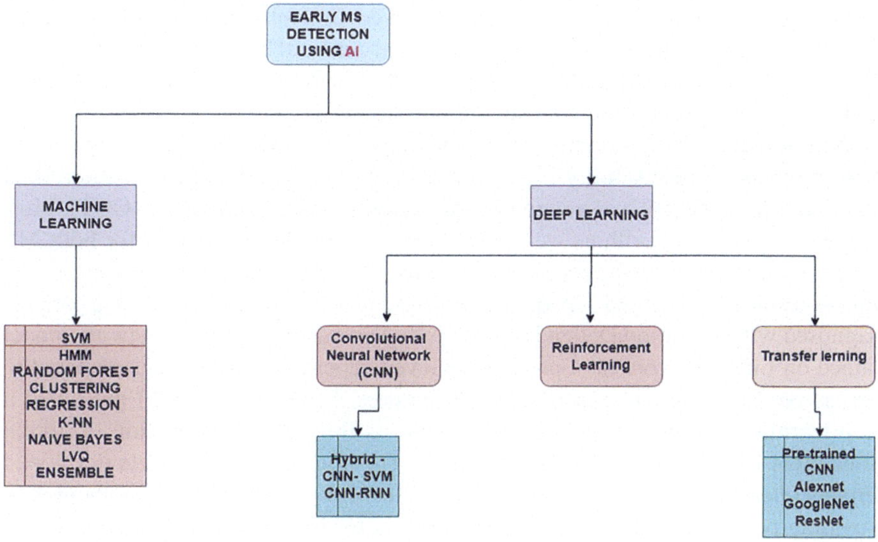

Fig. 2 Artificial Intelligence methodologies for MS detection

Approaches for the Early Detection of MS, and Sect. 3 describes the Challenges in Utilizing Deep Learning for MS Detection. The Opportunities, Advancements, and integration with other imaging modalities in Deep Learning for Early MS Detection are discussed in Sect. 4; finally, Sect. 5 gives the Future Directions and Research Opportunities followed by the conclusion.

2 Deep Learning Approaches for Early Detection of MS

Deep learning approaches for the early detection of MS leverage advanced neural network architectures and algorithms to analyze medical imaging data and identify MS-specific patterns. CNNs are widely used for image analysis and have shown great success in MS detection. These networks learn hierarchical representations of image features through convolutional layers and can effectively identify MS lesions in MRI scans. In their study, Eshaghi et al. [10] introduced a method for identifying different types of MS through unsupervised learning. They utilized different classifiers on an MRI dataset that is publicly accessible. The findings suggest that these MRI-based subtypes can accurately forecast the advancement of disability in individuals with MS and how they react to treatment. Furthermore, these subtypes can potentially serve as a means to categorize patients into specific groups for interventional trials. In the study referenced as [11], Ponnada et al. employed a CNN to categorize augmented lesions within MRI scans that hadn't been enhanced. The CNN analyzed individual slices, combining scores through a fully connected network to generate predictions for each participant. The research showcased CNN's effectiveness in terms of lesion detection ratios and the areas under the curve of the receiver operating characteristic. Julien et al. [12] put forth a study that employed Convolutional Neural Networks (CNNs) to autonomously segment both the spinal cord and lesions. The methodology efficiently tackled the difficulty arising from the relatively small volume of spinal cord and lesion voxels when compared to the rest of the dataset.

Montolío et al. [13] sought to refine the diagnosis of MS and forecast the long-term progression of disability using clinical data and the thickness of the retinal nerve fiber layer (RNFL) as gauged by optical coherence tomography (OCT). Multiple classification algorithms were tested to create predictive models for both MS diagnosis and predicting the course of disability. Casalino et al. [14] conducted a classification study to distinguish pediatric MS from healthy children, including patients diagnosed with Attention Deficit Hyperactivity Disorder (ADHD). A network model trained on miRNA expression profiles achieved superior performance compared to models based on human-expert-selected features. Schwab et al. [15] presented a deep learning technique aimed at MS diagnosis through the utilization of digital biomarkers obtained from smartphone data. The deep learning models developed demonstrated the ability to differentiate between individuals with and without MS, providing potential additional diagnostic criteria for MS. The study encompassed a variety of assessments designed to gauge different dimensions of participants' capacities and overall well-being. The following data were acquired using the smartphone in this study.

Mood Questionnaire: Participants were inquired about their present state of well-being. Their answers were assigned a mood score to monitor fluctuations in mood across time.

Symbol Matching: Participants were furnished with symbols linked to numbers and tasked with rapidly and precisely converting these symbols into numbers using an on-screen keyboard. The mean response time and the count of accurate responses were logged. Additionally, a baseline version devoid of mapping was included.

Walking: Participants were directed to take a two-minute stroll while their smartphones tallied the number of steps taken. This aimed to evaluate their walking capability.

U-turn assessment: Participants were instructed to swiftly walk between two designated points, while their smartphones documented the count of turns and the average speed of these turns, enabling an evaluation of their agility in changing direction.

Balance: Participants were obligated to maintain a stationary posture and uphold their equilibrium for a predetermined duration. Their postural sway was captured to appraise their capacity to remain stable.

Mobility: This assessment harnessed the location sensors in participants' smartphones to document their day-to-day spatial range. Unlike other evaluations, this test functioned inconspicuously without necessitating manual initiation.

Pinching: Participants were presented with virtual objects on their smartphone screens and instructed to promptly pinch and compress these objects using finger gestures. The app documented the number of successfully compressed objects and the hand employed for the pinching action, thus gauging pinching prowess.

Drawing: Participants were prompted to replicate shapes displayed on their screens by manually drawing them with their fingers. The app calculated the Hausdorff distance between the drawn and depicted shapes, thereby evaluating drawing precision.

The primary objective of these assessments was to comprehensively appraise diverse facets of participants' physical and cognitive abilities, encompassing mood, motor skills such as walking and turning, equilibrium, mobility, intricate motor skills like pinching, and the accuracy of drawings. This evaluation sought to yield insights into potential impairments linked to conditions like multiple sclerosis.

La Rosa et al. [16] contrasted superficial and intricate learning structures in their endeavor to automatically segment white matter lesions within magnetic resonance images of individuals with MS. The deep learning architecture exhibited a low false positive rate, while the shallow architecture excelled in accurately capturing lesion volume. Fabian et al. [17] investigated the image features utilized by a trained CNN for decision-making in MS diagnosis. They employed Layer-wise Relevance Propagation (LRP) to identify relevant image features aligning with established imaging markers in MS, validating the CNN model. In [18], the authors focused on accurately quantifying T2 lesions in MS using a 3D, multi-arm U-Net deep learning model. The model showed promising results in segmenting T2 lesions, achieving high accuracy and correlation with clinical disability scores. These studies collectively contribute to the advancement of MS diagnosis, treatment response prediction, lesion segmentation, and identification of relevant image features using various machine learning and deep learning techniques. In [19], Olivier et al. reported that detecting and segmenting new lesions in MS remains a challenging task. While automatic methods have shown increased sensitivity in detecting new lesions, they often produce more false positives compared to manual delineation by experts. However, recent advancements have narrowed the performance gap between automatic solutions and human experts, bringing them closer in accuracy. Table 1 discusses the comprehensive overview of recent studies of MS detection using deep learning.

To make these automatic methods viable for clinical routine, several steps still need to be taken. These include integrating computerized solutions into the hospital's information flow and quantifying the uncertainty associated with automatic lesion detection. Instead of providing a binary output (lesion or non-lesion), quantifying uncertainty can help clinicians by indicating the confidence level of the automated

Table 1 Summary of recent deep learning system for MS detection

Related work	Dataset	Methodology	Outcome
Yılmaz et al. [12]	LabIT	A CNN model with splitting	Slice—98% Patient—90.3%
La Rosa et al. [13]	Two 7 T datasets	U-net-based deep learning	TP—74% FP—30%
Shmueli et al. [14]	UMCL	EfficientNet5 and Y-net4	Accuracy—91%
López et al. [15]	SS-OCT images	Multiple CNN	Specificity—100% Sensitivity—100%
Aslani et al. [16]	ISBI	Encoder-decoder	69.80%
Afzal et al. [17]	MICCAI ISBI	Multiple CNN	DSC = 67%
McKinley [18]	MSSEG Insel90 Insel32	DeepSCAN	DSC = 60% F1-Score = 57%
Hu [19]	ISBI	U-Net	DSC = 63.45%
Gabr [20]	CombiRx	Multiclass U-Net FCNN	T2 Lesions DSC = 82%
Yildirim [30]	Publicly available dataset	Mask R-CNN	NA
Yildirim [31]	ISBI 2015-MICCAI 2008	Mask R-CNN	Dice similarity 86.30% and 81.32%
Creagh [32]	FLOODLIGHT (FL)	D-CNN	Digitally estimated
Salem [33]	ISBI2015	Encoder-Decoder U-NET	Score 91.44
Hashemi [34]	ISBI longitudinal MS	FC-DenseNet	Dice similarity 69.9% and 65.74%

detection. This way, the clinician's expertise can be utilized for challenging cases, while obvious lesions can be handled efficiently by the automated system. By addressing these steps, a new generation of computerized medical assistants can be designed to enhance care in MS. These assistants would leverage the expertise of clinicians, assisting them in diagnosing and monitoring the disease more effectively. With the integration of computerized solutions and the quantification of uncertainty, these assistants can contribute to improved workflows and better patient outcomes in clinical settings. The study presented by Sepahvand et al. in [20] introduces a deep learning framework specifically designed for the automated detection and segmentation of NE T2-weighted lesions in longitudinal brain MRIs of RRMS patients. The proposed method demonstrates high overall detection accuracy and outperforms other approaches, especially for small lesions. These findings contribute to the advancement of automated NE lesion analysis in MS, enabling improved monitoring of disease activity and treatment evaluation.

In this section, an analysis was conducted on prior studies from the last decade that focused on utilizing (DL) to diagnose (MS). Our objective was to determine the commonly employed techniques and data types utilized in the automated diagnosis of MS, as well as to identify the techniques that yielded noteworthy outcomes.

3 Challenges in Utilizing Deep Learning in the Detection of MS

The integration of deep learning methods has initiated a significant transformation in the field of medical diagnostics, encompassing the identification of intricate conditions like multiple sclerosis (MS). Deep learning presents an opportunity to revolutionize the precision and effectiveness of MS detection by capitalizing on neural networks' capability to extract complex patterns and correlations from medical data. Nonetheless, within these potential benefits, there exist obstacles that require thoughtful navigation to fully exploit deep learning's capabilities in MS detection. In this segment, we delve into these hurdles and illuminate the complexities entailed in employing deep learning for the purpose of detecting MS. Here are some challenges in utilizing deep learning for MS detection:

(A) Limited and heterogeneous datasets: Acquiring extensive and varied datasets for training deep learning models in the context of MS detection poses a significant challenge. The availability of such datasets that encompass a wide range of MS cases, imaging modalities, patient demographics, disease progression, and clinical characteristics is limited. One obstacle is the rarity of MS cases, making it difficult to amass a substantial amount of data from a single source. Additionally, the heterogeneity of MS, which manifests in various forms and progresses differently among individuals, necessitates the inclusion of diverse cases in the training data to capture the full spectrum of the disease. Moreover, obtaining high-quality labeled data for training deep learning models in MS detection requires meticulous annotation and

labeling of MS-related features or lesions in medical images. This process is typically performed manually by experts, and it can be time-consuming, labor-intensive, and subject to inter-observer variability.

Addressing the challenge of obtaining huge and divergent datasets for training deep learning models for MS detection is crucial for developing accurate and robust algorithms. Collaborative efforts among researchers, institutions, and medical centers can facilitate the pooling of data from multiple sources, thereby increasing the dataset size and diversity. Furthermore, advancements in data-sharing initiatives and privacy-preserving techniques can enable the development of larger and more representative datasets while safeguarding patient confidentiality and complying with ethical and legal requirements. To address this limitation, researchers might consider exploring the feasibility of utilizing magnetic resonance imaging (MRI) datasets from diverse ethnoracial groups. By incorporating MRI data from multiple ethnoracial backgrounds, several potential benefits and challenges emerge like Enhanced Diversity, Generalizability, and Uncovering Unique Features. MS data can vary in terms of imaging modalities, patient demographics, disease progression, and clinical characteristics. Ensuring an adequate representation of these factors in the training data is crucial but can be difficult to achieve. Table.2 lists some of the publicly available datasets for MS detection used in deep learning.

(B) Annotation and labeling of data: Deep learning models require annotated data for training, which often involves manual labeling of MS-related features or lesions in medical images. Training deep learning models for MS detection necessitates annotated data, typically achieved through manual labeling of MS-related features or lesions in medical images. Annotating medical images involves the meticulous identification and marking of specific regions or abnormalities relevant to MS diagnosis. Manual labeling of MS-related features or lesions is performed by experts, such as radiologists or neurologists, who possess the necessary expertise to identify and delineate the relevant regions accurately [41]. These experts carefully examine the medical images, identify MS-specific characteristics, and mark the areas of interest. The annotations serve as ground truth labels that guide the deep learning model during the training process. However, manual labeling of medical images for MS detection can be a time-consuming and labor-intensive task. It requires significant expertise, attention to detail, and domain-specific knowledge. Moreover, due to the subjective nature of lesion identification, there can be inter-observer variability, where different experts may provide slightly different annotations for the same image. The process of manual labeling also poses challenges when dealing with large datasets. The sheer volume of data, especially in the case of MS detection, can make manual annotation impractical or infeasible within a reasonable timeframe. Efforts are being made to alleviate these challenges by developing semi-automated or automated annotation tools. These tools leverage computer algorithms and image processing techniques to assist experts in the annotation process, reducing the manual effort required while maintaining accuracy. Additionally, initiatives for building standardized annotation guidelines and promoting consensus among experts help minimize inter-observer variability. Automating the annotation process or improving the efficiency of manual annotation is crucial for enabling the training of deep learning models on larger

Table 2 Open-source MRI dataset for MS detection

Study	Dataset	Description
Muslim Ali [35]	Brain MRI Dataset of MS	Within this dataset, the creators furnish a fresh compilation of multi-sequence MRI data encompassing 60 individuals with MS. The dataset incorporates consensus-derived manual lesion segmentation, along with essential patient details, Expanded Disability Status Scale (EDSS) ratings, and clinical particulars
eHealthLab [36]	MRI Lesion Segmentation in MS Database	MS lesions from 38 subjects, manually segmented by an experienced MS neurologist, on transverse T2-weighted images obtained from serial brain MR imaging scans
Lmsls [37]	Longitudinal MS Lesion Segmentation Challenge	Longitudinal MS Lesion Segmentation
LabIT [38]	A Novel Public MRI of MS Patients	MR Image Dataset of Multiple Sclerosis Patients With Lesion Segmentations Based on Multi-rater Consensus
[39]	Brain Web	SBD includes a collection of authentic MRI data volumes generated through an MRI simulator
[40]	UMCL	The UMCL's 3D MR image database for MS patients contains accurately segmented MR images identifying WMHs using a consensus and ground truth method

datasets and reducing the burden on experts. This, in turn, can enhance the development of robust and accurate algorithms for MS detection, facilitating early diagnosis and improving patient outcomes. The process of annotating large amounts of data can be time-consuming and subjective, leading to inter-observer variability and potential inconsistencies in the labeled data.

(C) Interpretability and explainability: The complex architectures of deep learning models often lead to their perception as opaque systems or black boxes. Understanding how and why a model makes certain predictions in MS detection can be challenging, limiting the ability of clinicians to trust and interpret the model's decisions. Gaining a comprehensive understanding of how and why a deep learning model makes specific predictions in the context of MS detection can be challenging. The inherent complexity of deep learning models, characterized by their intricate architectures and millions of interconnected parameters, often makes it difficult to interpret their decision-making process.

Deep learning models for MS detection are trained to recognize intricate patterns and relationships in medical images or other input data. They learn these patterns through an iterative optimization process, adjusting their parameters based on labeled training examples [42]. However, the inner workings of the model, the specific features it uses for prediction, and the reasoning behind its decisions are not readily transparent or easily explainable. This lack of transparency and interpretability raises concerns for clinicians and healthcare professionals who need to trust and interpret the model's decisions in a clinical setting. Understanding why a model arrives at a certain prediction is crucial for clinicians to have confidence in its recommendations and to effectively incorporate the model's outputs into their decision-making process. Without a clear understanding of the rationale behind the model's predictions, clinicians may hesitate to fully rely on the model's output, particularly when important clinical decisions are at stake. They may find it challenging to interpret the model's decisions in the context of individual patients, leading to a potential lack of trust and limited adoption of deep learning models in clinical practice.

Addressing this challenge, researchers are exploring methods such as attention mechanisms, feature visualization, and model-agnostic interpretability techniques to shed light on the salient features and reasoning process of the model. Developing post-hoc explanation methods that can provide insights into the model's decision-making process without compromising its performance is an active area of research. Improving the interpretability of deep learning models in MS detection not only builds trust between clinicians and the models but also enables more informed decision-making, facilitates knowledge transfer, and enhances the overall adoption and acceptance of these models in clinical practice.

(D) Limited generalization: Deep learning models that have been trained on specific datasets might encounter challenges in effectively generalizing to novel, unseen data. Variations in imaging protocols, equipment, or patient populations can affect the model's performance, making it important to validate and fine-tune models on diverse datasets to ensure robustness. Deep learning models trained on specific datasets often face challenges when it comes to generalizing their learned knowledge to new, unseen data. While these models can achieve remarkable performance on the training data they were exposed to, their ability to effectively handle novel examples or data from different sources is not guaranteed [43]. One of the primary factors of limited generalization capability is the presence of biases and peculiarities within the training dataset. If the training data is biased or does not adequately represent the true distribution of the target domain, the model may learn patterns or dependencies that are specific to the training data but do not hold in the broader context. Consequently, the model may struggle to make accurate predictions or exhibit unexpected behavior when faced with unseen data. Furthermore, variations in imaging protocols, equipment, or patient populations can impact the performance of deep learning models. These models rely on the assumption that the distribution of the training data aligns with the distribution of the target data they will encounter in real-world scenarios. However, if there are substantial differences between the training and target data, the model's performance may degrade significantly.

Addressing the challenge of generalization requires strategies to enhance the robustness and adaptability of deep learning models. Techniques such as data augmentation, transfer learning, and domain adaptation can help improve generalization by exposing the model to a more diverse range of examples and bridging the gap between the training and target domains. Regularization methods, such as dropout or weight decay, can also assist in reducing overfitting and promoting generalization. Additionally, continual model evaluation and validation on new datasets are crucial to monitor and assess the model's performance in real-world scenarios. Fine-tuning or retraining the model using new data from the target domain can help improve its generalization ability and ensure its reliability when deployed in practical settings. Overall, addressing the challenge of generalization is vital to ensure that deep learning models for tasks like MS detection can perform effectively and reliably on unseen data, enabling their broader applicability and usefulness in clinical practice.

(E) Lack of transparency in model decision-making: Deep learning models for MS detection often learn complex patterns and relationships in the data. However, the underlying decision-making process may not be transparent or easily interpretable, raising concerns about the potential biases or confounding factors the model might inadvertently learn from the training data. The opacity in the decision-making mechanism of deep learning models for detecting MS is a notable cause for concern. While these models are capable of learning complex patterns and relationships within the data, understanding how they arrive at specific predictions can be challenging and opaque.

Deep learning models are constructed with intricate architectures that consist of numerous interconnected layers and millions of parameters. They learn to make predictions by iteratively adjusting these parameters based on labeled training examples. However, this complexity often results in models that are considered "black boxes" since it can be difficult to discern the specific features or factors that contribute to their decisions. This lack of transparency raises valid concerns regarding potential biases or confounding factors that the model may inadvertently learn from the training data. If the training data contains biases, such as underrepresentation or overrepresentation of certain demographic groups or specific imaging characteristics, the model may make predictions based on these biases rather than the true underlying relationships. This can result in inaccurate or unfair predictions, exacerbating existing disparities in health care. Moreover, the lack of transparency hinders the interpretability of the model's decisions [44]. Clinicians and healthcare professionals need to understand the reasoning behind the model's predictions to trust and effectively utilize them in clinical practice. Without transparency, it becomes challenging to assess the reliability and robustness of the model's outputs, limiting its interpretability and hindering its adoption. Addressing the lack of transparency in model decision-making is an active area of research. Efforts are being made to develop methods and techniques that enhance the interpretability and explainability of deep learning models. These include approaches such as attention mechanisms, feature visualization, and model-agnostic interpretability methods. By providing insights into the salient features and decision processes of the model, these techniques aim to increase transparency and facilitate a better understanding of how the model arrives at its predictions. Transparency in model decision-making is crucial for ensuring the fairness, accountability, and trustworthiness of deep learning models in MS detection. By promoting transparency, biases and confounding factors can be identified and mitigated, facilitating the development of more reliable and unbiased models that can be effectively integrated into clinical practice.

(F) Integration into the clinical workflow: Incorporating deep learning models into the existing clinical workflow for MS detection poses logistical challenges. Integration may require specialized hardware, software, or expertise, and ensuring seamless integration without disrupting clinical operations can be complex. Incorporating deep learning models into the existing clinical workflow for MS detection introduces a set of logistical challenges. While deep learning models hold promise for improving diagnostic accuracy and efficiency, seamlessly integrating them into clinical practice requires careful consideration and adaptation. One significant challenge is the need for specialized hardware and software infrastructure to deploy and run deep learning models effectively. Deep learning models frequently necessitate significant computational resources, such as high-performance GPUs or dedicated hardware accelerators, to efficiently process medical images or data. Ensuring the availability and compatibility of such infrastructure within clinical settings can be a logistical hurdle. Moreover, integrating deep learning models into current clinical workflows may entail making modifications or additions to existing information systems. This encompasses ensuring compatibility with electronic health record (EHR) systems, picture archiving and communication systems (PACS), and other platforms for managing medical data. Establishing seamless interoperability and data exchange between these systems and the deep learning models can be complex and time-consuming. Moreover, the training and validation of deep learning models require access to large and diverse datasets. Acquiring and curating such datasets, which may involve data sharing agreements, privacy considerations, and compliance with regulatory frameworks, pose additional logistical challenges. Ensuring the availability of representative and high-quality data for model development and evaluation is crucial but can be resource-intensive and require collaboration among multiple institutions or research groups [45]. Training and updating deep learning models for MS detection also require expert involvement. Collaborating with clinicians, radiologists, or neurologists who possess domain expertise is essential to guide the development and validation process, ensure clinical relevance, and address any potential biases or limitations of the model. Facilitating effective communication and collaboration between data scientists and healthcare professionals can be challenging due to differences in terminology, workflow, and priorities. Finally, the incorporation of deep learning models into clinical practice necessitates thorough validation and adherence to regulatory standards. Demonstrating the safety, efficacy, and generalizability of the models through rigorous testing and validation studies is essential for gaining regulatory approvals and clinician acceptance.

Addressing these logistical challenges requires multidisciplinary collaboration and a systematic approach. It involves close coordination between data scientists, healthcare providers, and IT professionals to address hardware and software requirements, establish data governance frameworks, optimize model performance, and ensure seamless integration within the existing clinical workflow. By overcoming these logistical challenges, deep learning models for MS detection can potentially enhance diagnostic accuracy, efficiency, and patient care outcomes in clinical practice. However, careful planning, resource allocation, and effective collaboration are necessary to navigate these challenges and successfully integrate deep learning models into the clinical workflow.

(G) Ethical and privacy considerations: Deep learning models trained on medical data, including MS-related information, raise concerns regarding patient privacy and data security. Protecting patient confidentiality and complying with regulatory requirements while utilizing deep learning for MS detection is a critical challenge. Deep learning models trained on medical data, including information related to MS, raise significant concerns regarding patient privacy and data security. Protecting patient confidentiality and ensuring compliance with regulatory requirements are critical challenges that must be addressed when utilizing deep learning for MS detection. Medical data, including imaging scans, clinical records, and other patient-specific information, is highly sensitive and subject to strict privacy regulations. Deep learning models require access to such data to train and learn patterns that enable accurate MS detection. However, this access poses inherent risks to patient privacy if not handled with utmost care. One primary concern is the potential for unauthorized access or breaches of stored medical data. Deep learning models often require large datasets, which increases the amount of patient information stored and the potential attack surface for malicious actors. Enforcing strong security protocols such as encryption, access management, and secure data storage is essential to protect patient information from unauthorized entry and mitigate the chances of data breaches. Moreover, ensuring patient anonymity is vital when working with medical data. Personal identifiers such as names, addresses, and social security numbers must be appropriately de-identified or anonymized to protect patient privacy [46]. Striking a balance between preserving data utility for model training and removing identifying information is a delicate process that requires adherence to privacy regulations and ethical guidelines. To address these challenges, organizations and researchers must prioritize the implementation of robust privacy and security measures. This includes establishing secure data storage infrastructure, implementing strong access controls, conducting regular security audits, and adhering to privacy regulations and ethical guidelines. Additionally, employing privacy-preserving techniques, such as federated learning or differential privacy, can help minimize the risk of privacy breaches while training deep learning models. Collaboration between data scientists, healthcare providers, and legal experts is crucial in navigating the intricate landscape of patient privacy and data security. By prioritizing patient privacy and complying with regulatory requirements, deep learning models for MS detection can be developed and deployed responsibly, ensuring the protection of patient data and maintaining public trust in the healthcare system.

(H) Diagnosing MS poses difficulties since there are no definitive tests, symptoms, or physical findings for its confirmation. Nevertheless, the advent of deep learning models shows potential in accurately identifying MS and aiding clinicians in the diagnostic process. Traditional methods of diagnosing MS rely on a combination of clinical evaluation, patient history, neurological exams, and the exclusion of other possible causes. This diagnostic process can be time-consuming and subjective, leading to potential delays and misdiagnoses. AI, powered by DL and ML models, offers

a new approach to MS diagnosis. These models have the ability to learn from large datasets and identify complex patterns and relationships in medical images, clinical data, and other relevant information. By training on diverse and representative datasets, DL and ML models can potentially capture subtle indicators or patterns that are difficult for human observers to detect. By leveraging DL and ML models in MS diagnosis, clinicians can benefit from improved accuracy, efficiency, and consistency in identifying MS. These models can serve as decision support tools, assisting clinicians in their diagnostic process by providing additional insights and highlighting potential areas of concern. However, it's important to note that AI models should not replace the expertise and clinical judgment of healthcare professionals. Instead, they should be utilized as complementary tools to aid clinicians in their decision-making. Trained medical experts should always make the ultimate diagnosis and treatment choices through a thorough assessment of all accessible data.

In summary, while MS remains a challenging disease to diagnose, DL and ML models show promise in improving the accuracy and efficiency of MS identification. These AI tools have the potential to assist clinicians by providing valuable insights and aiding in the diagnostic process, ultimately leading to better patient outcomes. Ongoing research and development in this field hold great potential for advancing MS diagnosis and improving the lives of individuals affected by the disease.

Addressing these challenges is crucial to enhance the efficacy, reliability, and ethical implications of utilizing deep learning for MS detection and improve patient care outcomes (Fig. 3).

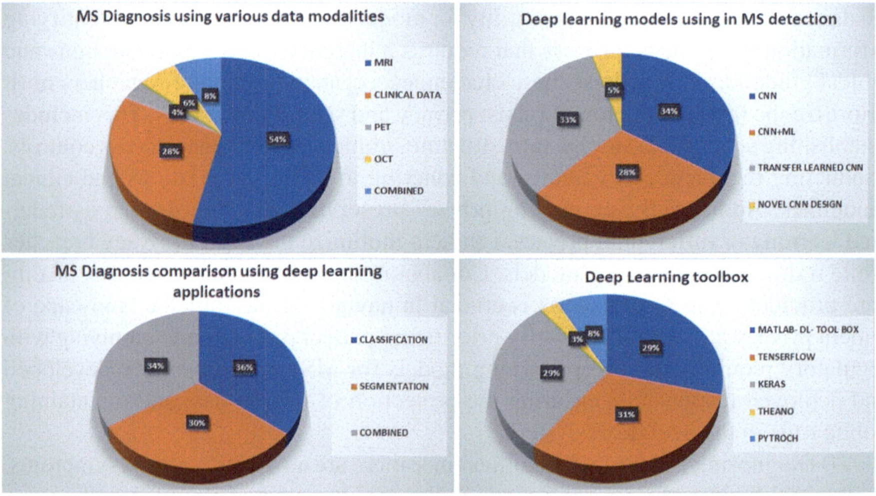

Fig. 3 Graphical summary of deep learning utilization in MS detection

4 Opportunities and Advancements in Deep Learning for Early MS Detection

Deep learning has introduced fresh possibilities and breakthroughs in the timely identification of MS. By harnessing the capabilities of deep neural networks and extensive data analysis, these techniques possess the ability to enhance the precision, swiftness, and effectiveness of early MS detection. Here are some key opportunities and advancements in this field:

(A) More Effective and Robust Algorithms: The utilization of AI-based methods in diagnosing MS is an area that hasn't been thoroughly explored, offering an exciting prospect for future research and development. While there's a shortage of research exploring AI's role in diagnosing MS, this absence of investigation presents encouraging avenues for crafting innovative and refined algorithms capable of enhancing the precision and effectiveness in detecting MS. The field of AI, particularly deep learning and machine learning, has demonstrated tremendous potential in various medical domains, including image analysis, pattern recognition, and predictive modeling [47]. This scarcity of research in AI-based MS diagnosis implies that there is a wealth of untapped potential for innovation and advancements in this field. Researchers have an opportunity to develop and refine algorithms tailored specifically to MS detection, leveraging the vast amount of available clinical, imaging, and genetic data. By designing new algorithms, researchers can aim to address the unique challenges associated with MS diagnosis, such as the lack of specific biomarkers and the complexity of disease manifestations. Moreover, the development of new algorithms can help overcome limitations in existing approaches and explore innovative ways to integrate different data modalities. For example, combining clinical data, imaging scans, genetic information, and other relevant variables can provide a more comprehensive and personalized view of MS, enabling earlier and more accurate diagnoses.

As researchers delve into this promising area, they can also focus on creating algorithms that are interpretable and transparent, enabling clinicians to understand and trust the reasoning behind AI-based MS diagnosis. This will be crucial for the successful integration of these algorithms into clinical practice, as it ensures that healthcare professionals can effectively utilize AI tools as decision support systems. To facilitate progress in this field, collaboration between researchers, clinicians, and data scientists is essential. By pooling expertise and resources, researchers can gather diverse datasets, establish robust evaluation frameworks, and validate the performance of AI-based algorithms for MS diagnosis. The limited number of studies on AI-based techniques for MS diagnosis presents an exciting opportunity for future research. By developing new and better algorithms specifically tailored to MS, researchers can contribute to improved diagnostic accuracy, early detection, and personalized treatment strategies. This area holds great potential for advancing MS care and ultimately improving the lives of individuals affected by the disease.

(B) Uncovering Novel Biomarkers with Deep Learning for Early MS Detection. Deep learning models have demonstrated the ability to uncover novel biomarkers by

mining complex patterns and relationships within diverse data sources. By analyzing various clinical and imaging data, these models can identify subtle indicators or combinations of features that may serve as early markers for MS. This holds tremendous potential for the development of predictive models that enable early detection and intervention. By training on diverse and representative datasets, deep learning models can learn intricate patterns and relationships that may be imperceptible to human observers. They can identify unique features or combinations of features across multiple data modalities, including clinical records, genetic information, and medical images such as MRI scans.

These deep learning models can capture and learn from complex interactions between clinical variables, imaging characteristics, and other relevant factors. They have the potential to identify early indicators or markers that correlate with the development or progression of MS. By recognizing these subtle patterns, deep learning models can contribute to the development of predictive models that enable early detection and intervention. Early detection of MS is crucial as it allows for timely intervention and treatment, potentially reducing the advancement of the disease and enhancing patient results. Deep learning models, with their ability to uncover novel biomarkers, have the potential to revolutionize the early detection process by providing clinicians with more accurate and reliable tools for MS diagnosis.

Molecular markers from affected individuals, such as cerebrospinal fluid (CSF) and blood tests, can play a crucial role in improving the accuracy and effectiveness of early detection models for MS. These markers can offer valuable insights into the biochemical changes that occur before the demyelination of myelinated neuron starts. Integrating molecular data into the training procedure can amplify the predictive capability of the models and potentially facilitate timelier and more precise MS diagnoses like Improved Sensitivity and Specificity, Individualized Diagnosis, Tracking Disease Progression, and Predicting Treatment Response [48]. However, it is important to note that the application of deep learning in uncovering biomarkers for MS is still an area of ongoing research and validation. Robust validation studies and collaboration between data scientists, clinicians, and researchers are necessary to ensure the clinical relevance and reliability of these identified biomarkers.

Deep learning models offer the ability to uncover novel biomarkers for early MS detection by mining complex patterns and relationships within diverse data sources. The development of predictive models based on these biomarkers has the potential to enable early intervention, improve diagnostic accuracy, and enhance patient outcomes. Continued research and validation efforts are necessary to fully harness the power of deep learning in identifying early markers for MS and realizing their clinical impact.

(C) Multimodal Data Integration: Deep learning has the remarkable capability to integrate multiple data modalities, such as clinical, genetic, and imaging data, to provide a more comprehensive and categorized understanding of MS. By combining these diverse sources of information, deep learning models can leverage the synergistic power of different data types, enhancing early detection accuracy and uncovering MS-related patterns that may not be readily apparent when analyzing individual data sources. MS is a complex disease with varied manifestations and underlying factors.

By integrating clinical data, which includes patient demographics, medical history, and symptoms, with genetic information and imaging scans such as magnetic resonance imaging (MRI), deep learning models can access a wealth of information. This multimodal integration enables a more holistic perspective on MS, allowing for a deeper understanding of the disease and its progression.

Clinical data provides essential context and background information about patients, such as risk factors, comorbidities, and disease history. Genetic data, on the other hand, can uncover genetic markers and variations that may predispose individuals to MS or influence disease progression. Imaging data reveals structural and functional changes in the brain and spinal cord, including the presence of lesions and abnormalities indicative of MS. Deep learning models can simultaneously analyze these diverse data modalities and learn complex relationships and patterns that exist among them. By fusing information from multiple sources, the models can uncover hidden connections and identify MS-related patterns that might not be evident when examining each data type independently. For example, a specific combination of clinical features, genetic markers, and imaging characteristics may be highly indicative of MS, providing valuable insights into early detection.

The integration of multiple data modalities in deep learning models not only enhances the accuracy of early MS detection but also contributes to a more personalized approach to disease management. By considering the unique characteristics and interactions among different data types, these models can tailor diagnostic and treatment strategies to individual patients, leading to more precise and effective interventions. However, it is important to note that the integration of multimodal data also presents challenges. Data quality, standardization, and interoperability across different sources must be carefully addressed to ensure reliable and meaningful integration. Furthermore, the interpretability and explainability of deep learning models when working with multiple data modalities are areas of ongoing research, as understanding the model's decision-making process is crucial for clinical adoption.

Deep learning's ability to integrate multiple data modalities empowers researchers and clinicians to gain a comprehensive view of MS. By leveraging the synergistic power of clinical, genetic, and imaging data, deep learning models can improve early detection accuracy and identify hidden patterns associated with MS. Continued research and collaboration between experts in various domains are essential to optimize the multimodal integration and unlock the full potential of deep learning in advancing our understanding and management of MS.

(D) Predictive Modeling: Deep learning models have the capacity to be trained on patient data, risk factors, and early indicators to predict the likelihood of developing MS. By analyzing a multitude of features and learning complex relationships within the data, these models can provide clinicians with valuable insights into the probability of MS development. This predictive capability facilitates early intervention and enables personalized treatment strategies. The ability to predict the likelihood of developing MS is of significant importance in clinical practice. Early detection and intervention can lead to timely and appropriate treatment, potentially slowing

down disease progression, minimizing long-term disability, and improving patient outcomes. Deep learning models offer a powerful tool to assist clinicians in this endeavor.

By training on large and diverse datasets that encompass patient demographics, medical history, genetic information, environmental factors, and other relevant variables, deep learning models can identify patterns and associations that contribute to MS development [49]. The models can analyze the complex interplay between these factors and identify early indicators that are often subtle and not easily detectable by conventional diagnostic methods. Deep learning models excel in capturing non-linear relationships and interactions within the data, allowing them to detect hidden patterns and predictive signals. They can learn from the vast number of features and their complex relationships, enabling the identification of risk factors and indicators that may not be apparent to human observers.

The predictive models developed through deep learning can offer clinicians valuable insights into the probability of MS development for individual patients. This information can aid in risk stratification, guiding decision-making regarding further diagnostic tests, monitoring strategies, and intervention plans. It allows for a proactive approach to patient care, facilitating early detection and personalized treatment strategies. Deep learning models possess the ability to forecast the probability of MS development using patient information, risk factors, and initial cues. By analyzing a multitude of features and learning complex relationships, these models provide clinicians with valuable insights into the probability of MS development. This facilitates early intervention, personalized treatment strategies, and improved patient outcomes. Continued research and validation efforts are vital to fully harness the potential of deep learning in predictive modeling for MS development.

(E) Data-driven Decision Support: Deep learning models can serve as decision support tools for healthcare professionals. By processing large amounts of data, these models can provide clinicians with evidence-based recommendations, assist in differential diagnosis, and suggest further diagnostic tests or interventions. This can enhance the efficiency and accuracy of early MS detection, leading to timely and targeted treatment plans.

(F) Real-time Monitoring: Deep learning models can analyze continuous data streams, such as wearable sensor data or electronic health records, to monitor disease progression and detect early signs of MS exacerbations. By leveraging temporal patterns and changes in patient data, these models can alert clinicians to potential relapses or disease progression, allowing for timely intervention and personalized care.

Overall, deep learning offers exciting opportunities for early MS detection, enabling more accurate and timely diagnosis, personalized treatment approaches, and improved patient outcomes. However, it is essential to validate and integrate these deep learning advancements into clinical practice through rigorous evaluation, collaboration between data scientists and clinicians, and adherence to ethical considerations and regulatory requirements.

5 Clinical Implications of Deep Learning-Based MS Diagnosis

Deep learning-based diagnosis has significant clinical implications for the detection and management of MS. The application of deep learning algorithms to MS diagnosis can provide clinicians with powerful tools to enhance accuracy, efficiency, and early detection, ultimately improving patient outcomes. One of the key clinical implications of deep learning-based MS diagnosis is increased diagnostic accuracy. Deep learning models can analyze diverse data sources, such as clinical records, medical images, genetic information, and other relevant variables, to identify subtle patterns and associations that may indicate the presence of MS. This improved accuracy can lead to earlier and more precise diagnoses, ensuring timely intervention and appropriate treatment strategies [50].

The efficiency and speed of deep learning-based diagnosis also have significant clinical implications. Deep learning models can process large volumes of data quickly and efficiently, enabling rapid analysis and interpretation of complex information. This can help reduce diagnostic delays and streamline the decision-making process, allowing clinicians to make informed decisions in a timely manner. Moreover, deep learning algorithms can assist in the integration of various data modalities. By combining clinical, genetic, and imaging data, deep learning models provide a more comprehensive view of MS, enabling a holistic approach to patient management. This integration of data modalities enhances the understanding of disease progression, individual variability, and treatment responses, leading to more personalized and targeted interventions. However, it is important to recognize that deep learning-based MS diagnosis is not meant to replace clinical expertise but rather to augment and support it. The role of deep learning algorithms is to provide clinicians with additional insights and decision support. Clinicians remain critical in interpreting the results, considering patient-specific factors, and making informed clinical judgments. Furthermore, the successful implementation of deep learning-based MS diagnosis requires addressing challenges such as model interpretability, data quality, privacy concerns, and regulatory compliance. Ensuring transparency, accountability, and ethical use of these algorithms is crucial for their clinical integration. Deep learning-based MS diagnosis offers numerous clinical implications, including improved diagnostic accuracy, identification of novel biomarkers, enhanced efficiency, and the integration of multiple data modalities. By harnessing the power of artificial intelligence, clinicians can benefit from more accurate and timely diagnoses, personalized treatment strategies, and ultimately improved patient care in the management of MS. Continued research, validation, and collaboration between data scientists and clinicians are essential to fully realize the clinical potential of deep learning in MS diagnosis.

6 Future Directions and Research Opportunities on Deep Learning for MS Detection

The application of deep learning in MS detection has shown promising results, but there are still numerous future directions and research opportunities that can further enhance its effectiveness and clinical impact. Here are some key areas for future exploration:

Improved interpretability and explainability: Deep learning models are commonly perceived as opaque, which poses difficulties in comprehending the underlying process of decision-making. Subsequent research efforts could concentrate on devising approaches to improve the interpretability and explainability of deep learning models specifically in the context of MS detection. Such endeavors would assist clinicians in developing confidence in the models and offer valuable insights into the characteristics and patterns that contribute to the model's predictions. Addressing data limitations: Deep learning models require large and diverse datasets for training. However, obtaining such datasets for MS detection can be challenging due to the scarcity of annotated data. Future research can explore techniques for data augmentation, transfer learning, and domain adaptation to mitigate the limitations of limited datasets and enhance the generalizability of deep learning models.

Multimodal fusion and integration: Integrating multiple data modalities, including clinical, imaging, genetic, and omics data, can provide a more comprehensive understanding of MS. Future research can focus on developing advanced techniques for multimodal fusion and integration, leveraging the synergistic power of different data types to improve diagnostic accuracy, identify novel biomarkers, and enable personalized treatment approaches. Longitudinal modeling and disease progression: MS is a chronic and progressive disease. Deep learning models can be leveraged to capture disease progression patterns and predict the course of the disease over time. Future research can explore longitudinal modeling techniques that incorporate temporal information and enable accurate predictions of disease progression, treatment response, and long-term outcomes.

Collaborative and multicenter studies: Collaborative efforts and multicenter studies can facilitate the pooling of large-scale datasets, allowing for the development of more robust and generalizable deep learning models for MS detection. Collaborations between institutions, researchers, and clinicians can also foster the sharing of expertise, knowledge, and best practices, accelerating advancements in the field. Clinical validation and real-world deployment: While deep learning models show promise in MS detection, their clinical validation and real-world deployment are crucial for widespread adoption. Future research should focus on conducting rigorous validation studies using diverse patient populations and comparing the performance of deep learning models against standard diagnostic methods. Additionally, investigating the integration of deep learning models into the existing clinical workflow and evaluating their impact on clinical decision-making and patient outcomes will be essential. Ethical considerations and bias mitigation: Deep learning models should be developed and deployed in a manner that addresses ethical considerations, such as patient privacy, data security, and fairness. Research should explore methods for mitigating biases and ensuring the equitable and unbiased performance of deep learning models across diverse populations.

In summary, future directions in deep learning for MS detection encompass improving interpretability, addressing data limitations, integrating multiple data modalities, modeling disease progression, promoting collaborative studies, validating models in clinical settings, and addressing ethical considerations. Advancements in these areas have the potential to further enhance the accuracy, reliability, and clinical utility of deep learning models in MS detection, ultimately benefiting both patients and clinicians in the fight against this complex disease.

7 Conclusion

This study brings to the forefront the potential of employing deep learning techniques, particularly CNNs, for the early detection of MS. By examining medical imaging data like magnetic resonance imaging (MRI), deep learning models have the capability to recognize patterns and features specific to MS, which can serve as early indicators of the disease's onset. However, several challenges need to be addressed to fully leverage deep learning for MS diagnosis, including the need for large annotated datasets, interpretability of models, and integration of multimodal data sources. The study emphasizes the importance of overcoming these challenges to ensure the generalizability and robustness of deep learning models across diverse patient populations and imaging protocols. It also highlights opportunities for advancements in deep learning approaches, such as transfer learning, data augmentation, and ensemble methods. Furthermore, integrating deep learning with other imaging modalities holds promise for enhancing diagnostic accuracy and sensitivity.

Importantly, the potential clinical implications of deep learning-based MS diagnosis are discussed, including improved early intervention, personalized treatment plans, and disease progression monitoring. The research discoveries subsidize a comprehensive understanding of the opportunities and challenges in utilizing deep learning for early detection of MS.

Through the creation of diagnostic tools that are both more precise and efficient, this research has the potential to significantly impact patient outcomes and advance the field of MS diagnosis and management. Further research and collaboration between clinicians and data scientists are essential to translate these findings into clinical practice, ensuring the safe and effective implementation of deep learning techniques for MS detection. Ultimately, the application of deep learning in MS diagnosis has the potential to improve patient care, enhance treatment strategies, and contribute to the ongoing fight against this complex autoimmune disease.

References

1. Klawiter EC (2013) Current and new directions in MRI in multiple sclerosis. Continuum (Minneap Minn). 2013 Aug; 19(4 Multiple Sclerosis):1058-73. https://doi.org/10.1212/01.CON.0000433283.00221.37. PMID: 23917101; PMCID: PMC4234130
2. Trip SA, Miller DH (2005) Imaging in multiple sclerosis. J Neurol, Neurosurg Psychiatry 76:iii11–iii18
3. Filippi M, Others (2019) Assessment of lesions on magnetic resonance imaging in multiple sclerosis: practical guidelines. Brain 142(7):1858–1875 (2019). https://doi.org/10.1093/brain/awz144
4. Siger M (2022) Magnetic resonance imaging in primary progressive multiple sclerosis patients. Clin Neuroradiol 32:625–641. https://doi.org/10.1007/s00062-022-01144-3
5. Moazami F, Lefevre-Utile A, Papaloukas C, Soumelis V (2021) Machine learning approaches in study of multiple sclerosis disease through magnetic resonance images. Front Immunol 12:700582. https://doi.org/10.3389/fimmu.2021.700582. PMID: 34456913; PMCID: PMC8385534
6. Forghani R, Savadjiev P, Chatterjee A, Muthukrishnan N, Reinhold C, Forghani B (2019) Radiomics and artificial intelligence for biomarker and prediction model development in oncology. Comput Struct Biotechnol J 17:995–1008. https://doi.org/10.1016/j.csbj.2019.07.001. PMID: 31388413; PMCID: PMC6667772
7. Ahmed Z, Mohamed K, Zeeshan S, Dong X (2020) Artificial intelligence with multi-functional machine learning platform development for better healthcare and precision medicine. Database (Oxford) 2020:baaa010. https://doi.org/10.1093/database/baaa010. PMID: 32185396; PMCID: PMC7078068
8. Mohammed Aarif KO, Mohamed Yousuff C, Mohammed Hashim BA, Mohamed Hashim C, Sivakumar P (2022) Smart bin: waste segregation system using deep learning-Internet of Things for sustainable smart cities. Concurrency Comput: Pract Exper 34(28):e7378
9. Mohamed Aarif KO, Sivakumar P, Mohamed Yousuff C, Mohammed Hashim BA (2021) Deep MammoNet: early diagnosis of breast cancer using multi-layer hierarchical features of deep transfer learned convolutional neural network. Advanced machine learning approaches in cancer prognosis: challenges and applications. Springer International Publishing, Cham, pp 317–339
10. Eshaghi A, Young AL, Wijeratne PA, Prados F, Arnold DL, Narayanan S, Ciccarelli O (2021) Identifying multiple sclerosis subtypes using unsupervised machine learning and MRI data. Nature Commun 12(1):2078
11. Narayana PA, Coronado I, Sujit SJ, Wolinsky JS, Lublin FD, Gabr RE (2020) Deep learning for predicting enhancing lesions in multiple sclerosis from noncontrast MRI. Radiology 294:398–404. https://doi.org/10.1148/radiol.2019191061
12. Gros C, De Leener B, Badji A, Maranzano J, Eden D, Dupont SM, Talbott J, Zhuoquiong R, Liu Y, Granberg T, Ouellette R Charley A, Gros C, De Leener B, Badji A, Maranzano J, Eden D, Dupont SM, Talbott J, Zhuoquiong R, Liu Y, Granberg T, Ouellette R, Tachibana Y, Hori M, Kamiya K, Chougar L, Stawiarz L, Hillert J, Bannier E, Kerbrat A, Julien GE (2019) Cohen-Adad utomatic segmentation of the spinal cord and intramedullary multiple sclerosis lesions with convolutional neural networks. NeuroImage 184:901–915. ISSN 1053-8119. https://doi.org/10.1016/j.neuroimage.2018.09.081
13. Montolío A, Martín-Gallego A, Cegoñino J, Orduna E, Vilades E, Garcia-Martin E, Palomar APD. Machine learning in diagnosis and disability prediction of multiple sclerosis using optical coherence tomography. Comput Biol Med 133:104416. https://doi.org/10.1016/j.compbiomed.2021.104416. Epub 2021 Apr 26. PMID: 33946022
14. Casalino G, Castellano G, Consiglio A et al (2021) MicroRNA expression classification for pediatric multiple sclerosis identification. J Ambient Intell Human Comput. https://doi.org/10.1007/s12652-021-03091-2
15. Schwab P, Karlen W (2020) A deep learning approach to diagnosing multiple sclerosis from smartphone data. IEEE J Biomed Health Inform 25:1284–1291

16. La Rosa F et al (2018) Shallow vs deep learning architectures for white matter lesion segmentation in the early stages of multiple sclerosis. BrainLes@MICCAI (2018)
17. Eitel F, Soehler E, Bellmann-Strobl J, Brandt AU, Ruprecht K, Giess RM, Kuchling J, Asseyer S, Weygandt M, Haynes JD, Scheel M, Paul F, Ritter K (2019) Uncovering convolutional neural network decisions for diagnosing multiple sclerosis on conventional MRI using layer-wise relevance propagation. NeuroImage: Clin 24:102003. ISSN 2213-1582. https://doi.org/10.1016/j.nicl.2019.102003
18. Krishnan AP, Song Z, Clayton D et al (2023) Multi-arm U-Net with dense input and skip connectivity for T2 lesion segmentation in clinical trials of multiple sclerosis. Sci Rep 13:4102. https://doi.org/10.1038/s41598-023-31207-5
19. Commowick O, Combès B, Cervenansky F, Dojat M (2023) Editorial: Automatic methods for multiple sclerosis new lesions detection and segmentation. Front Neurosci 17:1176625. https://doi.org/10.3389/fnins.2023.1176625
20. Sepahvand NM, Arnold DL, Arbel T (2020) CNN detection of new and enlarging multiple sclerosis lesions from longitudinal Mri using subtraction images. In: Proceedings of the international symposium on biomedical imaging, Iowa City, IA, USA, 4 April 2020
21. Yılmaz Acar Y, Bąşçiftçi F, Ekmekci AH, (2022) A convolutional neural network model for identifying multiple sclerosis on brain FLAIR MRI. Sustain Comput Inform Syst 35:100706
22. La Rosa F, Beck ES, Maranzano J, Todea RA, van Gelderen P, de Zwart JA, Luciano NJ, Duyn JH, Thiran JP, Granziera C et al (2022) Multiple sclerosis cortical lesion detection with deep learning at ultra-high-field MRI. NMR Biomed 35:e4730
23. Shmueli OZ, Solomon C, Ben-Eliezer N, Greenspan H (2022) Deep learning based multiple sclerosis lesion detection utilizing synthetic data generation and soft attention mechanism. In: Proceedings of the medical imaging 2022: computer-aided diagnosis, San Diego, CA, USA, 20 February–28 March 2022; vol. 12033, p 120330R
24. López-Dorado A, Ortiz M, Satue M, Rodrigo MJ, Barea R, Sánchez-Morla EM, Cavaliere C, Rodríguez-Ascariz JM, Orduna-Hospital E, Boquete L et al (2022) Early diagnosis of multiple sclerosis using swept-source optical coherence tomography and convolutional neural networks trained with data augmentation. Sensors 22:167
25. Aslani S, Murino V, Dayan M, Tam R, Sona D, Hamarneh G (2020) Scanner invariant multiple sclerosis lesion segmentation from MRI. In: 2020 IEEE 17th international symposium on biomedical imaging (ISBI). IEEE, pp 781–785
26. Afzal HM, Luo S, Ramadan S, Lechner-Scott J, Amin MR, Li J, Afzal MK (2021) Automatic and robust segmentation of multiple sclerosis lesions with convolutional neural networks. CMC Comput Mater Contin 66(1):977–991
27. McKinley R, Wepfer R, Aschwanden F, Grunder L, Muri R, Rummel C, Wiest R (2021) Simultaneous lesion and brain segmentation in multiple sclerosis using deep neural networks. Sci Rep 11(1):1–11
28. Kang G, Hou B, Ma Y, Labeau F, Su Z (2020) Acu-Net: a 3D attention context U-net for multiple sclerosis lesion segmentation. In ICASSP 2020-2020 IEEE international conference on acoustics, speech and signal processing (ICASSP). IEEE, pp 1384–1388
29. Gabr RE, Coronado I, Robinson M, Sujit SJ, Datta S, Sun X, Narayana PA (2020) Brain and lesion segmentation in multiple sclerosis using fully convolutional neural networks: a large-scale study. Multiple Scleros J 26(10):1217–1226
30. Yildirim MS, Dandil E (2021) DeepMSWeb: a web-based decision support system via deep learning for automatic detection of MS lesions. In: 2nd international informatics and software engineering conference (IISEC). Ankara, Turkey 2021, pp 1–6. https://doi.org/10.1109/IISEC54230.2021.9672360
31. Yıldırım MS, Dandıl E (2021) Automated multiple sclerosis lesion segmentation on MR images via mask R-CNN. In: 5th international symposium on multidisciplinary studies and innovative technologies (ISMSIT). Ankara, Turkey 2021, pp 570–577. https://doi.org/10.1109/ISMSIT52890.2021.9604593
32. Creagh AP, Dondelinger F, Lipsmeier F, Lindemann M, De Vos M (2022) Longitudinal trend monitoring of multiple sclerosis ambulation using smartphones. IEEE Open J Engin Med Biol 3:202–210. https://doi.org/10.1109/OJEMB.2022.3221306

33. Salem M et al (2019) Multiple sclerosis lesion synthesis in MRI using an encoder-decoder U-NET. IEEE Access 7:25171–25184. https://doi.org/10.1109/ACCESS.2019.2900198
34. Hashemi SR, Mohseni Salehi SS, Erdogmus D, Prabhu SP, Warfield SK, Gholipour A (2019) Asymmetric loss functions and deep densely-connected networks for highly-imbalanced medical image segmentation: application to multiple sclerosis lesion detection. IEEE Access 7:1721–1735. https://doi.org/10.1109/ACCESS.2018.2886371
35. Muslim AM (2022) Brain MRI dataset of multiple sclerosis with consensus manual lesion segmentation and patient meta information. Mendeley Data V1. https://doi.org/10.17632/8bctsm8jz7.1
36. Dataset. https://www.medinfo.cs.ucy.ac.cy/old/doc/Publications/Datasets/MRIFreeDataset.zip
37. Carass A et al (2017) Longitudinal multiple sclerosis lesion segmentation: resource and challenge. Neuroimage 148:77–102. https://doi.org/10.1016/j.neuroimage.2016.12.064
38. Lesjak Ž, Galimzianova A, Koren A, Lukin M, Pernuš F, Likar B, Špiclin Ž (2018) A novel public MR image dataset of multiple sclerosis patients with lesion segmentations based on multi-rater consensus. Neuroinformatics 16(1):51–63. https://doi.org/10.1007/s12021-017-9348-7. PMID: 29103086
39. Merzoug A, Benamrane N, Taleb-Ahmed A (2021) Lesions detection of multiple sclerosis in 3D brian MR images by using artificial immune systems and support vector machines. Int J Cogn Inform Nat Intell 15:97–110
40. Ucml laboratory of imaging technologies 3d Mr image database of multiple sclerosis patients with white matter lesion segmentations. http://lit.fe.uni-lj.si/tools.php?lang=eng. (Accessed: 20 October 2020)
41. Kwan RK-S, Evans AC, Pike GB (1996) An extensible MRI simulator for post-processing evaluation" visualization in biomedical computing (VBC'96). Lecture notes in computer science, vol 1131. Springer, pp 135–140
42. Kazancli E, Prchkovska V, Rodrigues P, Villoslada P, Igual L (2018) Multiple sclerosis lesion segmentation using improved convolutional neural networks. In: VISIGRAPP (4: VISAPP) (Portugal), pp 260–269. https://doi.org/10.5220/0006540902600269
43. Lublin FD, Reingold SC (1996) Defining the clinical course of multiple sclerosis: results of an international survey. National multiple sclerosis society (USA) advisory committee on clinical trials of new agents in multiple sclerosis. Neurology 46(4):907–911. https://doi.org/10.1212/wnl.46.4.907
44. Roca P, Attye A, Colas L, Tucholka A, Rubini P, Cackowski S, et al (2020) OFSEP investigators; steering committee; investigators; imaging group. Artificial intelligence to predict clinical disability in patients with multiple sclerosis using FLAIR MRI. Diagn Interv Imaging 101(12):795–802. https://doi.org/10.1016/j.diii.2020.05.009
45. Zhao WJ, Fu LR, Huang ZM, Zhu JQ, Ma BY (2019) Effectiveness evaluation of computer-aided diagnosis system for the diagnosis of thyroid nodules on ultrasound: A systematic review and meta-analysis. Medicine 98:e16379
46. Zhan A et al (2018) Using smartphones and machine learning to quantify Parkinson disease severity: the mobile Parkinson disease score. JAMA Neurol 75:876–880
47. Ronneberger O, Fischer P, Brox T (2015) U-Net: convolutional networks for biomedical image segmentation. In: Navab N, Hornegger J, Wells W, Frangi A (eds) Medical image computing and computer assisted intervention - MICCAI 2015. Springer, Cham. https://doi.org/10.1007/978-3-319-24574-428
48. Ziemssen T, Akgün K, Brück W (2019) Molecular biomarkers in multiple sclerosis. J Neuroinflammat 16:272. https://doi.org/10.1186/s12974-019-1674-2
49. Shanmuganathan M, Almutairi S, Aborokbah MM, Ganesan S, Ramachandran V (2020) Review of advanced computational approaches on multiple sclerosis segmentation and classification. IET Signal Process. 14:333–341. https://doi.org/10.1049/iet-spr.2019.0543
50. Danelakis A, Theoharis T, Verganelakis DA (2018) Survey of automated multiple sclerosis lesion segmentation techniques on magnetic resonance imaging. Comput Med Imaging Graph 70:83–100. https://doi.org/10.1016/j.compmedimag.2018.10.002

AI-Assisted Model for Risk Detection of Autoimmune Diseases

R. S. M. Lakshmi Patibandla, B. Tarakeswara Rao, and M. Ramakrishna Murthy

Abstract In autoimmune disorders, your immune system attacks your body. Included in this category are rheumatoid arthritis, Crohn's disease, and a few thyroid diseases. Typically, the immune system defends against pathogens and viruses. As soon as it detects these unfamiliar intruders, it dispatches a group of fighter cells to absorb them. It takes expertise and can be subjective in a medical setting to observe the slight variations in the disease's site of inflammation. In this situation, it would be quite helpful and helpful to the doctors if a model could be created to score the severity of the sickness. Deep learning and machine learning are two AI techniques that are increasingly active in computer-aided design systems. These systems help experts diagnose patients by assisting in the detection of irregularities in medical images. The severity of autoimmune diseases is still unknown, despite the popularity of AI-assisted techniques like Deep Learning and other intelligent methods in the detection of various diseases, and more specifically in the grading and classification of the types as well as symptoms of autoimmune diseases like Type 1 diabetes, psoriasis/psoriatic arthritis, etc. This chapter presents a revolutionary AI-assisted model for rating the severity of autoimmune illnesses to lower the danger of people being attacked.

Keywords Autoimmune diseases · Deep learning · Medical images

R. S. M. Lakshmi Patibandla (✉)
Koneru Lakshmaiah Education Foundation (Deemed to be University), Guntur, Andhra Pradesh, India
e-mail: patibandla.lakshmi@gmail.com

B. Tarakeswara Rao
Kallam Haranadhareddy Institute of Technology, Guntur, Andhra Pradesh, India

M. Ramakrishna Murthy
Anil Neerukonda Institute of Technology and Sciences, Visakhapatnam, Andhra Pradesh, India

K. Raza and S. Singh (eds.), *Artificial Intelligence and Autoimmune Diseases*, Studies in Computational Intelligence 1133, https://doi.org/10.1007/978-981-99-9029-0_9

List of Abbreviations

AI	Artificial Intelligence
AI-AM	AI-assisted Model
ATD	Autoimmune Thyroid Disease
DT	Decision Tree
ML	Machine Learning
NLP	Natural Language Processing
Prxs	Peroxiredoxins
RF	Random Forest
SVM	Support Vector Machine
T1D	Type 1 Diabetes

1 Introduction

The immune system affects healthy cells and tissues within the body, resulting in chronic inflammation and tissue injury. Early detection is essential to prevent long-term damage and enhance patient outcomes for these diseases, which can be challenging to diagnose and treat. To aid in the exposure and identification of autoimmune diseases, AI-based assisted models can be used [1, 2]. These models use machine-learning algorithms to explore huge extents of patient data, including medicinal histories, lab results, and imaging studies. By identifying patterns and correlations in this data, the AI model can assist healthcare professionals in making accurate diagnoses and developing effective treatment plans. One important aspect of AI-based assisted models for autoimmune disease detection is the ability to identify risk factors for these diseases. By analyzing patient data, the model can identify common risk factors such as genetic predisposition, environmental factors, and lifestyle choices that can increase the likelihood of developing an autoimmune disease [3].

Generally, the use of AI-based assisted models for autoimmune disease exposure has the imminent to mend patient consequences by assisting former verdicts and further targeted action plans. However, it is important to note that these models have to be used in coincidence by clinical capability and patient input to ensure the best possible outcomes [4, 5]. A risk detection AI-based assisted model for autoimmune diseases uses machine learning (ML) algorithms to scrutinize patient statistics and ascertain potential risk aspects for developing autoimmune disorders. The model is trained using large datasets of patient information, including medical history, genetic markers, environmental exposures, and lifestyle factors.

The ML systems can then isolate contours and correlations within the data to identify risk factors that may be associated with developing autoimmune diseases [6]. This can help healthcare professionals make more accurate diagnoses and develop targeted treatment plans for patients at high risk of developing autoimmune diseases. The AI-based model can also be used to monitor patients with autoimmune diseases and identify potential complications or disease progression [7]. By exploring patient statistics concluded stage, the model can detect changes in disease activity and predict future outcomes, enabling healthcare professionals to make more informed decisions about treatment options and disease management.

In recent years, the rapid advancements in AI and ML, particularly Deep Learning, have revolutionized various fields of medicine, including the diagnosis and management of complex conditions such as autoimmune diseases. AI-driven models have exhibited remarkable potential in deciphering intricate patterns within medical data and providing valuable insights that were previously inaccessible. Specifically, in the context of autoimmune diseases, AI models are being harnessed to uncover hidden correlations in large-scale datasets, enabling early detection, personalized treatment recommendations, and a deeper understanding of the underlying immunological mechanisms. This paper explores the application of AI, ML, and Deep Learning models in the realm of autoimmune diseases, highlighting their transformative role in improving diagnosis accuracy, treatment strategies, and ultimately, patient outcomes. A risk detection AI-assisted model for autoimmune diseases has the potential to enhance patient outcomes by facilitating earlier diagnosis and more targeted treatment plans. It is essential to note, however, that these models are not a substitute for clinical expertise and should be used in conjunction with patient input to ensure the most accurate conclusions.

2 Literature Survey

The paper by Valeria Calcaterra et al. [1] directed an efficient analysis of the existing works on Autoimmune Thyroid Diseases (ATDs) and then gut microbiota, focusing on studies conducted in pediatric populations. The review included studies that investigated the composition and diversity of gut microbiota in children with ATDs, as well as studies that explored the potential effects of probiotics on thyroid function and autoimmunity. The authors used a comprehensive search strategy to identify relevant studies, which were then assessed for eligibility and quality. The included studies were then analyzed to identify common themes and trends related to the relationship between gut microbiota and ATDs in children.

The authors found that it is an evolving indication to advise that gut microbiota dysbiosis might show a starring role in the expansion and progression of ATDs in children. Specifically, they found that children with ATDs tend to have lower diversity and altered composition of gut microbiota compared to healthy children. Additionally, they found that probiotics might have a beneficial effect on thyroid function and autoimmunity in children with ATDs, although extra exploration is desired to endorse these conclusions. This study concludes that additional research is required to better understand the association between gut microbiota and ATDs in children and to investigate the potential function of probiotics in the management of these conditions. More research is needed to determine the optimal dose, duration, and type of probiotic for this population [8].

They discovered that dysbiosis of the gastrointestinal microbiota may contribute to the development and progression of ATDs in children. It was discovered that probiotics, particularly Lactobacillus and Bifidobacterium strains, may have a beneficial influence on thyroid function and autoimmunity in children with ATDs. To determine the optimal dose, duration, and type of probiotic for this population, however, additional research is necessary. Overall, the review indicates that probiotics may provide a safe and effective adjunctive therapy for children with ATDs; however, additional research is required to confirm the results [9].

There are several limitations to Valeria Calcaterra et al.'s review. Firstly, most of the studies included in the review were conducted on adults, and there is limited research on the relationship between gut microbiota and ATDs specifically in children. Secondly, the studies reviewed had varying methodologies, making it difficult to draw definitive conclusions. Thirdly, the optimal dose, duration, and type of probiotic for the management of ATDs in children are not yet clear, and more research is needed to determine this. Fourthly, the studies included in the review used different criteria for defining ATDs, which could have affected the consistency of the findings. Lastly, the review only included studies published in English, which could have resulted in important studies being excluded.

Fuli Zhou et al.'s [4] article is a review that aims to summarize the recent consideration of the functions of peroxiredoxins (Prxs) in various autoimmune illnesses. They included articles published from 2000 to 2022 that investigated the roles of Prxs in autoimmune diseases. The authors then critically evaluated the articles and summarized their findings. The review covers several autoimmune illnesses amongst others. The authors also discuss the potential therapeutic applications of targeting Prxs in the management of autoimmune diseases.

In their review, Fuli Zhou et al. provide evidence that peroxiredoxins (Prxs) play vital parts in the pathogenesis of various autoimmune diseases. Prxs are antioxidant enzymes that normalize the intracellular redox balance and are elaborate in numerous cellular manners, comprising explosion, differentiation, and apoptosis. The authors found that the expression levels of Prxs are dysregulated in autoimmune diseases and that this dysregulation contributes to the progress and evolution of these syndromes [10]. For example, in rheumatoid arthritis, Prx2 and Prx4 are overexpressed and promote inflammation and joint destruction. In multiple sclerosis, Prx1 is involved in oligodendrocyte cell death and demyelination. The authors also discuss the potential therapeutic applications of targeting Prxs in the management of autoimmune diseases. For example, inhibiting Prx activity could reduce inflammation and tissue damage in rheumatoid arthritis. The authors conclude that auxiliary exploration is desired to fully understand the measures of Prxs in autoimmune diseases and to develop effective therapeutic strategies targeting Prxs [11–15].

One potential limitation of the review by Fuli Zhou et al. is that it primarily focuses on the roles of Prxs in a limited number of autoimmune diseases, such as rheumatoid arthritis and multiple sclerosis, and may not fully reflect the roles of Prxs in other autoimmune diseases. Additionally, while the authors discuss potential therapeutic applications of targeting Prxs in autoimmune diseases, they do not provide a detailed discussion of the potential side effects or safety concerns associated with Prx-targeted therapies. Furthermore, the review focuses mainly on the dysregulation of Prxs in autoimmune diseases and may not provide a comprehensive understanding of the complex mechanisms underlying the development and progression of these diseases. Finally, the authors primarily rely on studies conducted in animal models or cell cultures, and extra investigation is required to confirm the relevance of these findings to human autoimmune diseases [16].

The article by Cheryl F. Lichti and Xiaoxiao Wan [17] describes the use of mass spectrometry to classify neoantigens in autoimmune diseases, with a specific focus on type 1 diabetes as an example. The authors afford a detailed synopsis of the mass spectrometry methodology used to identify neoantigens, including sample preparation, protein extraction, digestion, and peptide analysis. They also discuss the challenges associated with identifying neoantigens, such as the low abundance of these antigens in samples and the difficulty of distinguishing them from self-antigens. To illustrate the utility of mass spectrometry in identifying neoantigens, the authors provide examples of studies in which this approach has been used to identify potential neoantigens in type 1 diabetes. They discuss the potential clinical implications of these findings, such as the development of personalized immunotherapies based on the specific neoantigens identified in individual patients.

Generally, the methodology presented in this article involves a comprehensive approach to mass spectrometry analysis for the identification of neoantigens in autoimmune diseases, with a precise emphasis on type 1 diabetes. The authors also provide insights into the challenges and potential clinical implications of using this approach. In their paper, discussed the use with a focus on type 1 diabetes (T1D). They explained that neoantigens are proteins that are not present in healthy cells but are generated by mutations, post-translational modifications, or other mechanisms. These neoantigens can be recognized by the immune system as foreign, leading to autoimmune responses. Several studies, including one that revealed new antigens also discussed the challenges associated with identifying neoantigens using mass spectrometry, such as the need for high-quality samples and the complexity of the data analysis [17].

Generally, Lichti and Wan [17] argued that mass spectrometry is a promising approach for identifying neoantigens in autoimmune diseases, including T1D, and that this approach can lead to the development of new diagnostic and relaxing policies. They suggested that future studies should focus on improving the sensitivity and specificity of mass spectrometry-based methods, as well as on validating the identified neoantigens in large patient cohorts.

The limitations of the study by Lichti and Wan [17] are not explicitly stated in the chapter. However, there are some potential limitations of expanding mass spectrometry to detect neoantigens in autoimmune diseases, which could apply to this study. One limitation is the availability of suitable samples for analysis, as high-quality tissue or cell samples may not always be accessible. Another limitation is the complexity of the data analysis required, as mass spectrometry generates huge expanses of data that are essential to be carefully explored and interpreted. Additionally, there may be technical limitations, such as issues with the sensitivity and specificity of the mass spectrometry equipment used. Moreover, the identification of neoantigens by mass spectrometry requires a comparison of the patient's peptides with healthy control tissues or cells, which may not be feasible in all cases, especially for rare diseases or diseases with no known healthy tissue or cells for comparison. Furthermore, the study focuses on neoantigens in T1D, and it is not clear whether the results could be generalized to other autoimmune diseases [18–22].

3 Methodologies

Various AI-based methodologies can be employed for risk detection and prediction of autoimmune diseases. One approach is to use ML algorithms to analyze large datasets of clinical and genetic data from patients with autoimmune diseases and healthy controls. ML algorithms can be trained to identify patterns and correlations in the data that can be used to develop predictive models for disease risk and progression. Another approach is to use natural language processing (NLP) techniques to analyze medical records, patient surveys, and social media data to identify risk factors and early warning signs of autoimmune diseases. NLP can be used to extract information from unstructured text data and identify relevant symptoms, comorbidities, and lifestyle factors that may be associated with an increased risk of autoimmune diseases.

Other AI-based methodologies that can be used for risk detection of autoimmune diseases include computer vision for analyzing medical images and robotics for automating diagnostic procedures and patient monitoring. For example, computer vision algorithms can be trained to detect subtle changes in medical images that may indicate the early stages of autoimmune diseases, while robotics can be used to perform repetitive diagnostic tests and monitor patients in real time. Generally, AI-based methodologies for risk detection of autoimmune diseases offer promising avenues for improving the early detection and prediction of these conditions. However, it is important to ensure that these methodologies are carefully validated and integrated into clinical practice to ensure their safety and efficacy. AI-Assisted Model for detecting the risk factors of Autoimmune disease-attacked persons is represented in Fig. 1.

Designing an AI-assisted model for rating the severity of autoimmune illnesses would require a comprehensive approach that involves multiple steps. Here is an outline of the possible steps involved in creating such a model that are data collection, this is the first step in designing an AI-assisted model for rating autoimmune illnesses' severity would involve collecting relevant data. This would include data on autoimmune diseases, their symptoms, and the severity of the symptoms. Other important factors that could be considered include patient demographics, lifestyle factors, genetic predispositions, and environmental factors that might be relevant to autoimmune disease. Once the data has been gathered, it must be cleaned and preprocessed to ensure that it is accurate, consistent, and in a format that an AI model can

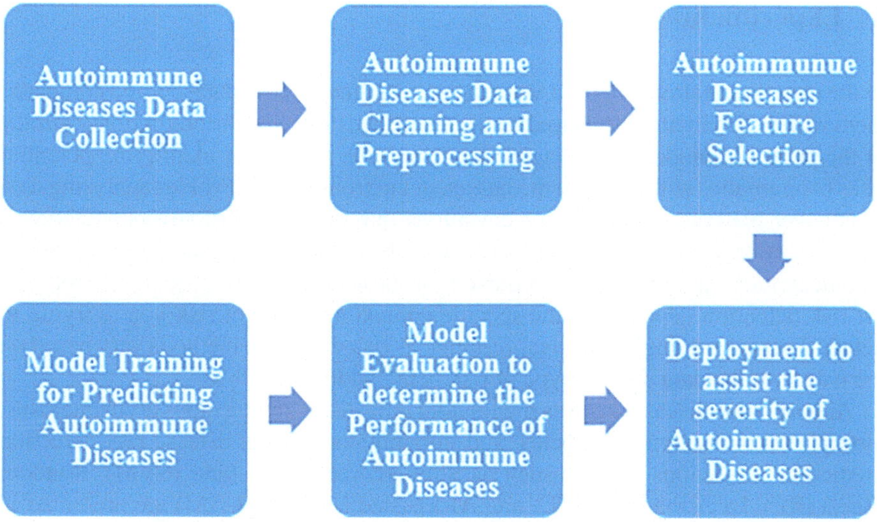

Fig. 1 AI-assisted model for autoimmune disease prediction

use. This would involve removing any incorrect or absent data and transforming the data into an analysis-ready format. The subsequent stage entails selecting the most pertinent features that can be used to train the AI model. Various techniques, such as correlation analysis, principal component analysis, and feature importance ranking algorithms, could be utilized for this purpose. After the features have been determined, the AI model must be trained on the data. Various machine-learning algorithms, such as support vector machines, random forests, and neural networks, may be used for this purpose. Based on the specified features, the model must be trained to accurately predict the severity of autoimmune diseases.

Once the model has been trained, it must be evaluated to determine its accuracy and effectiveness. This may involve employing a variety of evaluation metrics, such as precision, recall, F1 score, and ROC curve analysis. Finally, the model needs to be deployed so that healthcare providers to assist in rating the severity of autoimmune illnesses can use it. This could involve integrating the model into an electronic health record system, developing a web application, or building a mobile app. Generally, an AI-assisted model for rating the severity of autoimmune illnesses could be a powerful tool in lowering the danger of people being attacked. By accurately predicting the severity of autoimmune diseases, healthcare providers can better manage patients' symptoms and provide more targeted treatments, ultimately improving patient outcomes and quality of life.

4 Experimental Wok

In the experimentation, we used various autoimmune disease datasets and compared them with different models. Based on the results we observed the prediction accuracy of the proposed model. Risk detection refers to the process of identifying potential risks or anomalies within a system, dataset, or environment. It involves analyzing data to uncover patterns, behaviors, or deviations that could lead to adverse outcomes. Risk detection is commonly used in various fields such as finance, cybersecurity, healthcare, and quality control to prevent or mitigate negative events. The formula for risk detection depends on the specific context and type of risk you're trying to detect. There is no single universal formula, as risk detection methods vary based on the nature of the data and the type of risk being addressed.

Autoimmune diseases such as rheumatoid arthritis, systemic lupus erythematosus, multiple sclerosis, type I diabetes, and inflammatory bowel disease risk detection prediction on various models such as Support Vector Machine (SVM), Random Forest (RF), Decision Tree (DT), and AI-assisted Model (AI-AM) are presented in Table 1 and depicted in Fig. 2. Based on the results, we observed that proposed model shows the best accuracy than other existing models. Table 2 and Fig. 3 represent the experimentation conducted on some people on clinical characteristics like age, sex, performance status, and predictive index.

5 Conclusion and Future Scope

In conclusion, designing a revolutionary AI-assisted model for rating the severity of autoimmune illnesses could have a significant impact on improving patient outcomes and lowering the danger of people being attacked. Such a model would require a comprehensive approach that involves collecting relevant data, cleaning and pre-processing the data, selecting the most relevant features, training the AI model, evaluating its performance, validating it on new patient data, and finally deploying the model to be used by healthcare providers. By accurately predicting the severity of autoimmune illnesses, healthcare providers can better manage patients' symptoms and provide more targeted treatments, ultimately improving patient outcomes and quality of life. However, it is important to note that creating such a model would be a complex and time-consuming process that requires a multidisciplinary team of experts in medicine, data science, and machine learning. Nevertheless, the potential benefits of creating an AI-assisted model for rating the severity of autoimmune illnesses are immense, and such a model could have a significant impact on reducing the danger of people being attacked by autoimmune diseases. It is therefore essential that continued research and development efforts be focused on creating and improving such models to better serve patients and healthcare providers.

The future scope of an AI-assisted model for rating the severity of autoimmune illnesses is promising. Here are some potential areas where this technology could

Table 1 Autoimmune diseases prediction on different machine learning models

Autoimmune diseases	Machine learning models	Risk detection (%)
Rheumatoid arthritis	SVM	88
	Random forest	86
	Decision tree	89
	AI-AM	92
Systemic lupus erythematosus	SVM	87
	Random forest	79
	Decision tree	86
	AI-AM	89
Multiple sclerosis	SVM	87
	Random forest	79
	Decision tree	87
	AI-AM	90
Type 1 diabetes	SVM	88
	Random forest	85
	Decision tree	87
	AI-AM	91
Inflammatory bowel disease	SVM	89
	Random forest	89
	Decision tree	88
	AI-AM	94

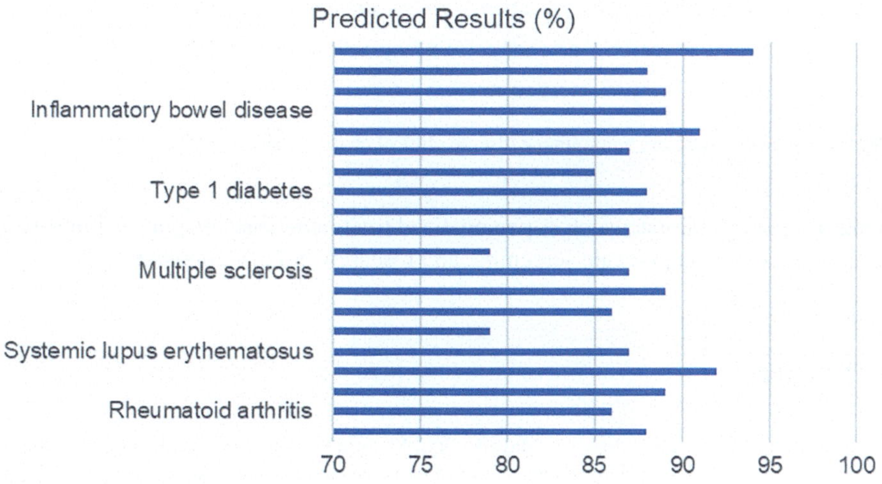

Fig. 2 Visualization of autoimmune diseases predicted results

Table 2 General characteristics for any autoimmune diseases

Characteristic		No autoimmune condition		Any autoimmune condition		
		N_1	%	N_2	%	P
Sex	Male	1318	67.0	122	51.3	<0.001
	Female	924	33.0	149	48.7	
Age	≤60 Years	1187	59.3	118	49.9	0.001
	>60 Years	989	40.7	153	51.1	
Performance status	<2	2102	96.1	259	92.9	0.16
	≥2	116	4.9	12	7.1	
Predictive index	Low-intermediate risk	1964	91.1	243	89.7	0.44
	High risk	164	8.9	28	10.3	

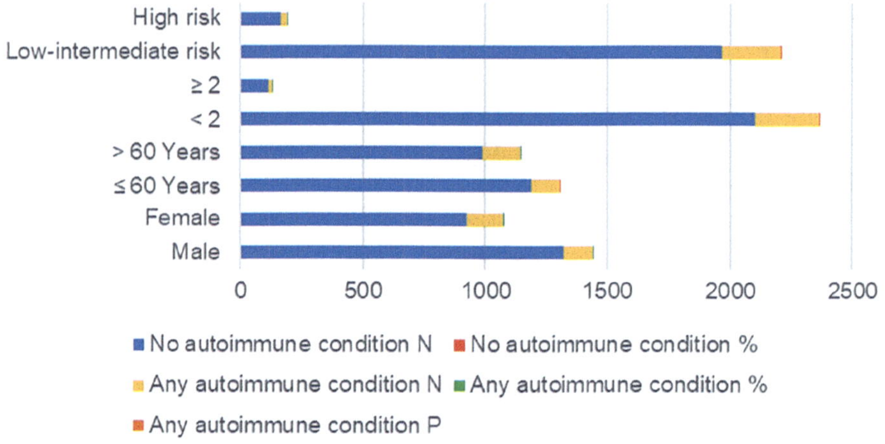

Fig. 3 Visualization of any autoimmune disease clinical characteristics

make a significant impact such as personalized treatment, early diagnosis, improved patient outcomes, large-scale screening, and research and development.

References

1. Calcaterra V, Mameli C, Rossi V, Magenes VC, Massini G, Perazzi C, Verduci E, Zuccotti G (2023) What we know about the relationship between autoimmune thyroid diseases and gut microbiota: a perspective on the role of probiotics on pediatric endocrinology. Minerva Pediatr 74:6. https://doi.org/10.23736/S2724-5276.22.06873-2
2. Bhuyan HK, Chakraborty C (2022) Explainable machine learning for data extraction across computational social system. In: IEEE transactions on computational social systems, pp 1–15. (Early Access publication)

3. Khuntia BK, Sharma V, Qazi S, Das S, Sharma S, Raza K, Sharma G (2021) Ayurvedic medicinal plants against COVID-19: an in silico analysis. Nat Prod Commun 16(11). 1934578X211056753
4. Zhou F, Chen F, Ouyang Z, Zhu R, Zhou R, Hu W, Lu, C (2023) Functions of peroxiredoxins and their roles in autoimmune diseases. Antioxid Redox Signal. https://doi.org/10.1089/ars.2022.0139
5. Bhuyan HK, Ravi V (2023) An integrated framework with deep learning for segmentation and classification of cancer disease. Int J Artif Intell Tools (IJAIT) 32(02):2340002
6. Wani N, Raza K (2018) Multiple kernel-learning approach for medical image analysis. In: Soft computing based medical image analysis. Academic Press, pp 31–47
7. Bhuyan HK, Chakraborty C, Pani SK, Ravi V (2023) Feature and sub-feature selection for classification using correlation coefficient and fuzzy model. IEEE Trans Eng Manag 70(5)
8. Qazi S, Raza K (2021) Phytochemicals from Ayurvedic plants as potential medicaments for ovarian cancer: an in silico analysis. J Mol Model 27:114. https://doi.org/10.1007/s00894-021-04736-x
9. Bhuyan HK, Ravi V, Brahma B, Kamila NK (2022) Disease analysis using machine learning approaches in healthcare system. Health Technol 12(5), 987–1005
10. Brzezicka KA, Paulson JC (2023) Impact of siglecs on autoimmune diseases. Mol Asp Med 90(101140). https://doi.org/10.1016/j.mam.2022.101140
11. Gupta TK, Raza K (2020) Optimizing deep feedforward neural network architecture: a tabu search based approach. Neural Process Lett 51:2855–2870. https://doi.org/10.1007/s11063-020-10234-7
12. Pan S, Gupta TK, Raza K (2023) BatTS: a hybrid method for optimizing deep feedforward neural network. Peer J Comput Sci 9:e1194. https://doi.org/10.7717/peerj-cs.1194
13. Chengoden R, Victor N, Huynh-The T, Yenduri G, Jhaveri RH, Alazab M, Gadekallu TR (2023) Metaverse for healthcare: a survey on potential applications, challenges and future directions. IEEE Access
14. Agrawal S, Sarkar S, Aouedi O, Yenduri G, Piamrat K, Alazab M, Gadekallu TR (2022) Federated learning for intrusion detection system: concepts, challenges and future directions. Comput Commun
15. Sahu A, Qazi S, Raza K, Singh A, Verma S (2022) Machine learning-based approach for early diagnosis of breast cancer using biomarkers and gene expression profiles. In: Raza K (ed) Computational intelligence in oncology. Studies in computational intelligence, vol 1016. Springer, Singapore. https://doi.org/10.1007/978-981-16-9221-5_17
16. Singh PK, Stan RC (2023) Febrile temperatures modulate the formation of immune complexes relevant for autoimmune diseases. J Therm Biol. https://doi.org/10.1016/j.jtherbio.2022.103425,111,(103425)
17. Lichti CF, Wan X (2023) Using mass spectrometry to identify neoantigens in autoimmune diseases: the type 1 diabetes example. Semin Immunol 66(101730).https://doi.org/10.1016/j.smim.2023.101730,66,(101730)
18. Yenduri G, Gadekallu TR (2022) A multiple criteria decision analysis based approach to remove uncertainty in SMP models. Sci Rep 12(1):22386
19. Khan FN, Yousef M, Raza K (2022) Machine learning-based models in the diagnosis, prognosis and effective cancer therapeutics: current state-of-the-art. In: Raza K (ed) Computational Intelligence in Oncology. Studies in Computational Intelligence, vol 1016. Springer, Singapore. https://doi.org/10.1007/978-981-16-9221-5_2
20. Bashir AK, Victor N, Bhattacharya S, Huynh-The T, Chengoden R, Yenduri G, Liyanage M (2023) A survey on federated learning for the healthcare metaverse: concepts, applications, challenges, and future directions. arXiv:2304.00524

21. Gupta TK, Raza K (2019) Chapter 7—optimization of ANN architecture: a review on nature-inspired techniques. In: Dey N, Borra S, Ashour AS, Shi F (eds) Machine learning in bio-signal analysis and diagnostic imaging. Academic Press, pp 159–182. https://doi.org/10.1016/B978-0-12-816086-2.00007-2
22. Yenduri G, Gadekallu TR (2022) A systematic literature review of soft computing techniques for software maintainability prediction: state-of-the-art, challenges and future directions. arXiv: 2209.10131

AI in Treatment Planning and Management

Artificial Intelligence in the Diagnosis and Treatment of Rheumatoid Arthritis: Current Status and Future Prospects

Fatima Nazish Khan, Mohammad Asim, and Mohammad Irfan Qureshi

Abstract Rheumatoid arthritis (RA) is a prevalent autoimmune disease with unknown causes, characterized by joint damage and chronic polyarthritis. The exact pathogenesis of RA remains unclear, leading to a need for advanced approaches. Artificial intelligence (AI), specifically machine learning and deep learning, has gained traction in healthcare and medicine. AI algorithms have shown promise in RA diagnosis, prognosis, treatment monitoring, drug discovery, and basic science research support. In addition to conventional treatments, alternative medicine, including traditional Indian, Korean, and Chinese herbs, is being explored for RA management. The integration of AI into real-world scenarios is a significant step forward, with the potential for the development of effective and novel RA treatments. Many studies showed that AI algorithms have the potential to provide personalized treatments based on individual disease profiles, including genomics, and are assisting in medical services. Numerous studies have also identified single-nucleotide polymorphisms (SNPs) associated with the risk of developing RA, as well as epistatic relationships among them. These advancements have the potential to revolutionize early detection and intervention strategies, ultimately leading to better outcomes for patients with RA. However, there are technical challenges to overcome. The application of AI in screening medicinal herbs and addressing these challenges is a future research direction. This chapter presents the role of AI in the diagnosis and treatment of RA, along with future prospects.

Keywords Artificial intelligence · Machine learning · Deep learning · Rheumatoid arthritis · Medicinal herbs

F. N. Khan · M. I. Qureshi (✉)
Department of Biotechnology, Jamia Millia Islamia, New Delhi 110025, India
e-mail: miqureshi@jmi.ac.in

F. N. Khan
e-mail: fatimanazishkhan@yahoo.com

M. Asim
Department of Clinical and Experimental Medicine, University of Surrey, Guildford GU2 7WG, UK
e-mail: m.asim@surrey.ac.uk

K. Raza and S. Singh (eds.), *Artificial Intelligence and Autoimmune Diseases*, Studies in Computational Intelligence 1133, https://doi.org/10.1007/978-981-99-9029-0_10

1 Introduction

Artificial intelligence (AI) is a rapidly advancing field that enables machines to replicate human-like intelligent behavior [1]. With technology becoming increasingly prevalent, AI is finding applications in various scientific and medical domains, including pathology, radiology, personalized medicine, drug discovery, and public health prediction [2]. Machine learning (ML), a subset of AI, allows machines to acquire skills through practice and learning, similar to humans. ML encompasses techniques that autonomously learn patterns and relationships in complex problems without explicit programming [3]. ML methods can be categorized into supervised learning, unsupervised learning, and reinforcement learning [3, 4]. During the early 2010s, deep learning (DL) emerged as an advancement in ML, combining multiple processes to accomplish tasks [1] (Fig. 1). Despite progress in ML, its widespread application in clinical prediction modeling and integration of administrative and clinical datasets for patients with rheumatoid arthritis (RA) is still limited.

RA, the second most prevalent chronic autoimmune disease of unknown origin, affects over 20 million people worldwide (Figs. 2 and 3). It primarily affects joints and bones and is associated with an increased risk of various comorbidities, including thromboembolism [5], cardiovascular diseases [6], periodontal diseases [7], lung diseases [8], diabetes [9], eye diseases [10], and non-melanoma skin cancer [11, 67, 69]. Cartilage erosion and chronic polyarthritis characterize RA, and although traditional medicine has been used, there is currently no specific cure for the disease. The integration of AI and ML technologies in RA research and diagnosis, along with the availability of large-scale data, holds great potential for enhancing treatment, diagnosis, and drug development in RA and related arthritis diseases [1]. Incorporating AI into clinical practice can improve healthcare quality and cost. However, diagnosing RA is challenging due to the absence of a definitive diagnostic method or gold standard test. Various classification methods have been proposed to differentiate

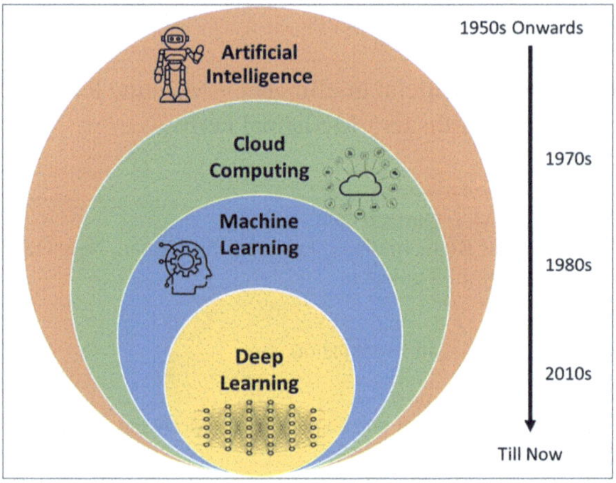

Fig. 1 Evolution of AI, cloud computing, machine learning, and deep learning

RA from other autoimmune diseases and classify patients based on disease characteristics [1, 65]. Current RA treatment aims to reduce inflammation and joint damage, involving the use of corticosteroids, nonsteroidal anti-inflammatory drugs (NSAIDs), and disease-modifying anti-rheumatic drugs (DMARDs) [12]. Utilizing publicly available big data, such as laboratory findings, medical images, omics datasets, electronic health records, and demographic data, is crucial for advancing RA research and treatment [13].

Currently, the most commonly used approach for pre-clinical detection of RA involves measuring autoantibodies like rheumatoid factor (RF) or anti-citrullinated protein antibodies (ACPAs), which are present before symptomatic disease onset. However, the positive predictive value of these tests is not consistently reliable [14]. In their study, O'Neil et al. developed regression models that utilize serum proteome as input to identify RA patients (i.e., progressors) among first-degree relatives of confirmed cases (i.e., at-risk population). By employing the least absolute shrinkage and selection operator (LASSO) regression, they achieved 100% accuracy in recognizing progressors among ACPA-negative cases using 17 proteins. Another model, which attained an accuracy of 86.9%, was developed for ACPA-positive individuals. Additionally, a third model utilizing 23 proteins as variables achieved an accuracy of

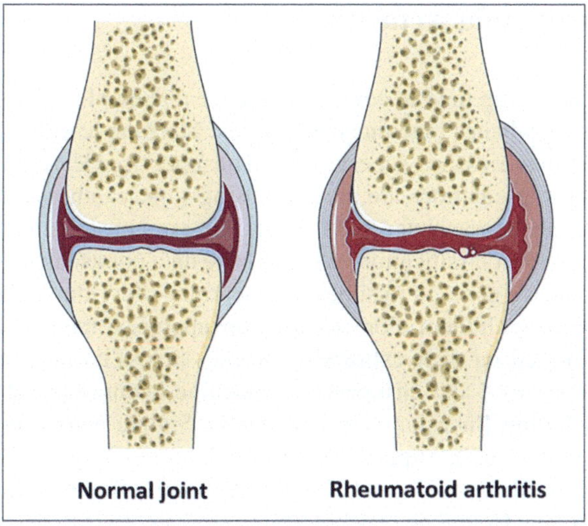

Fig. 2 Normal joint versus Rheumatoid arthritis

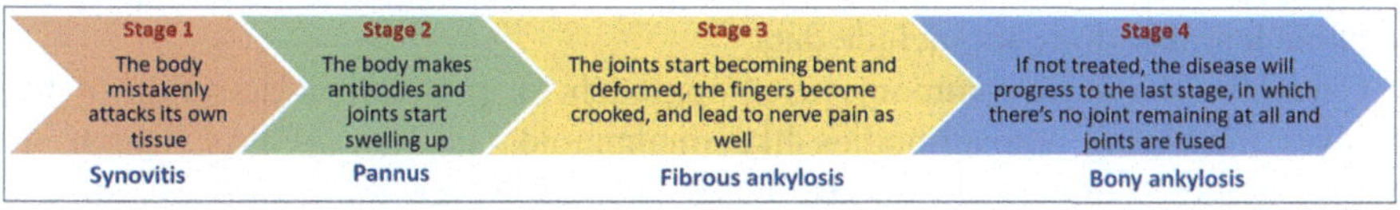

Fig. 3 Flow diagram showing stages of development of RA

91.2% in identifying progressors [14]. Numerous studies have also identified single-nucleotide polymorphisms (SNPs) associated with the risk of developing RA, as well as epistatic relationships among them. Kruppa et al. employed a random-forest model to identify a 496-SNP panel closely linked with RA (AUC = 0.89) [18]. Negi et al. identified four SNPs significantly associated with RA, with minimum and maximum odds ratios (OR) of 0.86 and 1.42, respectively [17]. Epistatic relationships between human leukocyte antigen (HLA) and non-HLA genes using Bayesian LASSO regression.

AI algorithms have the potential to provide personalized treatments based on individual disease profiles, including genomics, and are assisting in medical services [1, 67]. This chapter explores the practical applications of AI and traditional medicinal practices, such as Indian, Unani, Ayurvedic, Tibetan, Korean, and Chinese herbals, for treating and diagnosing RA. It also addresses the challenges and gaps in AI and medicinal plant research, providing future research directions. Incorporating ML and DL algorithms into real-world medical scenarios is a significant step in advancing AI in medicine, and it is expected that AI will contribute to the development of effective and innovative RA treatments and diagnostics in the future.

2 AI in Rheumatoid Arthritis

AI is a rapidly advancing field in computer science that employs various interdisciplinary methods to enhance machine capabilities. Machine learning algorithms are divided into two categories, i.e., supervised and unsupervised learning. In supervised learning algorithms, predictions are made by using some examples. In other words, data points have labels associated with them. For example, in an application of a supervised method, the classification of genes have data points labeled as 1 and 0 for control and responsive gene. In unsupervised learning algorithms, data points have no labels associated with them. For example, unsupervised methods could be used to cluster genes based on their expression profiles across tissues, cases, or conditions. Several supervised and unsupervised machine learning-based methods have been applied including Bayesian Networks (BN), Simple Naïve Bayesian (SNB), Naïve Random Forest (RF), Support Vector Machine (SVM), Decision Tree (DT), Logistic Regression (LR), k-Nearest Neighbourhood (kNN), Conditional Random Field (CRF), Artificial Neural Networks (ANN), etc. The study of decision-making is called reinforcement learning (RL). It involves understanding how to act in a situation to reap the most benefits. Data for RL is gathered from machine learning systems that employ a trial-and-error process. Input for either supervised or unsupervised machine learning does not include data.

Currently, the most commonly used approach for pre-clinical detection of RA involves measuring autoantibodies like rheumatoid factor or ACPAs, which are present before symptomatic disease onset [14]. However, the positive predictive value of these tests is not consistently reliable. This is where AI plays a crucial role by assisting in predicting the likelihood of future RA development using diverse

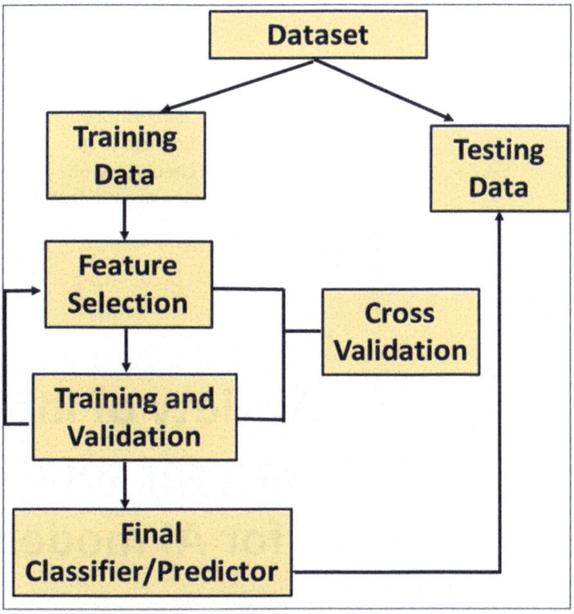

Fig. 4 Flow diagram showing steps involved in pre-processing of input datasets for predicting AI models for monitoring, diagnosis, and treatment of RA

datasets (Figs. 4 and 5). In their study, O'Neil et al. developed regression models that utilize serum proteome as input to identify RA patients (i.e., progressors) among first-degree relatives of confirmed cases (i.e., at-risk population) [14]. Numerous studies have also identified single-nucleotide polymorphisms (SNPs) associated with the risk of developing RA, as well as epistatic relationships among them. For the purpose of identifying those who have the disease and controls, numerous models for the diagnosis of autoimmune diseases have been developed. The majority demonstrated the usefulness of machine learning in diagnostics by achieving high classifier performance (any combination of the following metrics are over these thresholds: accuracy >81%, AUC > 0.95, Sensitivity > 82, Specificity > 84).

Table 1 provides a summary of studies incorporating ML for assessing the risk of RA development. In sum, by harnessing the power of AI and ML, we can significantly improve our ability to identify individuals at risk of developing RA and make more accurate predictions. These advancements have the potential to revolutionize early detection and intervention strategies, ultimately leading to better outcomes for patients with RA.

2.1 Diagnosis/Early Diagnosis

The early diagnosis of RA is crucial as it allows for timely interventions that can prevent further joint damage and lead to better outcomes [22]. The ACR/EULAR 2010 criteria classify RA based on biomarkers such as anti-cyclic citrullinated

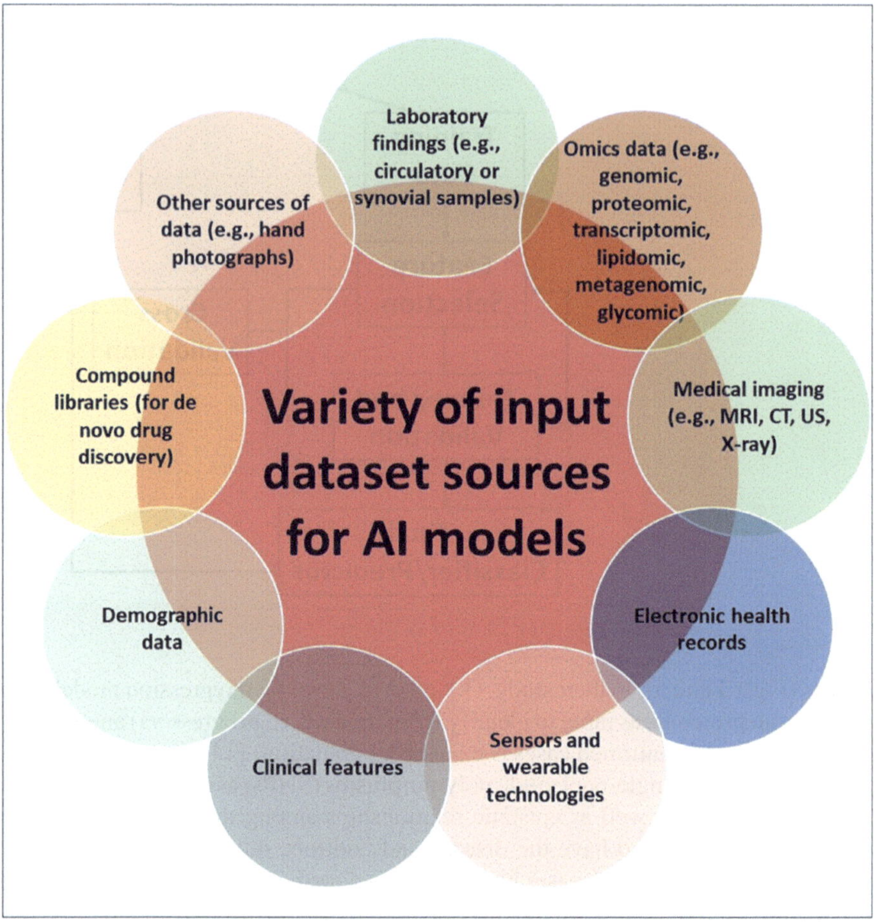

Fig. 5 Different types of input datasets for AI models for monitoring, diagnosis, and treatment of RA

peptide (anti-CCP) antibodies (often tested as ACPAs), rheumatoid factor (RF), C-reactive protein (CRP), and erythrocyte sedimentation rate (ESR) [23]. However, these biomarkers have limitations in terms of specificity and sensitivity. Therefore, there is a need to develop novel biomarker panels with optimal specificity and sensitivity for early detection of RA.

The analysis of large datasets, such as genomics, transcriptomics, proteomics, metabolomics, lipidomics, glycomics, or metagenomic datasets, using machine learning methods can facilitate the simultaneous assessment of the relationships between various biomolecules and RA [1]. For instance, imaging analysis, including synovitis evidence, combined with clinical and sensor data, plays a significant role in monitoring, managing, and diagnosing RA. The utilization of AI-driven data analysis enables early disease detection and efficient utilization of human resources. In

Table 1 Studies utilizing AI for assessment of the development risk of RA

ML Algorithms	Size of dataset	Validation/Testing	Objectives	References
Random forest; Model-based MDR; Elastic Net	RA (868); Control (1194)	Nested tenfold cross-validation	Prediction of disease	[9]
LASSO regression	Total at-risk (127); ACPA-negative (not progressor, 47); ACPA-positive (not progressor, 63); Progressors (17)	The dependent test set for 3rd model and whole data for models 1st and 2nd)	For identification of protein markers related to RA susceptibility	[14]
Random forest; Logistic regression	No arthritis (6151); Arthritis (2272)	N/A	Finding eye diseases that enhance the development risk of arthritis	[15]
SVM + NMF	RA (1007); Controls (921,192)	tenfold cross-validation	For identification of RA risk factors	[16]
SVM	Discovery: RA (706), Controls (761); Replication: RA (927), Controls (1148)	Cross-validation; replication set	SNPs linked with RA are identified	[17]
Logistic regression; LASSO regression, Random jungle	RA (707); Controls (738)	tenfold cross-validation, Dependent test set	For identifying associations between RA and SNPs	[18]
Logistic regression, Random Forest	NARAC1 (training): RA (908), Controls (1260); NARAC2 (validation): RA (952), Controls (1760)	Independent test set	For predicting RA and SNPs status	[19]
Logistic regression	Extension: RA (677), Controls (750); Replication: RA (947), Controls (1756)	Replication set	To identify epistatic relationships with the PTPN22 gene in RA susceptibility	[20]
Bayesian LASSO regression	RA (868); Controls (1194)	N/A	For identifying epistatic relationships between HLA and non-HLA SNPs linked with RA	[21]

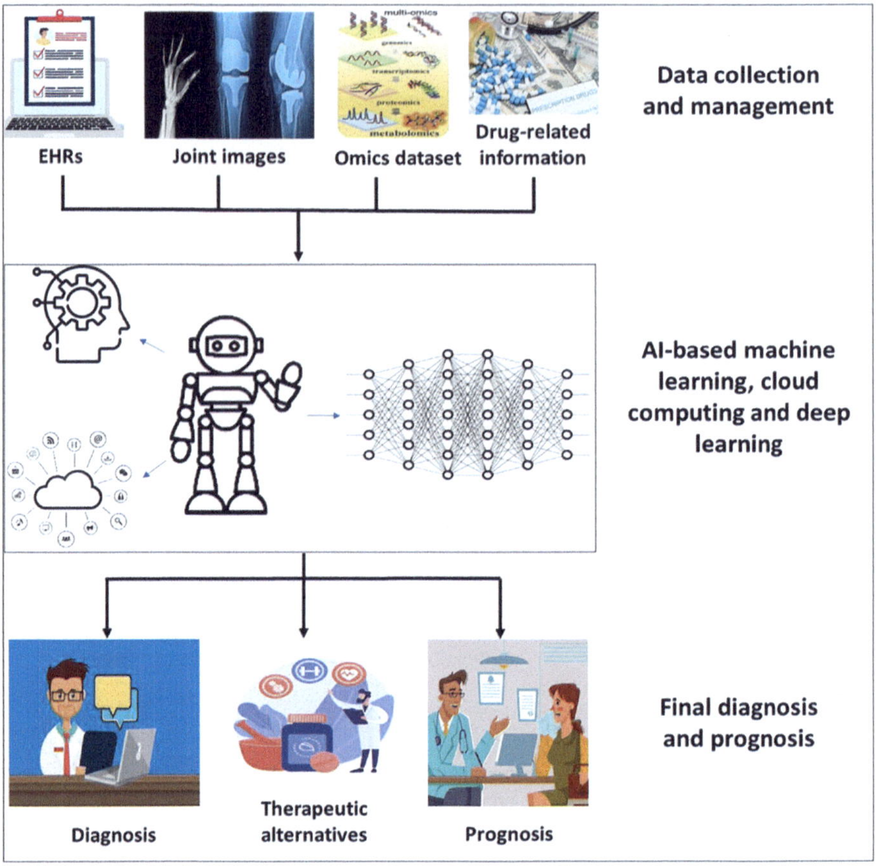

Fig. 6 AI-assisted machine learning, cloud computing, and deep learning model for diagnosis and treatment of RA

this context, we provide a summary of ML applications in RA diagnosis, utilizing omics, clinical, imaging, and sensor data (Fig. 6).

2.1.1 Using Omics Data in the Diagnosis of RA

Many studies have used multiple coding and non-coding RNAs to develop panels for establishing an accurate diagnosis of RA using ML methods. Recently, Liu et al. discovered the differential expression of 52 gene signatures in RA patients by analyzing gene expression profiles of peripheral blood cells [24]. Ormseth et al. developed a panel of microRNAs (miRNAs) using logistic regression and LASSO variable selection to differentiate RA patients from controls. They identified several upregulated miRNAs in RA patients, including miR-22-3p, miR-627-5p, miR-140-3p, miR-24-3p, miR-134-5p, and miR-96-5p [25]. Geurts et al. found that boosted decision trees outperformed other ML techniques such as k-nearest neighbors (kNN) and SVM. By using this method, they discovered protein peak patterns that can distinguish RA patients from controls as well as patients with other autoimmune diseases, with high specificity and sensitivity [3, 26].

Circulating levels of 38 cytokines have been analyzed using ANN to distinguish RA patients from controls and osteoarthritis (OA) patients, resulting in a model with 100% specificity and sensitivity [27]. Machine learning methods utilizing glycomics and metabolomics datasets have also shown promising results in RA diagnosis. Chocholova et al. trained ML-based diagnostic models using glycomics data and compared the diagnostic accuracy of LASSO regression and ANN models in seropositive patients. In detecting seronegative patients, ANN outperformed LASSO regression in their study [28]. Yeo et al. distinguished RA patients from controls by using ML approaches with 10 chemokine genes. They also reported that synovial biomarkers assist in the early identification of RA patients [29]. Wu et al. utilized a logistic regression algorithm to improve multiclass classification between RA patients, liver cirrhosis, type 2 diabetes mellitus, and controls. Their model achieved an AUC value of 0.95 [30]. Recently, Volkova et al. conducted a meta-analysis using random forest algorithms and observed that the gut microbiome can differentiate patients with RA from controls and other autoimmune diseases [31].

These studies demonstrate the potential of ML methods in utilizing coding and non-coding RNAs for the accurate diagnosis of RA and highlight the importance of considering various biomarkers and datasets in RA research.

2.1.2 Using Imaging Data in the Diagnosis of RA

Radiological observations play a critical role in the staging and diagnosis of RA. Among the commonly used methods, conventional radiography is widely utilized. Numerous models have been developed for RA diagnosis, including convolutional neural networks (CNN) that use hand X-ray datasets as input, achieving an accuracy of approximately 95%. When compared to computed tomography (CT) and conventional radiography, ultrasound and magnetic resonance imaging (MRI) are considered the best techniques for detecting early soft tissue changes [3, 26].

RA imaging features typically include bone erosions, joint space narrowing, synovitis, bone marrow edema, subcortical cysts, and joint effusion. AI models have been used to detect bone erosions, synovitis, joint space narrowing, and bone marrow edema. However, studies on subcortical cysts, late imaging findings, and joint effusion are relatively limited. Both supervised and unsupervised ML algorithms have been developed for detecting and quantifying synovitis using MRI images. Wu et al. recently proposed a DL-based model that assesses RA severity by classifying synovial proliferation. AI-based models have also been utilized to detect joint space narrowing in RA patients using plain X-rays [30].

Additionally, various clustering methods have been employed to detect and quantify bone marrow edema in RA patients using wrist MRI. Importantly, given the accessibility of acquiring the necessary data, such algorithms can serve as screening tools for RA [30].

2.1.3 Using Clinical and Sensor Data for Diagnosis of RA

Clinical rheumatologists have extensively utilized advanced algorithms, trained AI, and DL models in the processing of medical images, information acquisition, treatment, and diagnosis of various diseases, including RA. A large number of models have been developed for RA diagnosis using clinical datasets.

Singh et al. reported in their study that a fuzzy inference system demonstrated improved diagnostic performance by inputting a dataset of clinical symptoms (REF). Fukae et al. converted a clinical dataset into two-dimensional array images and employed a CNN (AlexNet) to differentiate RA patients based on these images. ML algorithms have utilized various features extracted from lymphocyte images captured by electronic image sensors for the classification of RA, achieving an accuracy of approximately 97.5%. Bardhan et al. developed a two-stage classification algorithm capable of labeling three-fourths of knee thermograph scans [3].

2.1.4 Phenotype Identification Using EHRs

For the identification of disease status using electronic health records (EHRs), both supervised and unsupervised machine learning models, as well as rule-based models, have been utilized. These algorithms leverage various information sources such as laboratory data, billing codes, natural language processing (NLP), and medication exposures to make accurate predictions. Several models have been developed for the identification of RA patients efficiently using ML and NLP techniques.

SVM is a commonly used algorithm for identifying phenotypes. Carroll et al. proposed an SVM model in 2010 that predicts the status of RA using novel and refined data, achieving an AUC value of 0.90. A recent performance assessment of Carroll et al.'s model using a 2017 dataset and different diagnostic techniques reported accurate and improved performance with rule-based algorithms. Maarseveen et al. recently reported that among SVM, random forest, naive Bayes, neural networks, gradient boosting, random classifier, and decision tree, SVM performed the best in identifying diseases using EHR [3].

Several supervised ML models have also been developed for phenotype identification. Zhou et al. used the random forests algorithm and proposed an algorithm that identifies RA status predictors by utilizing a large dataset from primary and secondary care settings, achieving an accuracy of 92.3% [32]. ML models not only help in predicting disease status but also aid in patient stratification. Cai et al. developed a supervised ML model in their study that assists in the selection of participants for clinical trials by providing an alternative solution to the time-consuming and costly procedure of review and screening. They combined logistic LASSO regression and random forest to develop a model from EHRs that identify potentially eligible RA patients for clinical trials [3].

The application of supervised models for phenotype identification faces a major challenge due to the need for a large amount of labeled training data. However, this challenge can be mitigated using unsupervised and semi-supervised models. For example, Chen et al. combined active learning (a type of semi-supervised learning method) and SVM to develop a model that performed well with fewer annotated samples, reducing the required labeled dataset by approximately two-thirds [33]. Gronsbell et al. proposed a two-step model in their study, where the first step used unsupervised clustering techniques, and the second step employed regression on unlabeled datasets to identify important features available in EHRs. This model improved efficiency with an AUC of 0.93 by reducing the number of labels needed [34].

3 Predicting Treatment Response Using AI

The initial treatment for RA is typically methotrexate (MTX), but in cases where the disease is not adequately controlled and treatment has failed, other more expensive anti-inflammatory drugs may be administered. ML-based algorithms have been developed to predict the response to MTX using clinical and demographic data, achieving an AUC value of approximately 0.84. Morid et al. conducted a study evaluating semi-supervised and supervised ML techniques to find an accurate treatment method step-up within one year among 120,237 patients. The one-class SVM model demonstrated the best performance with a specificity of 83% and sensitivity of 89% [35, 64].

Transcriptomics data have also been utilized for predicting the response to MTX among patients in the early stages of treatment, achieving an AUC value of 0.78. Omics data, including genomics, can be particularly useful for predicting the response to second or third-line biological DMARDs (bDMARDs) compared to MTX. For example, SVM algorithms have been reported to accurately identify patients who respond to infliximab using genomics data, achieving an AUC value of 0.92 [3]. Imaging data can also be incorporated into models for predicting treatment response. Kato et al. developed a scoring system using ultrasound images in RA patients. They employed an unsupervised random forest in conjunction with projection algorithms and uniform manifold approximation to divide patients into two clusters with different treatment responses [36]. However, the variety of evaluation methods used to determine treatment response makes it challenging to compare results across different studies. The identification of patients for whom non-biological DMARDs are effective and safe alternatives using AI algorithms can be beneficial for many patients [3] (Fig. 7).

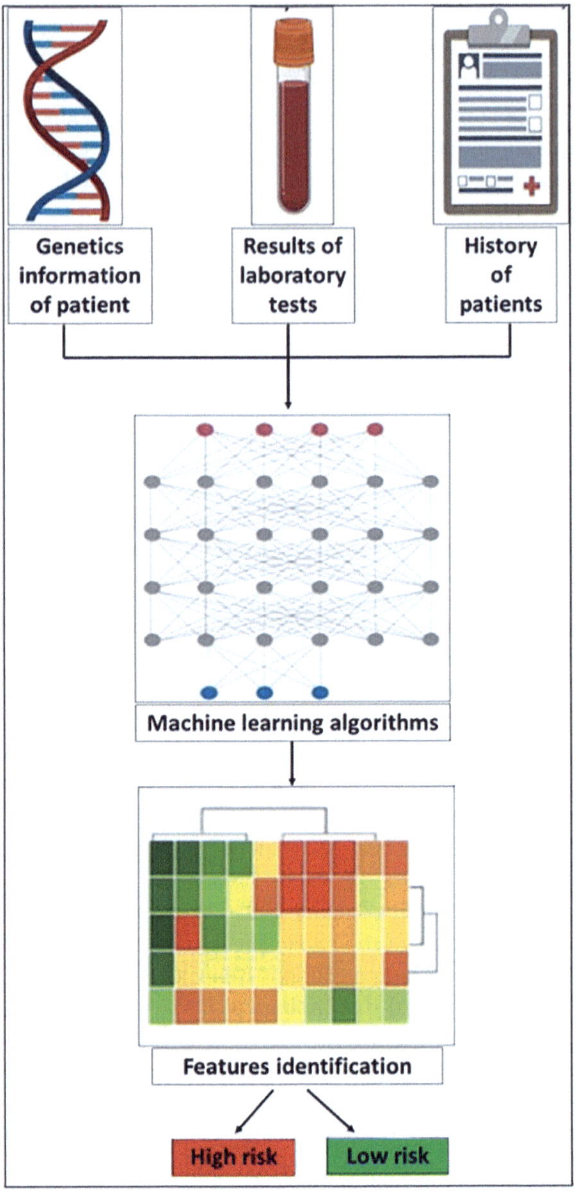

Fig. 7 Predicting treatment response of RA using AI

4 Monitoring Disease Course and Predicting Prognosis

Measuring disease activity is crucial for determining an appropriate treatment plan, evaluating therapy response, and predicting prognosis in RA. The Disease Activity Score in 28 joints (DAS28) is the most commonly used measure of RA severity.

An adaptive deep neural network, developed by Kalweit et al., outperformed non-deep learning methods in predicting DAS28-ESR (erythrocyte sedimentation rate) using clinical and demographic data. It achieved an AUC value of 0.73 and a mean standard error rate of 0.9 [37]. However, Rychkov et al. utilized omics datasets to predict DAS28 and found unsatisfactory results, indicating a weak correlation ($r = 0.33$) between the novel RA score and DAS28 [38].

Timely identification of patients at risk of disease complications is crucial. ML and DL algorithms have been utilized to enhance cardiovascular risk stratification in RA patients through image analysis. Wei et al. developed an ML algorithm using laboratory, clinical, and demographic data as input, predicting the incidence of coronary heart disease (CHD) in RA patients with an accuracy of 76% and an AUC of 0 [15]. Musculoskeletal complications are another major comorbidity in RA patients. Risk factors associated with bone loss in RA patients have been identified using LASSO regression, random forest, and conventional logistic regression methods. Age was found to have the lowest odds ratio (OR) associated with femoral neck bone loss ($OR = 1.17$), while TNF inhibitor use was associated with a decreased risk of lumbar spine bone loss ($OR = 0.27$). Gossec et al. developed a naive Bayes model that utilized physical activity as input to detect flares in RA patients. The results showed a specificity of 96.7% and a sensitivity of 95.7% [39].

5 Drug Discovery and Application of AI in Western Medicine and Traditional Medical Healthcare

Rheumatoid arthritis is a chronic autoimmune disease characterized by joint inflammation and destruction. Conventional synthetic disease-modifying antirheumatic drugs (csDMARDs) such as methotrexate are commonly used for RA treatment. However, when csDMARDs lose efficacy, biologic DMARDs (bDMARDs) like tumor necrosis factor inhibitors (TNFi) such as etanercept (ETN) and adalimumab (ADA) are prescribed [3].

The development of novel drugs for RA treatment is essential, considering the chronic nature of rheumatic diseases and the need for long-term medication. Machine learning models have been developed to improve the drug development process by selecting appropriate targets based on patients' expression profiles treated with potent drugs [40]. Gradient boosting machines and random forest algorithms were used to identify potential targets for RA treatment.

ML algorithms are particularly useful in handling the complex problems associated with the unknown pathways involved in RA pathogenesis. AI models have shown potential in various aspects of RA, including risk assessment, diagnosis using omics, clinical, sensor, and imaging data, patient detection through electronic health records (EHRs), treatment response prediction, prognosis determination, and disease monitoring. The global incidence of RA is approximately 1% of the total population, affecting nearly 700 million people worldwide, with women comprising about 80%

of the affected population. Inflammatory cytokines, such as IL-1, IL-6, and TNF-α, play a major role in RA development and disease occurrence. RA medications mainly involve non-steroidal anti-inflammatory drugs (NSAIDs), glucocorticoids, and anti-rheumatic drugs [1].

AI facilitates the identification of novel concepts and solutions for complex problems by mining large medical datasets, including clinical images, drug databases, and information related to disease causes, examinations, development, prognosis, and outcomes. The digitalization of medical images has provided a convenient avenue for AI applications. Traditional medicine, such as Traditional Chinese Medicine (TCM), which has been used for many years, focuses on the treatment and diagnosis of various diseases, including RA, diabetes, and cancer. AI plays a crucial role in improving the accuracy and reliability of diagnoses in traditional medicine and promotes the modernization of ancient medical practices. AI can also help establish the relationship between a patient's genotype and the disease phenotype network [41] (Fig. 8).

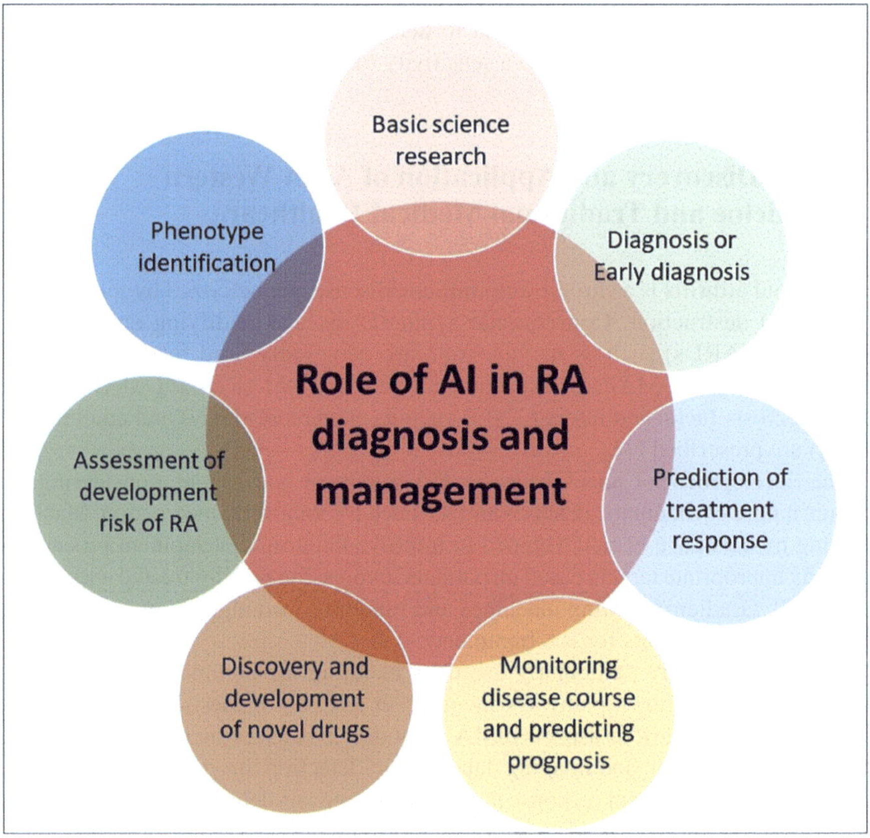

Fig. 8 Role of AI in the diagnosis and management of RA

6 Use of Herbal Drugs and Natural Product Extracts for RA Treatment

In addition to conventional medications, there are various approaches to treating RA, including the evaluation of medicinal plants for the development of novel drugs. Understanding the adverse effects and therapeutic potential of these plants is essential. Here, we explore the practical applications of AI in conjunction with traditional Indian, Unani, Ayurvedic, Tibetan, Korean, and Chinese herbal medicines for the treatment and diagnosis of RA [42]. The integration of ML and DL algorithms into real-world medical problems represents a significant advancement in the field of AI. It is anticipated that AI will play a role in the development of effective and novel drugs for the treatment and diagnosis of RA in the future. RA is a chronic autoimmune disease characterized by joint inflammation and the involvement of surrounding tissues. It can lead to joint deformity and affect various organs in the body, such as the eyes, skin, blood vessels, and lungs. RA is more prevalent in women and typically develops in the fourth and fifth decades of life, primarily affecting individuals between the ages of 35 and 50. The symptoms of RA can vary from person to person, with affected joints becoming tender, swollen, and warm. Morning stiffness lasting for several hours is common. Initially, the disease may present with fever, fatigue, and weight loss, which can later spread to the knees, wrists, ankles, hips, elbows, and shoulders. Over time, RA can cause joint deformities and displacement.

Many patients with RA turn to complementary and alternative medicine (CAM) for disease management. Medicinal herbs have gained importance in recent years for the treatment of RA. In earlier times, extracts from natural products, particularly those derived from various plant species, were widely used as folk medicines. In the nineteenth century, bioactive organic molecules were isolated from these natural sources for medicinal purposes. Numerous herbs with anti-arthritic properties have been historically used for the treatment of RA, and they can be employed both internally and externally as therapeutic agents [43]. By combining AI methodologies with the knowledge of traditional medicinal practices, there is great potential to explore the effectiveness of medicinal plants in treating RA and develop evidence-based treatment approaches. It is important to continue research efforts in this field to bridge the gap between traditional medicine and modern AI techniques, leading to the discovery of new treatment options for RA patients (Table 2).

7 Applying AI to Herbal Medicine for the Treatment of RA

Artificial intelligence can leverage the information about the medicinal properties of various plants, including those mentioned above to aid in the development of treatments for RA. Here's how AI can utilize this information:

Table 2 Herbal compounds and natural product extracts for treatment of RA and other diseases

Plant name	Chemical and therapeutic compounds	Applications	References
Myrobalan	Trans-cinnamic acid, aijunglucoside, triethyl ester of ehebulic acid, aljungenin, ajunic acid, daucosterol	Helps in treating asthma, hiccough, sore throat, diarrhea, vomiting, dysentery, bleeding piles, ulcers, and heart, gout, and bladder diseases	[44]
Deodar cedar	Himachalene, himachalol, himadarol, 9-himachalene, allohimachalol, isocentdarol, centdarol, ethyl stearate, 9-hydroxy-dodecanoic acid, methyl coniferin, ethyl laurate, 3-beta-hydroxy-oleanolic acid, beta-sitosterol, methyl ester, shikimic acid	Carminative, kidney stones, diaphoretic, urinary and pulmonary disorders, diuretic, rheumatism, piles, diabetes, insomnia, etc.	[45]
Teak	Astectoquinone, tectol, 5-hydroxylapachol, betulinic acid, squalene, aeetovanillone, betulinic aldehyde, e- isofuraldehyde, syringaresinol, evofolin, lariciresinol, medioresinol, balaphonin, zhebeiresinol, 1-hydroxypinoresinol	Anti-inflammatory, antibacterial, anti-oxidant, analgesic, anti-asthamatic, anti-fungal and anti-tumor	[55]
Black pepper	Piperene, sabinene, terpene, limonene, mercene, camphene, pinene, carypophylline, alpha-phellandrene, alpha-pinene, beta-bisbolene, beta-pinene, beta-farnesene, terpene-4-ol, linalool, thujone	Anti-inflammatory, anti-flatulent, riboflavin, niacin, thiamin, carminative and pyridoxine	[54]
Indian bay leaf	Geraniol, beta-caryophyllene, beta-pinene, camphene, limonene, alpha-pinene, cinnamaldehyde, p-cymene, eugenol	Anti-flatulent, carminative, diuretic, bladder disorder, anorexia, nausea and coryza	[53]
Ginger	Gingerols, zingiberol, zingiberine, bisabolene, sesquiphellandrene, dehydrogingerdione, curcumene, gingesulphonicacid, galanolactone, alpha curcumin, alpha farnesene	Anti-emetic, anti-viral, chemo-protective, anti-inflammatory, anti-ulcerogenic, migraine and anti-nauseant	[49]
Morning glory	Tetradecanyl palmitate, hexadecanyl p-hydroxycinnmate, stigmasteryl phydroxycinnamate, palminate, stearic, myristoleie, myristic, palmitic, linoleic, oleic acid, nonadecanoic	Antibacterial, immune-modulatory, anti-inflammatory, anti-convulsant, hypoglycemic, central nervous system activity	[52]

(continued)

Table 2 (continued)

Plant name	Chemical and therapeutic compounds	Applications	References
Aginbuti	Hentriacontine, ellagic acid, betulinic-acid, quercetin, dotriacontanol, lupeol, ellagic acid, lawsone, b-sitosterol	Anti-arthritic, rubifacient, anti-inflammatory, anti-urolithiasis, hypothermic, hypertensive, antibacterial	[46]
Tinospora gulancha	Tinocardifolin, columbin, colombine, picroretin, and tinocardifolioside, tinosponone, tinocardioside, cordioside	Jaundice, diabetes, rheumatoid arthritis, hypolipidemic, antineoplastic, antioxidant and hepatoprotective	[40]
Ram tulsi	Thymol, pentoses, gratissimol, uronic acid, hexoses, eugenol, cis-ocimene, pinene, trans-ocimene, cineole, linalool, methyl chavicol, eugenol, methyl eugenol	Relaxant and anti-nociceptive	[47]
Chanka piedra	Brevifolin, butyrolactone, butyrolactone, dibenzyl, deca-trans-2-cis-4-dienamide 24-isopropyl, corilagin, cymene	Asthma, anemia, eye disorders, astringent, cough, dropsy, conjunctivitis, menorrhagia, diarrhea, diabetes, bronchitis, dysentery, galactagogue, hepatitis, leucorrhea, jaundice	[44]
Bachelor's button	Parthenolide, germacranolides, eudesmanolides, guaianol ides, epoxyartemorin, epicanin, 3-beta-hydroxycostunolide, 1-beta-hydroxyarbusculin	Anticancer, cardio tonic, antispasmodic, an emmenagogue, anti-inflammatory activity, anti-cancer activity, migraine, headache	[48]
Indian mallow	Stigmasterol, adenine, scoparone, p-coumaric acid, scoparone, riboflavin, thymine, scopoletin, scopoletin, sitosterol, syringaldehyde, vanillic acid	Anti- arthritic, cold and fever, lung ailments, tuberculosis, urinary tract infection, tooth ache, bronchitis, gout	[44]

(continued)

Table 2 (continued)

Plant name	Chemical and therapeutic compounds	Applications	References
Clearing nut tree	Diaboline, sitosterol, isomotiol, stigmasterol, akuammidine, compesterol norharmane, loganin, sucrose, mannose, lignoceric, arachidonic, linoleic, oleic, palmitic acid	Microbial infections, analgesic, hepato-protective diarrhea and diabetes, anti-microbial, anti-inflammatory, anti-nociceptive, and anti-diarrhea activity	[50]
Shallaki	Boswellic-acid, p-cyinene-limonene, terpinolene, bomyl acetate, terpinolene, bomyl acetate, p-cymene-limonene, valencene, eudesmene o-phellandrene, cis-sabinol, y-murolene, terpinene	Inflammatory diseases, cervical spondylosis, osteoarthritis, ankylosing spondylitis	[51]

7.1 Pharmacological Data Analysis

AI algorithms can analyze and process large amounts of data, including research papers, clinical trials, and patient records, to identify patterns and correlations between the use of these plant species and RA treatment. This analysis can help researchers gain insights into the effectiveness of these plants in managing RA symptoms and potentially modifying the disease progression. The common understanding of RA pathogenesis currently places a lot of emphasis on immunological abnormalities brought on by internal and external surroundings. These inflammatory mediators will then concentrate on big joints, causing synovitis and bone destruction. From the dialectical type to symptomatic treatment, traditional Chinese medicine (TCM) has its own theories and approaches relating to the function of the disease; this is carried out in accordance with clinical criteria. Mentioned Chinese herbal medicines (CHM) compounds and their herbal extracts have an antagonistic effect on RA patients and experimental animal models, which can be explained by the inhibition of synovitis, vascular hyperplasia, bone disorders, and immune cells being out of balance [37]. TCM uses CHMs and their natural products to affect RA. It is well known that CHMs and their natural products have a wide range of biological activities; the main drivers of their pharmacological action are their anti-inflammatory and antioxidative stress properties. Although many of the results from the use of omics tools and approaches to examine the mechanism of RA in transgenic and induced arthritis animal models are good, these phenomena do not appear to be specific. It has been discovered that these herbal drugs and their natural products have inhibitory effects on these targets and pathways for diseases other than RA, such as NF-B, TNF-, and members of the interleukin family. We must immediately come up with a brand-new, extremely specific explanation for RA that is, of course, related to the most recent study techniques and findings [70]. Systemic biology research on the effects of herbal medicines on RA has revealed that these treatments have the potential to improve the pathological conditions of RA patients and experimental animal models by modulating the expression of inflammatory mediators to reduce oxidative stress, regulating the production of cytokines and chemicals, and reducing the proliferation of harmful genes and inducing apoptosis. Finally, joint inflammation is reduced, excessive synovial membrane and vascular wall cell proliferation is reduced, and the imbalance of osteoclasts is controlled to prevent bone destruction [71].

7.2 Drug Discovery

AI can assist in identifying the active compounds present in these plants, such as Boswellia serrata's boswellic acids, Tanacetum parthenium's parthenolide, and Ocimum gratissimum's thymol and eugenol. By simulating molecular interactions, AI can predict how these compounds interact with specific targets implicated in RA, such as inflammatory cytokines or immune cells. This information can guide the development of new drugs or repurposing existing ones for RA treatment [69]. Drugs may be tested on much smaller groups of patients who are more likely to respond favorably to the therapy and experience few adverse effects if drug developers were to grasp how genetic diversity affects a medicine's effectiveness. This may lower the price of drug trials and make medications that would not normally be considered worthwhile available to individuals who need them. The effectiveness of using DMARDs, particularly conventional DMARDs like MTX, sulfasalazine (SSZ), and leflunomide, to treat RA is well documented. These so-called biologic medicines, which target several cytokines, interleukins, and cell receptors essential in autoimmunity, have been developed over the past few years and may improve the outcomes for RA patients when administered alone or in combination. The anti-tumor necrosis factor (TNF) drugs etanercept, infliximab, adalimumab, certolizumab, and golimumab; an IL-1 receptor antagonist: anakinra; a CTLA4-Ig fusion protein: abatacept; and the antiCD20 antibody: rituximab is among the biologics that have received FDA approval. A number of anti-TNF substances are also in development, including tocilizumab, an antibody that targets the IL-6 receptor [72]. Unpredictable toxicities and various response rates have placed restrictions on both the use of these medicines alone and in combination with conventional DMARDs. Below is a discussion of how new developments in pharmacogenomics (knowledge of toxicity, severity profile, and cost) may impact our choice of treatments. The course and progression of joint destruction in RA are highly variable; therefore, it is important to identify individuals who will advance quickly in order to avert irreparable damage, disability, and shortened survival. It has been challenging to find predictors of disease activity or response due to the disease's variable course and the separation of the clinical symptoms from the advancement of bone deterioration. Clinical, environmental, laboratory, and genetic markers are examples of potential predictors. The Health Assessment Questionnaire (HAQ), the amount of swollen and sore joints, and the failure to respond to conventional DMARDs within 6 months are some of the clinical factors that have previously been discovered. Smoking, having less education, having a lower socioeconomic status, having anti-cyclic citrullinated peptide (antiCCP) antibodies, having higher erythrocyte sedimentation rate (ESR) or C-reactive protein (CRP) levels, and having erosions at baseline have all been identified as environmental and laboratory factors that predict the progression of the disease. Furthermore, it has been established that the shared epitope between HLA-DRB1 and illness susceptibility and severity [37].

7.3 *Personalized Medicine*

AI algorithms can analyze patient data, including genetic information, medical history, and treatment response, to identify biomarkers or genetic variants associated with RA and response to specific plant-based treatments. This enables the development of personalized treatment plans tailored to individual patients, optimizing their chances of successful outcomes. There are now many instances of using genetics to foretell whether a patient would respond better to particular medications. For instance, the prescription of thiopurine medications like 6-mercaptopurine (6-MP) and azathioprine (AZA) is pertinent to genetic testing of thiopurine S-methyltransferase (TPMT), the enzyme that catalyzes the S methylation of these drugs. Common polymorphisms that have been investigated in relation to AZA toxicity regulate the activity of TPMT in red blood cells. Patients with the wild-type TPMT alleles had better treatment tolerance than those with the mutant alleles, who typically experienced low leukocyte counts. Patients could be screened in this situation and others before the medicine is prescribed; those who are unlikely to benefit are spared the expenditure and potential toxicity. On the other hand, patients who are likely to benefit from them accept them with a high level of assurance that they will have a positive outcome. This strategy may even make it possible to safely administer medications to people who are unlikely to have an unfavorable reaction, even if they could otherwise be removed from the market due to their negative effects. In fact, the development and marketing of medications are being impacted by the role that genetic variation plays in effective pharmacological therapy [70]. The first step in choosing a course of treatment is to understand the severity profile of RA patients based on particular predictions; in addition, it is vital to identify the predictors of efficacy and toxicity to both conventional DMARDs and biologic medicines. Given the high cost, increased use, and development of new drugs aimed at particular target molecules in the RA pathway, it is crucial to be able to recognize the patients who will benefit from biologics the most. All medications have the potential to cause side effects.

7.4 Clinical Decision Support

AI-powered clinical decision support systems can integrate patient-specific information, research data, and treatment guidelines to assist healthcare professionals in making informed decisions about RA treatment options. These systems can provide recommendations on the use of plant-based treatments as part of a comprehensive treatment plan for RA patients. A clinical decision support system (CDSS) can act as an advisor for clinicians, patients, or other users. In its advisory capacity, the CDSS can prescribe a best practice for postsurgical patient discharge that might include suggested medication and doses, exercise routines, and recurring follow-up examinations and tests to guarantee the best outcomes. In addition to assisting with the safest and most cost-effective escalation and treatment of emergent problems, CDSS can assist patients in choosing alternative forms of therapy or rehabilitation. In terms of lowering medical errors, especially patient errors, CDSS can be very helpful. To protect patients, several EHR software systems incorporate capable medication error subsystems. These CDSSs will evaluate prescribed medications for known drug interactions with existing medication regimens, potential drug-drug interactions with known patient allergies, and/or suggest better or less expensive medicine options for consideration. Clinicians, hospital administrators, and practice managers can all benefit from CDSS in numerous ways. To help them adopt new procedures and regulations, for instance, doctors and nurses may add or amend rules [72].

7.5 Monitoring and Prediction

AI can analyze real-time patient data, such as symptoms, medication adherence, and lifestyle factors, to monitor disease progression and predict flare-ups or treatment responses. By continuously learning from new data, AI algorithms can refine and adapt treatment plans to optimize outcomes for RA patients. In order to select the best course of treatment, gauge a patient's response to therapy, and assess prognosis, it is essential to measure disease activity [69]. Furthermore, early illness severity prediction could help with prompt administration of the best treatments. One of the most used RA severity metrics is the Disease Activity Score in 28 Joints (DAS28). ESR or CRP are just two examples of the different inflammatory indicators that might be used to generate this score. An adaptive deep neural network was able to predict DAS28-ESR from clinical and demographic data with an AUC of 0.73 (categorical prediction) and mean standard error of 0.9 (numerical prediction) that outperformed non-DL approaches. Another example of how AI is being used to track the progression of RA disease is to predict the likelihood that patients who do not react to the first therapy may need to move up to tocilizumab as their next line of treatment. Numerous comorbidities, in particular cardiovascular, atherosclerotic, musculoskeletal, and neurological conditions, are linked to rheumatoid arthritis [37]. The early identification of people who are at risk is necessary for preventing these consequences. An effective and non-invasive method to evaluate atherosclerotic plaques is carotid ultrasonography. By analyzing these images, ML and DL algorithms offer improved cardiovascular risk classification in RA patients. Surprisingly, ML classifiers performed better than the traditional cardiovascular disease risk score in a recent study when they were fed cardiovascular risk indicators, including traditional risk factors, laboratory-based blood biomarkers, and ultrasound images. The monitoring of disease activity is another area where wearable and portable technology might be very helpful. The majority of the medical equipment used nowadays is portable, such as cardiac Holter monitors and pulse oximeters. The most useful outputs can be encoded into newer wearable technology, which measures a wide range of indications. Tracking physical activity is perhaps the most popular application for wearable sensors, and it has recently started to appear in medical fields. Throughout the course of their illness, RA patients may suffer flares, which will probably make it difficult for them to engage in physical activity because of the acute inflammation. Furthermore, even in people with minimal disease activity, flares are linked to disease progression and worse outcomes [71].

It's important to note that while AI can provide valuable insights and assist in treatment development, it should always be used in conjunction with human expertise and rigorous scientific research. The development of new treatments for RA requires a multidisciplinary approach and extensive clinical validation to ensure safety and efficacy.

8 Challenges and Limitations of Implementing AI in the Diagnosis and Treatment of RA

The utilization of AI models in patient care for the treatment of RA faces several technical challenges that can cause delays. One major challenge is the requirement for large and well-labeled datasets for training supervised models. Insufficient training datasets can lead to over-fitted models, so it is crucial to create high-quality and extensive databases to overcome this issue and improve the performance of the models. For instance, the datasets from the osteoarthritis initiative study have been employed to train and test various AI models for enhancing the diagnosis and predicting the progression of pain and osteoarthritis [56]. Another limiting factor in implementing AI models is the variability of input datasets. Datasets obtained from different healthcare sectors may differ in coding, data acquisition approaches, and patient populations. Consequently, each model may perform differently when provided with different input datasets. Additionally, these models tend to utilize any available signals that contribute to achieving optimal performance. However, these signals may include unknown confounders that can compromise the model's generalizability. For example, a model designed to detect hip fractures might employ confounding features such as the scanner model used for classifying the input dataset. Moreover, manipulating data can have a detrimental effect on AI model performance.

The retrospective study design also presents limitations for the real-world application of AI models. In the medical field, only a few studies have utilized AI applications [57]. In many neural network studies, conveying intuitive notions of the model can be a challenging task, making the interpretation of results complex and referring to them as the "black box". There are also numerous social and ethical challenges associated with decisions made by AI models. Lack of transparency in the model may lead to a loss of user trust, and the absence of understanding behind the decisions and error sources can increase the chances of errors, particularly when using new datasets obtained from different experiments. Algorithmic bias is another ethical challenge encountered when using AI models, as it can exacerbate existing inequities in society, including sexual and racial discrimination [58].

Despite these challenges, AI applications involving several algorithms have demonstrated advantages in addressing problems associated with the diagnosis, treatment, prognosis, identification, drug efficacy, and risk assessment of RA. For example, combining X-ray images of joint segmentation datasets with active shape models has shown promising results in assessing and diagnosing the progression of osteoarthritis. Fuzzy inference systems and ANN models linked with inflammatory factors have been utilized for early identification and diagnosis of arthritis [27]. ML algorithms, such as naïve Bayes, SVM, and random forest, can provide information about parameters associated with cartilage damage in RA patients [59]. AI-driven algorithms based on artificial neural networks have been developed to assess joint space width for quantitative arthritis assessment instead of relying on radiographical semi-quantitative scoring systems. These algorithms have demonstrated sensitivity in assessing RA, as they are fully automated with minimal user interaction. However, interpreting results from active appearance models for analyzing contour disorders in medical images can be challenging. Electromyographic response (ER) measurement during gait is not significant for the clinical diagnosis of RA. Hierarchical learning algorithms, such as MegaSNPHunter, have been developed to identify and quantify local interactions among numerous SNPs in RA patients. Furthermore, ML platforms can predict faulty interacting genes and assess risks to prevent their occurrence [18]. With the integration of multiple machine learning models, it is anticipated that more candidate drugs will be discovered and developed in the future, providing efficient methods for RA treatment drug development. Currently, the combination of ML and glycomics has proven helpful in screening potential serum markers for individuals with RA [28, 60]. Moreover, an AI-driven biopharmaceutical company has announced the development of an integrative AI-driven bioinformatics drug discovery platform. This platform aims to rapidly identify and validate novel drug candidates for RA treatment and gain a better understanding of RA pathophysiology for various other treatments [61, 62]. By leveraging machine learning algorithms and integrating different data sources, AI can contribute to improved patient care, personalized treatment approaches, and the discovery of novel therapeutic options for individuals with RA. Continued research and development in this field hold the potential to revolutionize RA management and improve patient outcomes.

9 Future Horizons

AI, an evolving field in the medical domain, presents new opportunities for the diagnosis, treatment, prognosis, and drug development of RA, which are listed as follows:

- Although, conventional methods for RA diagnosis, drug development, and utilization of machine learning, data mining, and AI exist in their early stages for diagnosing and prognosing RA [61, 62]. Yet, the long-term prospects of computer-assisted methods in preclinical and clinical studies hold great potential for advancing current medical practices within the next two to three decades.
- There is ample scope for future research and investigations in the field of rheumatoid arthritis. It is crucial to follow guidelines to achieve the best results in AI-related studies. Guidelines such as those released by the National Health Service (NHS) and the Checklist for Artificial Intelligence in Medical Imaging (CLAIM) recommend the use of digital and data-driven health technologies [63].
- Open communication regarding source codes is important to ensure result reproducibility and allow for verification using external datasets. Additionally, to assess the performance of AI models, it is essential to conduct external validation in real-world settings.
- The future investigation of any disease, including RA, necessitates high-quality datasets in large quantities to effectively train AI models. This can be achieved by creating comprehensive multimodal datasets that encompass clinical, demographic, genomic, laboratory, imaging, and lifestyle features of patients.
- Furthermore, future studies should consider the potential risk of algorithmic bias during model development. It is important to include data points representing minorities to mitigate bias risks.
- Ultimately, the real-world implementation and widespread application of AI algorithms will rely on prospective trial designs, randomized and multi-center studies, and achieving the best performance from AI models.
- AI enhances our understanding of RA pathophysiology through increased basic science research. However, there are challenges that need to be addressed, such as the need for large and well-labeled datasets, variability of input datasets, interpretability of AI models, and ethical considerations, including algorithmic bias. Collaboration between computer science and medical professionals is essential to leverage medical datasets effectively for the advancement of RA care.

10 Conclusions

In conclusion, artificial intelligence has laid the foundation for advancements in scientific and technological areas, particularly in the diagnosis, prognosis, and treatment of rheumatoid arthritis in both Western and ancient medicine. AI offers tremendous potential in various aspects of RA management, including diagnosis, screening, prognosis determination, monitoring, risk assessment, treatment outcomes, and drug development. It also enhances our understanding of RA pathophysiology through increased basic science research. Despite significant challenges in managing the vast amount of medical information obtained from sources such as electronic medical records, medical insurance systems, disease registries, public health monitoring, genomics databases, and other health management databases, ML models, data mining, deep learning, and cloud computing have shown promise in the diagnosis and treatment of RA, further optimization and improvement of these models are still expected. Integrating ML and DL algorithms into real-world environments should be the primary focus to progress AI in healthcare. Future research should prioritize the development of generalizable and reliable algorithms, addressing potential biases and ethical concerns. With continued advancements, AI has the potential to revolutionize RA management and provide personalized care for individuals affected by this chronic condition.

Acknowledgements Authors would like to express their gratitude to Jamia Millia Islamia, New Delhi.

References

1. Wang S, Hou Y, Li X, Meng X, Zhang Y, Wang X (2021) Practical implementation of artificial intelligence-based deep learning and cloud computing on the application of traditional medicine and western medicine in the diagnosis and treatment of rheumatoid arthritis. Front Pharmacol 23(12):765435
2. Xu Y, Liu X, Cao X, Huang C, Liu E, Qian S, Liu X, Wu Y, Dong F, Qiu CW, Qiu J (2021) Artificial intelligence: a powerful paradigm for scientific research. Innovation 28(4):2(4)
3. Momtazmanesh S, Nowroozi A, Rezaei N (2022) Artificial intelligence in rheumatoid arthritis: current status and future perspectives: a state-of-the-art review. Rheumatol Ther 9(5):1249–1304
4. Khan FN, Yousef M, Raza K (2022) Machine learning-based models in the diagnosis, prognosis and effective cancer therapeutics: current state-of-the-art. In: Computational intelligence in oncology: applications in diagnosis, prognosis and therapeutics of cancers 2 Mar 2022. Singapore: Springer Singapore, pp 19–54
5. Molander V, Bower H, Frisell T, Askling J (2021) Risk of venous thromboembolism in rheumatoid arthritis, and its association with disease activity: a nationwide cohort study from Sweden. Ann Rheum Dis 80(2):169–175
6. Semb AG, Ikdahl E, Wibetoe G, Crowson C, Rollefstad S (2020) Atherosclerotic cardiovascular disease prevention in rheumatoid arthritis. Nat Rev Rheumatol 16(7):361–379
7. Courbon G, Rinaudo-Gaujous M, Blasco-Baque V, Auger I, Caire R, Mijola L, Vico L, Paul S, Marotte H (2019) Porphyromonas gingivalis experimentally induces periodontis and an anti-CCP2-associated arthritis in the rat. Ann Rheum Dis 78(5):594–599
8. Juge PA, Lee JS, Ebstein E, Furukawa H, Dobrinskikh E, Gazal S, Kannengiesser C, Ottaviani S, Oka S, Tohma S, Tsuchiya N (2018) MUC5B promoter variant and rheumatoid arthritis with interstitial lung disease. N Engl J Med 379(23):2209–2219
9. Inamo J, Kochi Y, Takeuchi T (2021) Is type 2 diabetes mellitus an inverse risk factor for the development of rheumatoid arthritis? J Hum Genet 66(2):219–223
10. Artifoni M, Rothschild PR, Brezin A, Guillevin L, Puechal X (2014) Ocular inflammatory diseases associated with rheumatoid arthritis. Nat Rev Rheumatol 10(2):108–116

11. Raaschou P, Simard JF, Hagelberg CA, Askling J (2016) Rheumatoid arthritis, anti-tumour necrosis factor treatment, and risk of squamous cell and basal cell skin cancer: cohort study based on nationwide prospectively recorded data from Sweden. BMJ 28:352
12. Ozen G, Pedro S, Wolfe F, Michaud K (2019) Medications associated with fracture risk in patients with rheumatoid arthritis. Ann Rheum Dis 78(8):1041–1047
13. Ramlal A, Ahmad S, Kumar L, Khan FN, Chongtham R (2021) From molecules to patients: the clinical applications of biological databases and electronic health records. In: Translational bioinformatics in healthcare and medicine 1 Jan 2021. Academic Press, pp 107–125
14. O'Neil LJ, Spicer V, Smolik I, Meng X, Goel RR, Anaparti V, Wilkins J, El-Gabalawy HS (2021) Association of a serum protein signature with rheumatoid arthritis development. Arthritis Rheumatol 73(1):78–88
15. Wei T, Yang B, Liu H, Xin F, Fu L (2020) Development and validation of a nomogram to predict coronary heart disease in patients with rheumatoid arthritis in northern China. Aging (Albany NY) 12(4):3190
16. Wu H, Cai L, Li D, Wang X, Zhao S, Zou F, Zhou K (2018) Metagenomics biomarkers selected for prediction of three different diseases in Chinese population. BioMed Res Int
17. Negi S, Juyal G, Senapati S, Prasad P, Gupta A, Singh S, Kashyap S, Kumar A, Kumar U, Gupta R, Kaur S (2013) A genome-wide association study reveals ARL15, a novel non-HLA susceptibility gene for rheumatoid arthritis in North Indians. Arthritis Rheum 65(12):3026–3035
18. Kruppa J, Ziegler A, König IR (2012) Risk estimation and risk prediction using machine-learning methods. Hum Genet 131:1639–1654
19. Liu C, Ackerman HH, Carulli JP (2011) A genome-wide screen of gene–gene interactions for rheumatoid arthritis susceptibility. Hum Genet 129:473–485
20. Ekambaram S, Perumal SS, Subramanian V (2010) Evaluation of antiarthritic activity of Strychnos potatorum Linn seeds in Freund's adjuvant induced arthritic rat model. BMC Complement Altern Med 10:1–9
21. González-Recio O, De Maturana EL, Vega AT, Engelman CD, Broman KW (2009) Detecting single-nucleotide polymorphism by single-nucleotide polymorphism interactions in rheumatoid arthritis using a two-step approach with machine learning and a Bayesian threshold least absolute shrinkage and selection operator (LASSO) model. In: BMC proceedings 2009, vol 3, no 7. BioMed Central, pp 1–5
22. Kumar LD, Karthik R, Gayathri N, Sivasudha T (2016) Advancement in contemporary diagnostic and therapeutic approaches for rheumatoid arthritis. Biomed Pharmacother 1(79):52–61
23. Kay J, Upchurch KS (2012) ACR/EULAR 2010 rheumatoid arthritis classification criteria. Rheumatology. 1 Dec 2012. 51(suppl_6):vi5-9
24. Agarwal K, Varma R (2014) Ocimum gratissimum L.: A medicinal plant with promising antiurolithiatic activity. Int J Pharm Sci Drug Res 6(1):78–81
25. Ormseth MJ, Solus JF, Sheng Q, Ye F, Wu Q, Guo Y, Oeser AM, Allen RM, Vickers KC, Stein CM (2020) Development and validation of a microRNA panel to differentiate between patients with rheumatoid arthritis or systemic lupus erythematosus and controls. J Rheumatol 47(2):188–196
26. Geurts P, Fillet M, De Seny D, Meuwis MA, Malaise M, Merville MP, Wehenkel L (2005) Proteomic mass spectra classification using decision tree based ensemble methods. Bioinformatics 21(14):3138–3145
27. Heard BJ, Rosvold JM, Fritzler MJ, El-Gabalawy H, Wiley JP, Krawetz RJ (2014) A computational method to differentiate normal individuals, osteoarthritis and rheumatoid arthritis patients using serum biomarkers. J R Soc Interface 11(97):20140428
28. Chocholova E, Bertok T, Jane E, Lorencova L, Holazova A, Belicka L, Belicky S, Mislovicova D, Vikartovska A, Imrich R, Kasak P (2018) Glycomics meets artificial intelligence–potential of glycan analysis for identification of seropositive and seronegative rheumatoid arthritis patients revealed. Clin Chim Acta 1(481):49–55

29. Yeo L, Adlard N, Biehl M, Juarez M, Smallie T, Snow M, Buckley CD, Raza K, Filer A, Scheel-Toellner D (2016) Expression of chemokines CXCL4 and CXCL7 by synovial macrophages defines an early stage of rheumatoid arthritis. Ann Rheum Dis 75(4):763–771
30. Wu M, Wu H, Wu L, Cui C, Shi S, Xu J, Liu Y, Dong F (2022) A deep learning classification of metacarpophalangeal joints synovial proliferation in rheumatoid arthritis by ultrasound images. J Clin Ultrasound 50(2):296–301
31. Volkova A, Ruggles KV (2021) Predictive metagenomic analysis of autoimmune disease identifies robust autoimmunity and disease specific microbial signatures. Front Microbiol 4(12):621310
32. Zhou SM, Fernandez-Gutierrez F, Kennedy J, Cooksey R, Atkinson M, Denaxas S, Siebert S, Dixon WG, O'Neill TW, Choy E, Sudlow C (2016) Defining disease phenotypes in primary care electronic health records by a machine learning approach: a case study in identifying rheumatoid arthritis. PLoS ONE 11(5):e0154515
33. Chen Y, Carroll RJ, Hinz ER, Shah A, Eyler AE, Denny JC, Xu H (2013) Applying active learning to high-throughput phenotyping algorithms for electronic health records data. J Am Med Inform Assoc 20(e2):e253–e259
34. Gronsbell J, Minnier J, Yu S, Liao K, Cai T (2019) Automated feature selection of predictors in electronic medical records data. Biometrics 75(1):268–277
35. Morid MA, Lau M, Del Fiol G (2021) Predictive analytics for step-up therapy: supervised or semi-supervised learning? J Biomed Inform 1(119):103842
36. Kato M, Ikeda K, Sugiyama T, Tanaka S, Iida K, Suga K, Nishimura N, Mimura N, Kasuya T, Kumagai T, Furuya H (2021) Associations of ultrasound-based inflammation patterns with peripheral innate lymphoid cell populations, serum cytokines/chemokines, and treatment response to methotrexate in rheumatoid arthritis and spondyloarthritis. PLoS ONE 16(5):e0252116
37. Kalweit M, Walker UA, Finckh A, Müller R, Kalweit G, Scherer A, Boedecker J, Hügle T (2021) Personalized prediction of disease activity in patients with rheumatoid arthritis using an adaptive deep neural network. PLoS ONE 16(6):e0252289
38. Rychkov D, Neely J, Oskotsky T, Yu S, Perlmutter N, Nititham J, Carvidi A, Krueger M, Gross A, Criswell LA, Ashouri JF (2021) Cross-tissue transcriptomic analysis leveraging machine learning approaches identifies new biomarkers for rheumatoid arthritis. Front Immunol 8(12):638066
39. Gossec L, Guyard F, Leroy D, Lafargue T, Seiler M, Jacquemin C, Molto A, Sellam J, Foltz V, Gandjbakhch F, Hudry C (2019) Detection of flares by decrease in physical activity, collected using wearable activity trackers in rheumatoid arthritis or axial spondyloarthritis: an application of machine learning analyses in rheumatology. Arthritis Care Res 71(10):1336–1343
40. Zhao X, Kim YR, Min Y, Zhao Y, Do K, Son YO (2021) Natural plant extracts and compounds for rheumatoid arthritis therapy. Medicina 57(3):266
41. Xiang Y, Shujin L, Hongfang C, Yinping W, Dawei Y, Zhou D, Zhiqing L (2021) Artificial intelligence-based diagnosis of diabetes mellitus: combining fundus photography with traditional Chinese medicine diagnostic methodology. Biomed Res Int 20(2021):1–7
42. Khan FN, Khanam AA, Ramlal A, Ahmad S (2021) A review on predictive systems and data models for covid-19. In: Computational intelligence methods in COVID-19: surveillance, prevention, prediction and diagnosis, 123–164
43. Das D, Jaiswal M, Khan FN, Ahamad S, Kumar S (2020) PlantPepDB: s manually curated plant peptide database. Sci Rep 10(1):2194
44. Kumar SS, Bhosle D, Janghel A, Deo S, Raut P, Verma C, Agrawal M, Amit N, Sharma M, Giri T, Tripathi DK (2015) Indian medicinal plants used for treatment of rheumatoid arthritis. Res J Pharm Technol 8(5):597–610
45. Jain S, Jain A, Vaidya A, Kumar D, Jain V (2014) Preliminary phytochemical, pharmacognostical and physico-chemical evaluation of Cedrus deodara heartwood. J Pharmacogn Phytochem 3(1):91–95
46. Nidavani RB, Mahalakshmi AM (2014) Teak (Tectona grandis Linn.): a renowned timber plant with potential medicinal values. Int J Pharm Pharm Sci 6(1):48–54

47. Joseph A, Mathew S, Skaria BP, Sheeja EC (2011) Medicinal uses and biological activities of Argyreia speciosa sweet (Hawaiian baby woodrose)-an overview
48. Pareek A, Suthar M, Rathore GS, Bansal V (2011) Feverfew (Tanacetum parthenium L.): a systematic review. Pharmacogn Rev 5(9):103
49. Mu CX, Liu GL, Tian H, Li YC, Huang YL (2014) Effect of tetramethyl pyrazine on serum levels of IL-1beta, IL-6, and IL-2, and NO and PGE2 in the synovial fluid of CIA rats: an experimental research. Zhongguo Zhong xi yi jie he za zhi Zhongguo Zhongxiyi Jiehe Zazhi = Chinese J Integr Tradit West Med 1 Feb 2014 34(2):214–217
50. Yu HH, Li M, Li YB, Lei BB, Yuan X, Xing XK, Xie YF, Wang M, Wang L, Yang HJ, Feng ZW (2020) Benzoylaconitine inhibits production of IL-6 and IL-8 via MAPK, Akt, NF-κB signaling in IL-1β-induced human synovial cells. Biol Pharm Bull 43(2):334–339
51. Zhou YZ, Zhao LD, Chen H, Zhang Y, Wang DF, Huang LF, Lv QW, Liu B, Li Z, Wei W, Li H (2018) Comparison of the impact of Tripterygium wilfordii Hook F and Methotrexate treatment on radiological progression in active rheumatoid arthritis: 2-year follow up of a randomized, non-blinded, controlled study. Arthritis Res Ther 20:1–2
52. Hosseini A, Hosseinzadeh H (2018) Antidotal or protective effects of Curcuma longa (turmeric) and its active ingredient, curcumin, against natural and chemical toxicities: a review. Biomed Pharmacother 1(99):411–421
53. Chen JJ, Dai L, Zhao LX, Zhu X, Cao S, Gao YJ (2015) Intrathecal curcumin attenuates pain hypersensitivity and decreases spinal neuroinflammation in rat model of monoarthritis. Sci Rep 5(1):10278
54. Zhang L, Wei W (2020) Anti-inflammatory and immunoregulatory effects of paeoniflorin and total glucosides of paeony. Pharmacol Ther 1(207):107452
55. Zheng W, Lu X, Fu Z, Zhang L, Li X, Xu X, Ren Y, Lu Y, Fu H, Tian J (1864) Identification of candidate synovial membrane biomarkers after Achyranthes aspera treatment for rheumatoid arthritis. Biochim Biophys Acta (BBA)-Proteins Proteomics 1 Mar 2016 1864(3):308–316
56. Leung K, Zhang B, Tan J, Shen Y, Geras KJ, Babb JS, Cho K, Chang G, Deniz CM (2020) Prediction of total knee replacement and diagnosis of osteoarthritis by using deep learning on knee radiographs: data from the osteoarthritis initiative. Radiology 296(3):584–593
57. Badgeley MA, Zech JR, Oakden-Rayner L, Glicksberg BS, Liu M, Gale W, McConnell MV, Percha B, Snyder TM, Dudley JT (2019) Deep learning predicts hip fracture using confounding patient and healthcare variables. NPJ Digit Med 2(1):31
58. Panch T, Mattie H, Atun R (2019) Artificial intelligence and algorithmic bias: implications for health systems. J Glob Health 9(2)
59. Du Y, Almajalid R, Shan J, Zhang M (2018) A novel method to predict knee osteoarthritis progression on MRI using machine learning methods. IEEE Trans Nanobiosci 17(3):228–236
60. Khan FN, Ahmad S, Raza K (2021) Clinical applications of next-generation sequence analysis in acute myelogenous leukemia. In: Translational bioinformatics applications in healthcare. CRC Press, Boca Raton. 19 Apr 19. https://doi.org/10.1201/9781003146988-4
61. Langmead B, Nellore A (2018) Cloud computing for genomic data analysis and collaboration. Nat Rev Genet 19(4):208–219
62. Koppad S, Gkoutos GV, Acharjee A (2021) Cloud computing enabled big multi-omics data analytics. Bioinform Biol Insights 15:11779322211035920
63. Wang SY, Pershing S, Lee AY (2020) Big data requirements for artificial intelligence. Curr Opin Ophthalmol 31(5):318
64. Hafezi-Nejad N, Guermazi A, Roemer FW, Hunter DJ, Dam EB, Zikria B, Kwoh CK, Demehri S (2017) Prediction of medial tibiofemoral compartment joint space loss progression using volumetric cartilage measurements: data from the FNIH OA biomarkers consortium. Eur Radiol 27:464–473
65. Jabeen A, Ahmad N, Raza K (2018) Machine learning-based state-of-the-art methods for the classification of rna-seq data. Cllfication BioApps: Autom Decis Mak 133–172
66. Khan FN, Asim M, Qureshi MI (2022) Overview and classification of swarm intelligence-based nature-inspired computing algorithms and their applications in cancer detection and diagnosis. In: Nature-inspired intelligent computing techniques in bioinformatics 1 Nov 2022. Springer Nature Singapore, Singapore, pp 119–145

67. Qazi S, Iqbal N, Raza K (2021) Machine learning in cancer diagnosis, prognosis and therapy. Artif Intell Data-Driven Med Diagn 8(3):103
68. Sahu A, Qazi S, Raza K, Singh A, Verma S (2022) Machine learning-based approach for early diagnosis of breast cancer using biomarkers and gene expression profiles. In: Computational intelligence in oncology: applications in diagnosis, prognosis and therapeutics of cancers 2 Mar 2022. Springer Singapore, Singapore, pp 285–306
69. Li TP, Zhang AH, Miao JH, Sun H, Yan GL, Wu FF, Wang XJ (2019) Applications and potential mechanisms of herbal medicines for rheumatoid arthritis treatment: a systematic review. RSC Adv 9(45):26381–26392
70. Smuck M, Odonkor CA, Wilt JK, Schmidt N, Swiernik MA (2021) The emerging clinical role of wearables: factors for successful implementation in healthcare. NPJ Digit Med 4(1):45
71. Burgos PI, Danila MI, Kelley JM, Hughes LB, Bridges SL Jr (2009) Understanding personalized medicine in rheumatoid arthritis: a clinician's guide to the future. Ther Adv Musculoskelet Dis 1(2):97–105
72. Sloane EB, Silva RJ (2020) Artificial intelligence in medical devices and clinical decision support systems. In: Clinical engineering handbook 1 Jan 2020. Academic Press, pp 556–568

AI-Enhanced Data Analytics Framework for Autoimmune Disease: Revolutionizing Diagnosis, Monitoring, and Treatment Strategy

Arif Md. Sattar, Mritunjay Kr. Ranjan, and Sanjay Kr. Tiwari

Abstract AI and precision medicine have advanced to improve patient diagnosis, prognosis, and treatment for autoimmune diseases like multiple sclerosis (MS). However, evaluations of AI efficacy, cost, and scalability are needed to fully enhance autoimmune rCTD care. Data scientists use healthcare analytics to help doctors make accurate diagnoses and choose the best treatments. Predictive and prescriptive analytics can forecast and monitor illness, and AI and machine learning pipelines can examine and learn from various data sources. These techniques can help diagnose and treat autoimmune diseases like MS, reduce illness severity, and optimize care plans, drugs, treatments, and resources for high-cost patients. Our analytics platform extends the same technology, procedures, and experience to population-level information to detect autoimmune and associated disorders in large patient groups.

Keywords NIH · AI · Predictive analytics · Autoimmune diseases · Datasets · rCTD · Multiple sclerosis · Demographic

1 Introduction

The average human lifespan has experienced a substantial increase as a result of the progress in medical technology and enhancements in public health witnessed during the last two centuries. The aforementioned advancement has played a pivotal role in addressing noncommunicable diseases (NCDs), which are alternatively referred to as

A. Md. Sattar (✉)
Department of Computer Science, Anugrah Memorial College, Gaya, India
e-mail: amsattargaya@gmail.com

M. Kr. Ranjan
School of Computer Science &, Engineering Sandip University, Nashik, MH, India
e-mail: mritunjaykranjan@gmail.com

S. Kr. Tiwari
P.G. Department of Mathematics, Magadh University, Bodh-Gaya, India
e-mail: tiwaridrsanjay@gmail.com

K. Raza and S. Singh (eds.), *Artificial Intelligence and Autoimmune Diseases*, Studies in Computational Intelligence 1133, https://doi.org/10.1007/978-981-99-9029-0_11

chronic ailments. Recent research has revealed that chronic inflammatory diseases contribute to approximately 50% of global mortality rates. The diseases in question encompass a range of conditions, including type 2 diabetes, obesity, cardiovascular disease (CVD), metabolically associated fatty liver disease (MAFLD), cancer, chronic lung and renal disease, autoimmune disorders, and neurodegenerative illnesses [3]. In contemporary times, the genetic makeup of individuals operates within a markedly dissimilar milieu compared to its original evolutionary context, as evidenced by substantial transformations that have transpired within the past century. Numerous studies have consistently demonstrated that a significant proportion, ranging from 80 to 90%, of the risk attributed to specific diseases can be attributed to non-genetic factors [27]. Research conducted by the Global Burden of Disease (GBD) between 1990 and 2016 across 195 countries has provided evidence that a significant proportion, approximately 60%, of global fatalities can be attributed to modifiable risk factors. Chronic illnesses are distinguished by disruptions in the body's equilibrium, known as homeostasis, and persistent metabolic inflammation, frequently originating from lifestyle decisions. The dynamic relationship between inflammation and homeostasis serves as a fundamental aspect of the biological mechanisms underlying chronic diseases, which are influenced by a combination of genetic and environmental factors. The term "exposome" pertains to the cumulative effect of non-heritable environmental exposures experienced by an individual over their lifespan. This encompasses a wide range of factors including nutrition, psychological stress, physical impacts, and biological reactions. The field of exposomics utilizes a combination of internal and external evaluation techniques [21]. Precision medicine is a medical approach that takes into account an individual's genetic information, lifestyle choices, and environmental factors in order to inform and tailor patient treatments. This methodology individualizes the provision of treatment and preventive measures through a comprehensive comprehension of the factors that contribute to the likelihood of developing a disease. The utilization of "OMICS" or "EXPOsOMICS" and wearable sensors results in the generation of substantial quantities of data, commonly referred to as big data. Consequently, the analysis, integration, and interpretation of this data necessitate the development of novel digital methodologies and tools [36, 44]. Artificial intelligence (AI) is a contemporary scientific field that empowers computer systems to autonomously execute tasks. AI algorithms necessitate well-structured and annotated data for training, and subsequent to this training, they exhibit a high level of proficiency in scrutinizing and discerning patterns within extensive datasets. Machine learning, deep learning, and artificial neural networks are integral constituents of artificial intelligence (AI). The integration of artificial intelligence (AI) with high-performance computing has yielded substantial advancements in disease risk prediction [38]. Furthermore, the incorporation of AI into precision medicine has the capacity to enhance our comprehension of recurrent diseases [40]. Autoimmune diseases (ADs) occur as a result of the immune system's inability to differentiate between self and non-self cells, leading to the recognition and attack of the body's own cells. Currently, more than 80 distinct autoimmune diseases have been identified. ADs are distinguished by the presence of adaptive immunity, which encompasses the participation of T and B cells

[42]. The utilization of serological methods that involve the detection of antibodies has significantly progressed the detection and classification of Alzheimer's disease (AD). The impact of ads can extend to various bodily systems, encompassing both the entire body and specific organs, such as the gastrointestinal tract (GI). The GI tract is affected by a range of contributors and systemic diseases. Among the autoimmune diseases that commonly affect the GI tract are achalasia, atrophic autoimmune gastritis (AAG), celiac disease (CD), eosinophilic esophagitis (EoE), and inflammatory bowel disorders (IBD) such as Crohn's disease and ulcerative colitis (UC), among others. The present chapter provides an in-depth analysis of the conceptualization and origins of autoimmune diseases, the association between autoimmunity and inflammatory processes, a comprehensive overview of five distinct diseases, the significance of predictive antibodies, the interconnection between the gut and brain, considerations regarding nutrition, and various available treatment modalities. Autoimmune diseases are characterized by the immune system's aberrant targeting of healthy cells. The title "AI-Enhanced Data Analytics Framework for Autoimmune Disease: Revolutionising Diagnosis, Monitoring, and Treatment Strategy" highlights the significance of comprehending the relationship between chronic diseases, exposomics, precision medicine, and artificial intelligence. This understanding emphasizes the potential for groundbreaking progress in the diagnosis, monitoring, and treatment of autoimmune diseases.

2 Literature Review

The article "The interferon signature in autoimmune diseases" written by [32] investigates the function of interferons in relation to autoimmune diseases. There is a discussion of the processes through which interferons contribute to autoimmunity. Some of these mechanisms include stimulating the activation of autoreactive immune cells, boosting B cell responses, and changing the balance of immune cell subsets. Additionally, the potential therapeutic consequences of targeting interferon pathways in the treatment of autoimmune illnesses are brought to light by this study.

The article written by [12] presents an expert view on the current treatment techniques for primary Sjogren's Syndrome (pSS), which is a chronic autoimmune condition that is characterized by dryness of the mouth and eyes. This article examines the many therapy alternatives that are now available and explores the efficacy, safety, and possible future directions of these approaches. In addition to this, it highlights the significance of patient education, supportive treatment, and routine monitoring in the long-term management of pSS. The study is useful for healthcare professionals who are involved in the care of patients who have pSS because it provides insights into the management of this complicated autoimmune condition.

The article by [20] presents an overview of the progress achieved in understanding and perhaps preventing the development of clinical rheumatoid arthritis in those who are at risk for developing the condition. This article describes the pathophysiology of RA, the finding of biomarkers, as well as continuing research efforts in the development of preventative therapies. The article places an emphasis on the need for interdisciplinary approaches that involve researchers, primary care physicians, and rheumatologists in order to effectively identify patients who are at risk, monitor the course of the condition, and put preventative measures into place. In addition to this, it emphasizes the need for interdisciplinary methods that involve researchers, primary care physicians, and rheumatologists in order to effectively identify patients who are at risk, monitor the course of the illness, and apply preventative measures.

A literature overview of the diagnostic techniques that are employed in autoimmune rheumatic diseases (ARDs) can be found in [5], which highlights how important it is to get an accurate diagnosis as early as possible in ARDs in order to start the proper therapy and enhance patient outcomes. This article also discusses the function that clinical evaluation, laboratory tests, imaging modalities, and histology play in the diagnosis procedure. It places an emphasis on the teamwork that must take place between rheumatologists, laboratory experts, radiologists, and pathologists in order to integrate clinical observations, laboratory data, and imaging investigations in order to arrive at an appropriate diagnosis.

Orme and Scorza [25] present a literature review of the current techniques for diagnosing and managing MS and the future of these fields. It also underscores the need for continued study and collaboration to further enhance diagnosis accuracy, further explore innovative therapeutic techniques, and refine treatment tactics. Meroni et al. [23] discuss the impact that pregnancy can have on a variety of autoimmune diseases. It examines the hormonal and immunological changes that occur during pregnancy, the influence that these changes have on disease activity, the issues that come with managing autoimmune disorders during pregnancy, and the long-term consequences of pregnancy on autoimmune diseases. It is an extremely helpful resource for medical professionals who are involved in the treatment of women who suffer from autoimmune illnesses.

A literature review on the connection between infections and autoimmune disease can be found in De la et al. [6]. This article presents the role infectious agents, like bacteria, viruses, and parasites can have in the pathogenesis of a variety of autoimmune disorders and how they can either initiate these conditions or contribute to their development. The authors discuss the different ways that infections might be used to promote autoimmunity. Some of these strategies include molecular mimicry and bystander activation. In addition to this, they explore the influence that infections have on the progression and severity of autoimmune disorders, as well as the possible therapeutic implications of targeting infections in autoimmune diseases. Reddy and Desai [28] present an overview of the most current research and advancements in the area of lupus nephritis, which is a severe form of systemic lupus erythematosus (SLE). It discusses the epidemiology, clinical, pathogenesis, histological features, importance of biomarkers, and the classification of lupus nephritis. It also presents current treatment approaches for lupus nephritis.

3 Autoimmune Diseases: What It is, How It Works, and Where It Comes from?

The average lifespan of humans has increased throughout the course of the previous two centuries as a direct result of advancements in medical technology as well as improvements in public health. Over the course of a person's lifetime, they are at an increased risk of getting noncommunicable diseases (NCDs), also known as chronic illnesses as they are more popularly known. According to the findings of the most recent study, chronic inflammatory diseases are responsible for around half of all fatalities that occur across the globe. The conditions of type 2 diabetes, obesity, cardiovascular disease (CVD), metabolic associated fatty liver disease (MAFLD), cancer, chronic lung and renal disease, autoimmune illness, and neurodegenerative illness are all included in the scope of this research as per [34]. Our genes are able to function in a world that is significantly different from the one for which they were made, and individuals living in today's world are surrounded by an environment that has experienced tremendous alteration over the course of the previous century. Non-genetic variables are responsible for eighty to ninety percent of the illness risk that is associated with certain conditions. Sixty percent of fatalities throughout the world may be attributed to modifiable risk factors, according to the findings of research that were carried out by the Global Burden of Disease (GBD) between the years 1990 and 2016 in 195 different countries [8]. Chronic illnesses are generally characterized by abnormalities in homeostasis, in addition to chronic metabolic inflammation. These diseases are often the result of lifestyle decisions. Because of this, the biology of chronic illness establishes a connection between inflammation and the upkeep of homeostasis. It is already established that both hereditary genes and environmental variables can play a role in the progression of illness. The term "exposome" refers to the accumulation of non-inherited environmental exposures that occur over the course of a person's lifetime. An individual's "exposome" is an illustration of the complexity of their exposures to potentially hazardous factors, such as their nutrition, mental stresses, physical repercussions, and biological reactions to those elements. The "exposome" also includes their biological responses. According to [24] within the context of the study on the exposome, both internal and external assessment strategies are utilized. Patients are given treatments based on precision medicine, which takes into consideration the patient's DNA, the lifestyle choices they make, and the settings in which they live. By having an understanding of the variables that put a person at risk for getting a specific disease as well as the underlying biological processes that are the fundamental cause of that sickness, precision medicine makes it possible to individualize treatment and preventative methods. This may be accomplished by gaining a knowledge of precision medicine. "OMICS" or "EXPOsOMICS" and wearable sensors as measurement/assessment techniques may create tremendous amounts of data (big data), which needs the development of new digital methods and resources for analyzing, integrating, and interpreting the data. OMICS and wearable sensors as measurement/assessment techniques may produce enormous volumes of data (big data). The field of study known as AI is a scientific discipline in which computer systems may carry out activities without the need for direct supervision from humans. The data must first be organized and categorized before AI algorithms may be successfully produced by computer systems. When the algorithm has been provided with an adequate number of data points and labels, the resulting output is subjected to quality assurance testing to validate its accuracy. Algorithms used in AI are capable of monitoring, analyzing, and locating patterns in large volumes of data in a time and energy-efficient manner. In this context, AI encompasses a wide range of concepts, including machine learning, deep learning, and artificial neural networks. AI and high-performance computers now have the ability to analyze individual data and determine whether or not a person is at risk of contracting a disease. Machine learning and AI technology transform massive amounts of data into therapeutic knowledge. Because of these platforms, our ability to forecast the likelihood of becoming ill has been significantly improved. It is feasible that as AI gets increasingly incorporated into precision medicine, it will aid corporations in capitalizing on it and expanding our awareness of recurrent illnesses. Both of these outcomes are plausible.

Autoimmune illnesses are problems that manifest themselves when the body is unable to differentiate between its cells and other cells in the body. Over 80 different autoimmune disorders have been identified. The immune system is considered to be one of the physiological systems that has the least amount of knowledge associated with it. New information on the immune system has been available as a result of COVID-19. It's possible that a mix of environmental and genetic factors are to blame for ADs. This group of disorders is distinguished by a characteristic known as adaptive immunity, which is demonstrated by T and B cells. The utilization of antibody-detecting serological approaches has contributed to improvements in both the detection and categorization of AD. There is an autoimmunity that affects the entire body as well as organs specifically. The mouth, esophagus, stomach, small intestine, and large intestine are all part of the digestive system, often known as the gastrointestinal (GI) tract of the human body. A number of contributors to the etiology of the sickness have an effect on the GI tract, which is also affected by a number of systemic diseases. Achalasia, atrophic autoimmune gastritis (AAG), celiac disease (CD), eosinophilia esophagitis (EoE), and inflammatory bowel disorders (IBD), which include Crohn disease and ulcerative colitis (UC), are examples of common autoimmune illnesses that affect the gastrointestinal system. Other IBDs include celiac disease. Systemic lupus erythematosus (SLE), systemic mastocytosis, systematic sclerosis, CREST syndrome, autoimmune enteropathy, autoimmune hepatitis, autoimmune pancreatitis, mixed connective tissues disease, primary and autoimmune sclerosing cholangitis, and autoimmune enteropathy are all diseases that have the potential to cause symptoms in the gastrointestinal tract. This chapter does not go into the GI manifestation at all.

In this chapter, we will discuss the definition and etiology of autoimmune diseases, the relationship between autoimmunity and inflammation, an overview of the five diseases, the common antibodies that are used as predictor factors for the disease, the gut-brain axis and the psychological link in GI tract autoimmune diseases, nutrition in GI tract autoimmune diseases, and treatment options. Autoimmune diseases are characterized by the body's immune system mistakenly attacking its own healthy cells.

4 Inflammation to Autoinflammation and Epithelial Barrier Dysfunction: A Brief Look into the Developmental Stage

The most difficult part of immunological disorders such as autoinflammatory and autoimmune diseases is to identify the early events that initiate immune dysregulation [1]. This is the case because immunological diseases are caused by the body's own immune system attacking itself. The terms "autoinflammatory" and "autoimmunity" are often used interchangeably, perhaps because of their close relationship. Despite the fact that they have certain characteristics and may potentially exist on a continuum together, these two phrases do not necessarily refer to the same entity. The most important distinction that can be made between autoinflammatory disease and autoimmune disease is that autoinflammatory refers to the dysregulations related to adaptive immunity while autoimmunity is defined as the dysregulation in innate immunity [4]. This is the most important line of differentiation that can be drawn between autoinflammatory disease and autoimmune disease. This description is not completely true and is also a little bit out of date, as we will demonstrate in the next section how the innate immune system and the adaptive immune system are engaged in both autoinflammation and autoimmunity and what the connections are between the two. The self-destructive and systematic character of the two pathogenic processes, encompass monogenic and polygenic disorders. In any of these processes, which ultimately result in inflammation or injury to the tissue, the immune system becomes chronically activated.

4.1 The Role of Innate and Adaptive Immunity

Immunologic defenses in vertebrates consist of two immunologic subsystems—innate and adaptive immunities. Innate is the natural immunity by birth while adaptive immunity is the acquired immunity (Fig. 1).

4.1.1 Innate Immunity

When it comes to an individual's immune system, the innate immune system is considered to be the primary defensive mechanism. As a consequence of this, it is

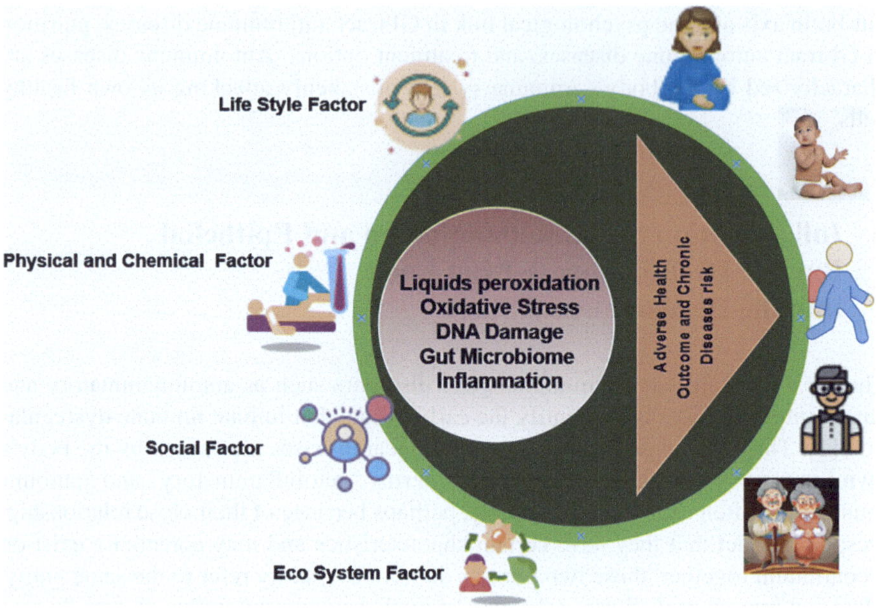

Fig. 1 The cycle of innate and adaptive immunity

able to identify infections in addition to other noxious stimuli that have the potential to produce inflammation and activate adaptive immunity. Macrophages, dendritic cells, and antigen-presenting cells (APCs) are all examples of effector cells that are a part of the innate immune system [10]. The molecular patterns that are expressed by pathogens (also known as pathogen-associated molecular patterns, or PAMPs) or by damaged cells (also known as damage-associated molecular patterns, or DAMPs) are recognized and identified by the innate immune system. TLRs, also known as Toll-like receptors, RLRs, also known as RIG-I-like receptors, and NLRs, also known as nucleotide-binding oligomerization domain-like receptors, are the three different kinds of pattern recognition receptors (PRR) that exist. It is believed that the induction of intracellular signal transduction pathways occurs upon the detection of foreign molecules. This, in turn, causes the development of interferon-alpha (IFN) sequences, IFN- sequences, TNF sequences, and interleukin 1 (IL-1) Immunology of the GI Tract 4 sequences. The dysregulation of these receptors, which most often manifests as excessive or protracted activation [15], has been implicated as a potential cause of autoinflammatory disorders as well as autoimmune diseases.

4.1.2 Adaptive Immunity

It takes between three and five days for adaptive immunity to reach its full maturity stage. In adaptive immunity, lymphocytes known as B cells, T cells, and cytotoxic

T cells all play a role [10]. Antigens are recognized by highly specialized antigen receptors, the majority of which are found on B and T cells (referred to respectively as BCR and TCR). Innate immunity serves as the body's initial line of defense against both harm and illness. Adaptive immunity, on the other hand, confers a resistance that is more powerful but also more gradual.

4.2 The Immunological Disease

IFN is more often connected with autoimmune illnesses, notably systemic lupus erythematosus (SLE), while IL-1 is associated with pure innate immunity. Continuum IL-1 1 and type I interferon (IFN) are also polarised cytokines that are related to innate immunity. The relevance of recognizing Type I IFN dysregulation as a driving factor in autoimmunity, as well as NLR dysfunction as a driving factor in conventional autoinflammatory disorders without autoantibody creation, has led to a polarization in the categorization of immunological illnesses. This polarization has been brought about as a result of the importance of recognizing autoantibody formation. Due to the fact that it was first recognized that autoinflammatory illnesses were connected to NLR cytoplasmic localized innate immune receptors (NLRP3 in particular), this discovery was made. Several studies have been published that establish a connection between innate immune-mediated diseases and inflammasomes, one of which is NLRC4. The fact that members of the NLR family exhibit a consistent link with both monogenic and polygenic autoinflammatory illness is notable. On the other hand, TLRs do not show this association, which may be due to the fact that TLRs have redundant functions.

4.3 The Epithelial Barrier Dysfunction

A third factor in pathogenesis is the presence of a leaky gut. The epithelium of the gastrointestinal system, also known as the epithelial barrier, is the biggest mucosal lining that provides contact between a mammalian host and the external environment. This epithelium is also widely referred to as the mucosal barrier. The epithelium barrier's principal responsibility is to defend the body from invading microorganisms and other external substances. Processes such as digestion, absorption, and the network of neuroendocrine glands, in addition to the balancing of immunological function, all take place inside the anatomical structure of the GI tract. The lumen of the gut is home to a diverse community of microbes numbering in the trillions. These microorganisms are very necessary for digestion, as well as the regulation of the immune system according to [17].

5 The Five Common GI Autoimmune Diseases

Autoimmune disorders are situations in which the immune system erroneously assaults and destroys the body's own tissues. These diseases can manifest in a variety of ways. In cases of GI autoimmune illnesses, the immune system mistakenly attacks the cells and tissues of the digestive system, which results in inflammation, damage to the tissues, and a variety of symptoms. These disorders have the potential to impact several areas of the gastrointestinal system, such as the esophagus, stomach, small intestine, large intestine, and other organs that are involved in the digestive process. The particular symptoms that are present as well as the degree to which GI autoimmune disorders affect a person might change based on the ailment as well as the person. Here are descriptions of five prevalent GI autoimmune diseases.

5.1 *Achalasia*

Achalasia is a rare autoimmune motility illness that is caused by the degeneration of the myenteric neuronal esophageal plexus According to [30]. This condition affects the muscles that move food through the digestive tract. As a result of the condition, this degradation leads to a peristalsis, a defective partial relaxation of the lower esophageal sphincter (LES), and ineffectual contractions in the body of the esophagus. Achalasia can be managed with medicines, but there is currently no cure for the condition. Achalasia is distinguished by a functional loss of myenteric plexus ganglion cells or chronic ganglionitis in the distal esophagus and the lower esophageal sphincter. This condition can also be caused by a combination of these two factors. Ganglionitis, a persistent inflammatory condition, is another potential reason for this loss. Because there is no known reason for the first loss of inhibitory neurons in those who suffer from achalasia, it is probable that achalasia is an idiopathic illness.

5.2 *Atrophic Autoimmune Gastritis (AAG)*

A disorder that is mediated by the immune system and that is marked by nonspecific symptoms is referred to as atrophic autoimmune gastritis, or AAG for short according to [22]. It is necessary to demonstrate the existence of circulating antibodies against the adenosine triphosphate enzyme H/K in order to verify a diagnosis of AAG. These antibodies are referred to as parietal cell antibodies (PCA). Antibodies with the same specificity have also been shown to react with anti-intrinsic factor (anti-IF) (Wiley Online [43]). During the progression of AAG, the native gastric glands that are located inside the mucosa of a patient's stomach gradually atrophy or disappear. This occurs in people who have the condition. The antrum is spared as a result of this, but the mucosal tissue begins to deteriorate as a consequence of this. In addition to this, a large amount of pseudopyloric or intestinal metaplasia occurs. It is possible that both the antrum and the corpus are implicated, but the only portion that has evident functional and clinical ramifications is the corpus according to [18]. There is a possibility that both the antrum and the corpus are involved. Prior to atrophy, there may be a variety of abnormalities, such as localized atrophy, lymphoplasmacytic infiltration in the lamina propria, parietal cells pseudohypertrophy, and enterochromaffin-like (ECL) cell hyperplasia. It has been known for a considerable amount of time that AAG, in addition to other autoimmune disorders, frequently occurs in clusters within families, which may imply that there is a genetic component to the disease.

5.3 *Celiac Disease*

Enteropathy is one of the many symptoms that are associated with celiac disease (CD), which is an illness that affects several body systems. When the immune system responds incorrectly to a T cell-mediated immunological response, people who are genetically predisposed to the illness can develop CD. Some studies suggest that extra-intestinal symptoms may occur more frequently than gastrointestinal symptoms According to [13], Celiac illness may have an effect on practically every organ system in the body. Between half and two-thirds of people with celiac disease experience symptoms outside of the digestive tract. Patients who have CD can be separated into two distinct groups: those who have symptoms and those who do not. A patient with Crohn's disease is regarded to be asymptomatic if, at the time of their initial diagnosis of Crohn's disease, they do not exhibit any symptoms, regardless of whether or not they are explicitly questioned about their illness. Patients with Crohn's disease can be asymptomatic even if they are questioned about their illness. People are reported to have symptomatic celiac disease if they have clinically obvious gastrointestinal and/or extraintestinal symptoms linked with the use of gluten. People who fall into this category are classified as having symptomatic CD. Classical celiac disease and nonclassical celiac disease are two forms of symptomatic celiac disease that may be differentiated from one another. Classical celiac disease is the more common of the two.

5.4 *Eosinophilic Esophagitis*

Eosinophilic esophagitis, sometimes referred to as EoE and commonly abbreviated as EoE, is an immune-mediated condition that leads to signs of dysfunction in the esophagus According to [29]. EoE happens when eosinophils penetrate the esophagus mucosa and create symptoms of esophageal dysfunction. This is also known as eosinophilic esophagitis. When there is no evidence of secondary causes, medical professionals consider this disorder to be a part of the spectrum of eosinophilic gastrointestinal diseases. Eosinophilic esophagitis, if left untreated, can lead to fibrosis of the esophagus, the formation of strictures, and esophageal constriction, all of which can lead to dysfunction of the esophagus. EoE is a major factor in the development of upper gastrointestinal morbidity, and it puts a load on the healthcare systems of nations all over the world.

5.5 Inflammatory Bowel Diseases

Other non-infectious inflammations of the bowel that are suggestive of recurring chronic illnesses of the bowel are also included in the definition of "inflammatory bowel diseases" (IBDs), which is why the term "inflammatory bowel diseases" (IBDs) is used to refer to both ulcerative colitis (UC) and Crohn's disease. The most prevalent of the two disorders is called inflammatory colitis, abbreviated as UC. There has been a general increase in the number of persons who are afflicted with inflammatory bowel disease (often referred to as IBD) all over the world. There is a consensus among researchers that a genetic predisposition, the external environment, the microbial flora of the gut, and immune responses are all elements that contribute to the pathophysiology of inflammatory bowel disease according to [33]. IBD affects 4.2 million people all over the world, including 1.5 million people in the United States and 2.2 million people in Europe. In the United States alone, 1.5 million people suffer from the condition. When compared to those who do not have IBD, individuals who have a first-degree relative who suffers from inflammatory bowel disease (IBD) have a fivefold greater chance of having the disorder themselves. It is probable that certain genes are shared between Crohn's disease and ulcerative colitis due to the fact that both disorders can afflict members of the same family. Environmental variables are ultimately what produce the precipitating events that both diseases are characterized by.

5.5.1 Crohn's Disease

Inflammatory bowel disease, also known as Crohn's disease, is distinguished by skip lesions and transmural inflammation, both of which lead to inflammation across the entirety of the gastrointestinal tract, all the way from the mouth to the anus. Crohn's disease is an example of an inflammatory bowel illness. There are three key areas of the digestive tract that are impacted by Crohn's disease: the terminal ileum, the colon, and the small intestine. In around 55% of patients, the condition affects the terminal ileum, whereas in approximately 20% of instances, the condition affects the colon. Along with fissures and fistulas in the gastrointestinal tract, an upper gastrointestinal disease or extraintestinal symptoms may also develop in up to 25 percent of patients. This is in addition to the gastrointestinal tract fissures and fistulas. In 10% of people, the development of isolated perianal symptoms has a distinct potential according to [39].

5.5.2 Ulcerative Colitis

Ulcerative colitis (UC) is a chronic inflammatory condition of the colon that is defined by a continuous mucosal inflammation that extends from the rectum to the proximal colon with a variation in the degree to which the inflammation extends. UC is characterized by a continuous mucosal inflammation that extends from the rectum to the proximal colon with a variance in the degree to which the inflammation extends. Colitis of the colon and rectum can be diagnosed when there is continuous inflammation and ulceration throughout the affected areas. Due to the fact that colitis affects the whole colon as well as the rectum, the afflicted regions do not contain any normal tissue. In the majority of instances, it just affects the most superficial layer of the lining. Two of the most prominent symptoms of UC are tenesmus and bloody diarrhea. Tenesmus and bloody diarrhea are two of the most typical symptoms of UC. Patients frequently report feeling tired and complaining of slight discomfort as a consequence of the loss of blood. Cramps in the lower abdominal region are another common symptom. There is an increasing body of data that suggests UC may be an autoimmune condition [41]. Although the precise reason why UC occurs has not yet been identified and the ailment can appear in individuals of any age, those under the age of 30 are often the ones who are diagnosed with it.

6 Role of Psychological Association with GI Tract Autoimmunity

When the requirements of a person's surroundings are higher than their ability to adapt to those demands, that person will suffer stress. Hans Selye coined the term "stress" in 1936, and it refers to an organism's attempt to maintain homeostasis in the face of either a genuine risk (physical) or a perceived threat (psychological), both of which need the organism to adjust its behavior in order to live. Selye was the first person to use the term "stress," and it has been used ever since. The word "eustress" refers to the positive impacts that stress may have in some situations, such as when it assists individuals in being more motivated and enhances their performance in life in general. Eustress may also occur when stress helps people become more productive in their work. A negative consequence is not always linked to stress in all cases. Nearly everyone will, at some point in their lives, encounter some form of traumatic event or significant life stressor, such as the passing of a loved one or the aftermath of a natural disaster. These kinds of events may have a significant impact on a person's mental health and well-being. A decrease in an individual's aptitude to adapt to the elements of their environment could result in events that are unpleasant and cause pain according to [7]. An acute stressor is one that only lasts for a few minutes, a brief stressor is one that only lasts for a short amount of time, and a chronic stressor is one that only lasts for a significant amount of time. Each of these three categories of stresses has the potential to cause a disturbance in the system. After being subjected to these stimuli over an extended period of time, some people may develop severe psychological reactions, one of which is posttraumatic stress disorder (also known as PTSD). In addition, the acute stress reaction is a reaction that is triggered by a life event that causes a considerable level of stress or a change in life that initiates an acute stress reaction. It is possible that this is the best way to describe the acute stress response. As a consequence of this, it should not come as a surprise that mental illness and stress would be able to bring about changes in the physiological condition of an individual. There is a good chance that the hypothalamic–pituitary–adrenal axis and the autonomic nerve system are both disrupted, which leads to an altered immune function and an increased sensitivity to a wide range of illnesses that can affect the body. There are a number of autoimmune diseases for which the underlying etiology is still unknown. It has been hypothesized that the psychological responses to the numerous pressures in one's life, as well as the impact such emotions have on autoimmune disorders, are heavily impacted by one another and work together to form a feedback loop. There has been a significant amount of investigation carried out on animals, and the findings tend to hint in the direction of a relationship between the two. Despite this, there is not a great deal of study carried out on human subjects [35].

6.1 Pathways for Stress and Related Disorders

The activation of endocrine systems, which stress is responsible for, is an essential stage in the sequence of events that ultimately results in detrimental effects on one's health. There are two principal endocrine systems that are at work here: the hypothalamic-pituitary-adrenocortical (HPA) axis and the sympathetic-adrenal-medullary (SAM) axis. Cortisol is the major agent responsible for a variety of physiological processes, including anti-inflammatory actions, the metabolism of lipids, carbohydrates, and proteins, and gluconeogenesis. Because activation of the HPA controls these processes, cortisol is the primary agent responsible for these processes. In a way that is comparable, catecholamine, which is formed as a result of SAM activation, works in combination with the autonomic nervous system to govern a variety of activities. These activities include the control of the cardiovascular, pulmonary, hepatic, skeletal muscle, and immunological systems, among others. The exposure of these endocrine systems to a variety of stimuli causes them to begin producing hormones and other hormone-like substances. When the HPA and SAM are stimulated for a prolonged length of time, the outcome is a disruption in the control of the physiological systems that are accountable for both physical and mental illness. This can be a direct cause of one or both of these conditions.

6.2 Stress as a Trigger for Autoimmune Diseases

According to the findings of several studies, stress may be the root cause of glandular disorders, such as autoimmune endocrine illnesses. An important etiological element in autoimmune diseases is the close connection that exists between stress and essential stress hormones. This connection can be demonstrated in the form of a causal relationship between the two events. Immunological dysregulation may be to blame for the infiltration of cytokine production as well as increased host defense, both of which may ultimately result in atopic autoimmune illnesses. It is possible that prolonged and repeated exposure to stress might result in an acute phase response, which could later progress into a chronic inflammatory disease according to [14]. Due to the fact that the inflammatory response is a component of the stress response, indicates that stress may have an influence on the innate immune system of the body, which may then lead to the emergence of an inflammatory response. There is a link between experiencing some form of psychological stress, including post-traumatic stress disorder (PTSD) and having an increase in the number of T cells in the body. This might result in hyperreactive immunological responses, higher levels of immunoglobulin M, and lower levels of dehydroepiandrosterone, all of which are reported in a range of autoimmune and cardiovascular disorders.

6.3 Phycological Associations with GI Autoimmune Diseases

Comorbid mental conditions such as anxiety, stress, and depression affect a significant number of people who suffer from GI autoimmune diseases. Anxiety, stress, and depression might be an etiology in addition to comorbidities that are associated with autoimmune illnesses. This suggests that the interaction between them could go in both directions.

6.3.1 Psychological Association with Achalasia

After a prolonged time of being subjected to chronic stress, there is a possibility that an individual may acquire achalasia. There has not been a lot of research done to study the relationship between stress and anxiety and achalasia because achalasia is such an uncommon disorder. In the year 2020, Kalantari and colleagues conducted a study with the intention of mapping the experience of achalasia patients, beginning with the development of symptoms and continuing through the treatment of symptoms. They observed that those who had achalasia prior to getting a diagnosis had anxiety as a consequence of the lack of clarity surrounding their disease. The findings of their research showed that this anxiety was caused by the lack of clarity surrounding their condition. According to the findings of a study that was carried out in Germany, those who had previously been diagnosed with achalasia had a considerably increased risk of developing depression at rates that were significantly higher than those of individuals who did not have the condition. According to the findings of their investigation According to [19], achalasia is associated with a greater likelihood of experiencing depression. This is the case regardless of whether or not additional comorbidities or the clinical characteristics of the patients are taken into consideration. It has not been determined if stress, anxiety, or depression is a cause or trigger for achalasia, whether they are a subsequent outcome of achalasia, or whether they are a subsequent result of achalasia. This is an open question that needs to be investigated further.

6.3.2 AAG

Acute stress has also been suggested as a probable factor in the development of acute amyloid angiopathy. More evidence shows that AAG may result in a deficiency of vitamin B12, which may in turn produce neuropsychiatric illnesses such as emotional instability, cognitive deficits, depression, and changes in personality. In 2015, Tenca and colleagues came to the realization that the psychopathological profile did, play a role in the occurrence of symptoms in AAG [37]. It was also shown that those with AG had a considerably increased chance of experiencing psychological distress, with younger females being at a significantly increased risk. This was the case regardless of age.

6.3.3 Celiac Disease

There is strong evidence to support the hypothesis that celiac disease (CD) is causally related to psychological distress, including stress, anxiety, and depression. The controversy is still open, the same as it is for the other autoimmune disorders of the gastrointestinal tract. On the other hand, there is evidence that suggests CD plays a part in these manifestations. Changes in behavior are obvious in instances of anxiety, depression, short-term memory loss, sleep difficulties, cognitive impairment, psychosis, and attention deficit disorder. CD manifests itself in a wide variety of clinical manifestations, most of which are not well understood. A significant number of CD patients have reported experiencing CD symptoms after traumatic life experiences. In a longitudinal research, Addolorato et al. revealed that 71% of persons with celiac disease suffered from high levels of anxiety. In comparison, the levels of anxiety were high in 24% of the control participants, and 26% of newly diagnosed celiac patients exhibited anxiety. Children who have CD have a higher chance of acquiring mental illnesses as adults, according to the findings of research that was conducted in Sweden and studied patients with CD between the years 1973 and 2016 [16].

6.4 Eosinophilic Esophagitis

There is some evidence to show that both Eosinophilic Esophagitis (EoE) and the treatments for it can significantly impair psychological functioning, which can result in increased levels of anxiety and depression. Those who are younger than 35 years old have a higher risk of experiencing substantial anxiety according to [31], which is a factor that contributes to the prevalence of mental distress among adult EoE patients. Those who are older than 35 years old have a lower likelihood of experiencing considerable anxiety. If we look at it from a mechanistic standpoint, the protein known as Eotaxin-1/CCL11, which is involved in the recruitment of eosinophils, could be the reason for the pathopsychological involvement in EoE patients. There is evidence to show that eotaxin has an impact on the central nervous system. Additionally, it was revealed that eotaxin-1/CCL11 is able to pass through the blood–brain barrier without being altered.

6.5 Inflammatory Bowel Disease

Celiac disease and ulcerative colitis The presentation of symptoms in people who have Crohn's disease may be impacted by stresses, often known as environmental events. This is because Crohn's disease is an autoimmune disorder. Crohn put up the idea himself in the 1949 edition of his book Regional ileitis, which was published the previous year. The idea that the condition is caused by traumatic experiences in one's life has been a popular one since the year 1960 According to [11]. Since 1969, research has demonstrated that UC is a mental disorder rather than a physical one. It has been demonstrated that psychological stress can trigger systemic and mucosal proinflammatory responses, both of which may contribute to the exacerbation of UC in day-to-day. People who have UC will continue to exhibit antagonistic behavior, somatization, anxiety, and melancholy even when the condition is in remission. Given that the sickness may be cured entirely, this shouldn't come as much of a surprise.

6.5.1 The Bidirectionality in IBD

Individuals who reported having the greatest amount of stress over time were those who had symptoms that were consistently active, as shown by the findings of a study that investigated how people assessed their level of stress over the course of two years in three distinct subgroups. Researchers found that those who experienced symptoms that remained passive throughout time had the lowest levels of perceived stress in their lives. The participants whose symptoms fluctuated between inactive and active over the course of the two years had ratings for felt stress that fell somewhere in the center of the spectrum. In these studies, determining the directionality of the connection between poor mental health and active indicators of sickness was not possible. Poor mental health was linked to active signs of illness. They do, however, provide the impression that persons whose disease has clinical signs have a problem with their mental health, which is a concern. According to [2], research has shown that the prevalence of psychological comorbidity among those who suffer from inflammatory bowel disease is three times greater than the prevalence in the general population.

7 Microbiome and Autoimmune Diseases: The Gut-Brain Axis in GI Autoimmune Diseases

The mammalian microbiota is made up of a diverse collection of microorganisms, including bacterial, archaeal, fungal, and viral species. There is a mutually beneficial interaction that occurs between people and bacteria, the majority of which are found in the digestive tract. The collection of intestinal bacteria that live throughout the GI tract is known as the gut microbiota. This microbiota plays an important role in the health and well-being of the host. During birth, the gut microbiome is first assembled, mostly from the vaginal and fecal microbiomes of the mother if the baby is normally born, or from the skin and environmental bacteria if the baby is delivered through cesarean section [9]. The digestive tract is home to more than a hundred trillion different kinds of microbes, all of which come together to create the microbiota, an intricate biosystem. The term "microbiota" refers to a diverse group of creatures that span all three kingdoms of life: eukaryotes, bacteria, and archaea. These microuniverse's primary constituents are all members of the bacterial kingdom, which is further subdivided into the four phyla of Actinobacteria, Proteobacteria, Bacteroidetes, and Firmicutes.

8 AI-Driven Approaches to Autoimmune Disease Diagnosis, Tracking, and Treatment

The term "modular approach" refers to a method that divides the process of diagnosing, monitoring, and treating autoimmune diseases into different "modules" or "components." Each of these "modules" or "components" addresses a certain facet of the condition. Each module makes use of AI technology in order to increase its accuracy, efficiency, and ability to provide personalized care. The following is an overview of the modular approach in general (Fig. 2).

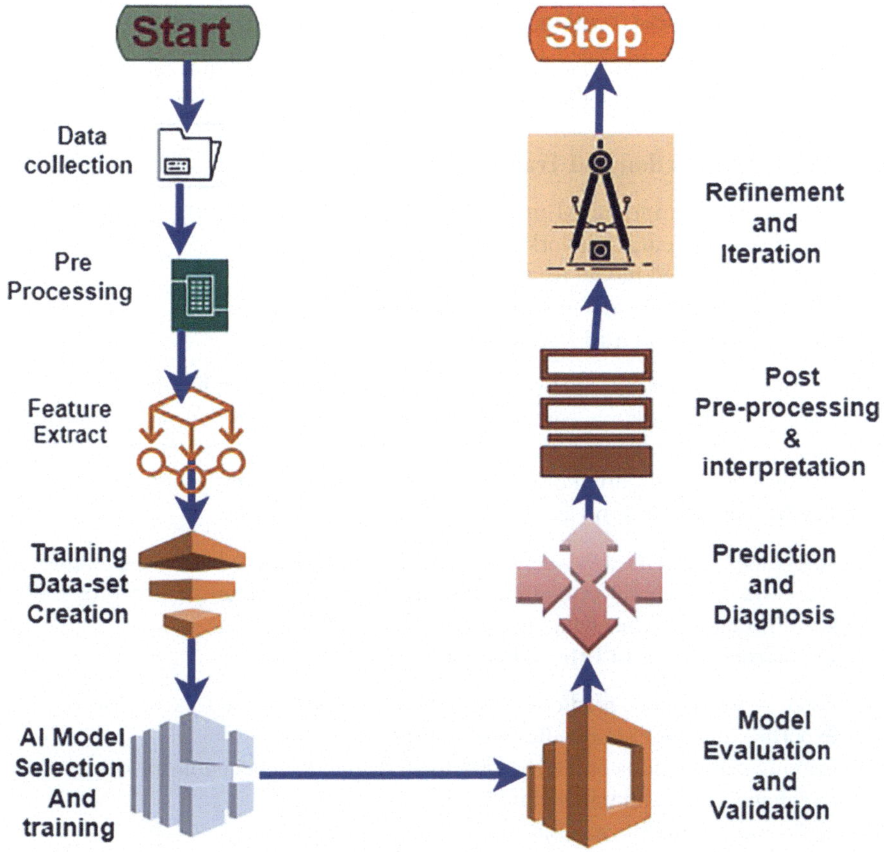

Fig. 2 Flow chart of Autoimmune Disease diagnosis using AI

8.1 Algorithm of Autoimmune Diseases Diagnosis Using AI

#1. **Data Collection**:
  a. Gather patient information, including medical history, symptoms, and laboratory test results.
  b. Collect relevant biomarkers and genetic data if available.

#2. **Preprocessing**:
  a. Clean and preprocess the collected data to remove noise and inconsistencies
  b. Normalize the data to ensure uniformity across different features.

#3. **Feature Extraction**:
  a. Extract meaningful features from the preprocessed data.
  b. This can involve statistical methods, dimensionality reduction techniques, or domain-specific knowledge.

#4. **Training Dataset Creation**:

a. Split the preprocessed data into a training set and a validation set.
b. Ensure an adequate representation of different autoimmune diseases in the training data.

#5. **AI Model Selection and Training**:

a. Choose an appropriate AI model, such as a machine learning algorithm or a deep learning neural network.
b. Train the selected model using the training dataset.
c. Optimize model parameters to achieve better performance.

#6. **Model Evaluation and Validation**:

a. Evaluate the trained model's performance using the validation dataset.
b. Assess metrics like accuracy, precision, recall, and F1-score to measure diagnostic performance.
c. Perform cross-validation or use other techniques to ensure generalizability.

#7. **Prediction and Diagnosis**:

a. Apply the trained model to new, unseen patient data for prediction and diagnosis.
b. The model will analyze the input data and provide a diagnosis or a probability score for each autoimmune disease.

#8. **Post-processing and Interpretation**:

a. Analyze the model's predictions and consider additional factors, such as clinical expertise and patient-specific information.
b. Provide explanations or interpretability of the model's decision-making process to enhance trust and understanding.

#9. **Refinement and Iteration**:

a. Continuously update and refine the AI model based on new data and feedback from healthcare professionals.
b. Incorporate new features, improve the model's performance, and address any limitations or biases.

8.2 Algorithm of Autoimmune Diseases Tracking Using AI

#1. **Data Collection**:
- Gather patient data, including medical history, symptoms, laboratory test results, and treatment information.
- Collect additional data sources like wearable devices, patient-reported outcomes, and electronic health records (EHRs).

#2. **Data Integration and Preprocessing**:
- Integrate the collected data from multiple sources into a unified database or data storage.

- Preprocess the data by cleaning, filtering, and normalizing it to ensure consistency and remove noise or outliers.

#3. **Feature Extraction and Selection**:
- Extract relevant features from the preprocessed data, such as biomarkers, clinical indicators, and disease-specific measurements.
- Perform feature selection techniques to identify the most informative and discriminative features.

#4. **AI Model Development**:
- Choose an appropriate AI model, such as machine learning algorithms (e.g., decision trees, random forests, or support vector machines) or deep learning models (e.g., convolutional neural networks or recurrent neural networks).
- Train the AI model using historical data with known disease progression and outcomes.
- Optimize the model's hyperparameters to improve its performance.

#5. **Real-Time Data Acquisition and Monitoring**:
- Continuously collect real-time data from patients, including symptoms, vital signs, medication adherence, and patient-reported data.
- Use IoT devices, wearables, or mobile applications to capture and transmit data to the tracking system.

#6. **Data Integration and Model Updating**:
- Integrate real-time patient data with the existing database.
- Update the AI model periodically or in real-time by retraining it using new data to improve its accuracy and adaptability.

#7. **Disease Progression Prediction and Tracking**:
- Apply the trained AI model to the collected and updated data to predict disease progression.
- Track changes in symptoms, disease severity, and response to treatments over time.
- Generate alerts or notifications for healthcare providers and patients **based on predicted disease trajectories or critical events**.

#8. **Visualization and Reporting**:
- Visualize the tracked disease progression using charts, graphs, or dashboards.
- Provide comprehensive reports to healthcare providers and patients summarizing the disease status, treatment effectiveness, and recommendations.

#9. **Clinical Decision Support**:
- Use the AI model's predictions and insights to support clinical decision-making for personalized treatment plans and interventions.
- Assist healthcare providers in optimizing therapies, adjusting medication dosages, or recommending lifestyle modifications.

#10. **Refinement and Improvement**:
- Continuously evaluate and refine the AI model's performance based on feedback from healthcare professionals and patient outcomes.
- Incorporate new data sources, update feature selection, and improve the model's accuracy and usability (Fig. 3).

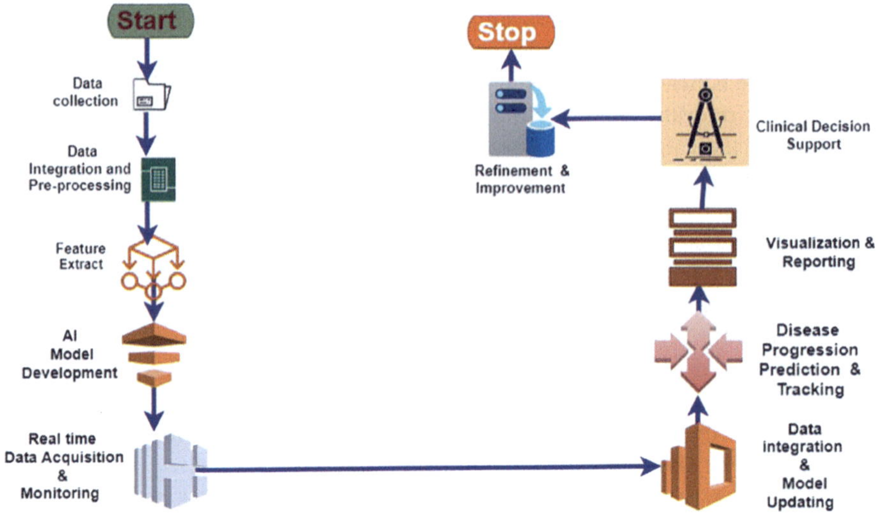

Fig. 3 Flow chart of Autoimmune diseases tracking using AI

8.3 Algorithm of Autoimmune Diseases Treatment Planning Tracking Using AI

#1. **Data Collection**:
- Gather patient data, including medical history, diagnostic test results, disease severity assessments, and treatment records.
- Collect additional data sources like genetic information, lifestyle factors, and patient-reported outcomes.

#2. **Data Integration and Preprocessing**:
- Integrate the collected data into a centralized database or data storage system.
- Preprocess the data by cleaning, normalizing, and standardizing it to ensure consistency and remove noise or outliers.

#3. **AI Model Development**:
- Choose an appropriate AI model or combination of models for treatment planning and tracking.
- Develop models that can handle various aspects, such as predicting treatment responses, optimizing therapy plans, and assessing disease progression.

#4. **Treatment Planning**:
- Apply AI models to the patient data to predict optimal treatment options.
- Consider factors like disease subtype, patient characteristics, available medications, and potential side effects.
- Generate personalized treatment plans based on AI-driven recommendations.

#5. **Treatment Tracking and Monitoring**:
- Continuously monitor patients' responses to treatments.

- Collect real-time data, including symptoms, medication adherence, adverse events, and patient-reported outcomes.
- Integrate data from wearable devices, mobile apps, or remote monitoring systems.

#6. **Real-Time Data Integration and Analysis**:
- Integrate real-time patient data with the existing database.
- Apply AI models to analyze and interpret the collected data, identifying patterns, trends, and treatment effectiveness.
- Continuously update and refine the treatment plans based on new insights.

#7. **Decision Support and Alerting**:
- Provide decision support to healthcare providers by alerting them to treatment adjustments or changes based on AI-driven analysis.
- Generate alerts or notifications for healthcare providers and patients to address critical events, adverse reactions, or treatment non-compliance.

#8. **Treatment Evaluation and Optimization**:
- Continuously evaluate treatment outcomes using AI models.
- Assess treatment effectiveness, disease progression, and patient quality of life.
- Optimize treatment plans by incorporating feedback from patients and healthcare providers.

#9. **Visualization and Reporting**:
- Visualize treatment progress and outcomes using charts, graphs, or dashboards.
- Generate comprehensive reports summarizing treatment response, disease management, and recommendations for healthcare providers and patients.

#10. **Refinement and Improvement**:
- Continuously refine the AI models based on feedback, new research, and emerging treatment strategies.
- Incorporate additional data sources, update treatment algorithms, and enhance the model's accuracy and effectiveness (Fig. 4).

8.4 Data Analytics Autoimmune Diseases Diagnosis Using AI

Data analytics and AI may help diagnose autoimmune illnesses. Autoimmune disorders are difficult to identify owing to their varied symptoms and comorbidity with other ailments.

#1. Data collection and integration: AI algorithms may analyze data from electronic health records, medical imaging, lab tests, patient-reported symptoms, and genetic information. This extensive data collecting helps detect patterns and connections in the patient's condition.

#2. Pattern recognition: AI systems can find hidden patterns in massive datasets. AI algorithms can identify autoimmune disease trends in massive patient data sets, including symptoms, test findings, and medical histories. Early detection and action may result.

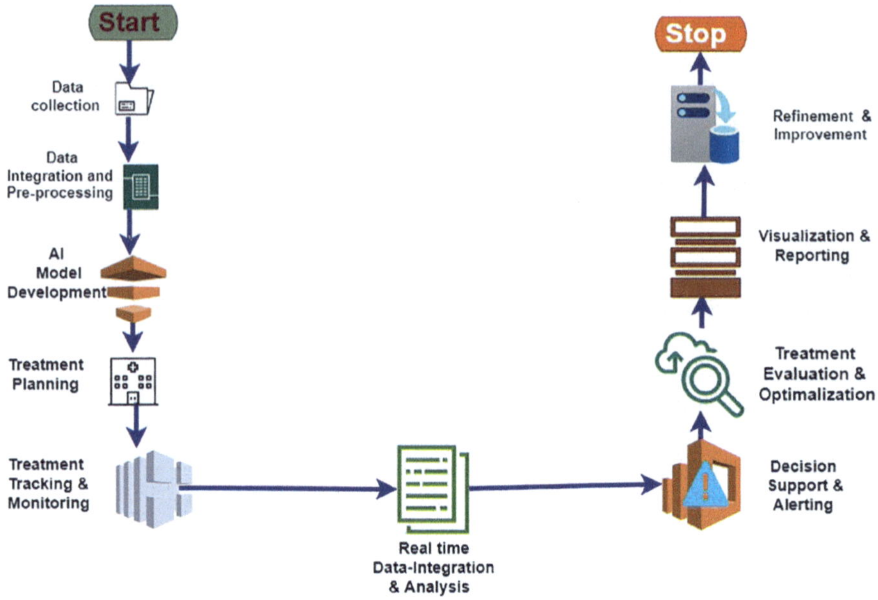

Fig. 4 Flowchart of Autoimmune diseases treatment Planning tracking using AI

#3. AI-powered decision support tools: Help doctors diagnose autoimmune disorders. Machine learning algorithms analyze patient's data and provide diagnostic recommendations or predictions. This may help doctors diagnose more accurately and quickly, decreasing misdiagnosis and delay.

#4. Image analysis: AI may help diagnose autoimmune illnesses analyzing X-rays, MRIs, and histopathology slides. Radiologists and pathologists may improve their interpretations by training machine learning algorithms recognize autoimmune disease patterns.

#5. Predictive modeling: AI can analyze vast datasets to assess the risk of autoimmune illnesses based on genetics, lifestyle, environmental exposure, and comorbidities. These models help identify and treat autoimmune diseases early (Fig. 5).

AI optimize autoimmune disease treatment regimens. AI algorithms may offer personalized treatments and forecast intervention efficacy by analyzing data from comparable instances and evaluating patient features, biomarkers, and treatment results. It's important to note that while AI can offer valuable insights and support in the diagnosis of autoimmune diseases, it should not replace the expertise and judgment of healthcare professionals. AI technologies should be considered as complementary tools to aid in the diagnostic process and improve patient outcomes.

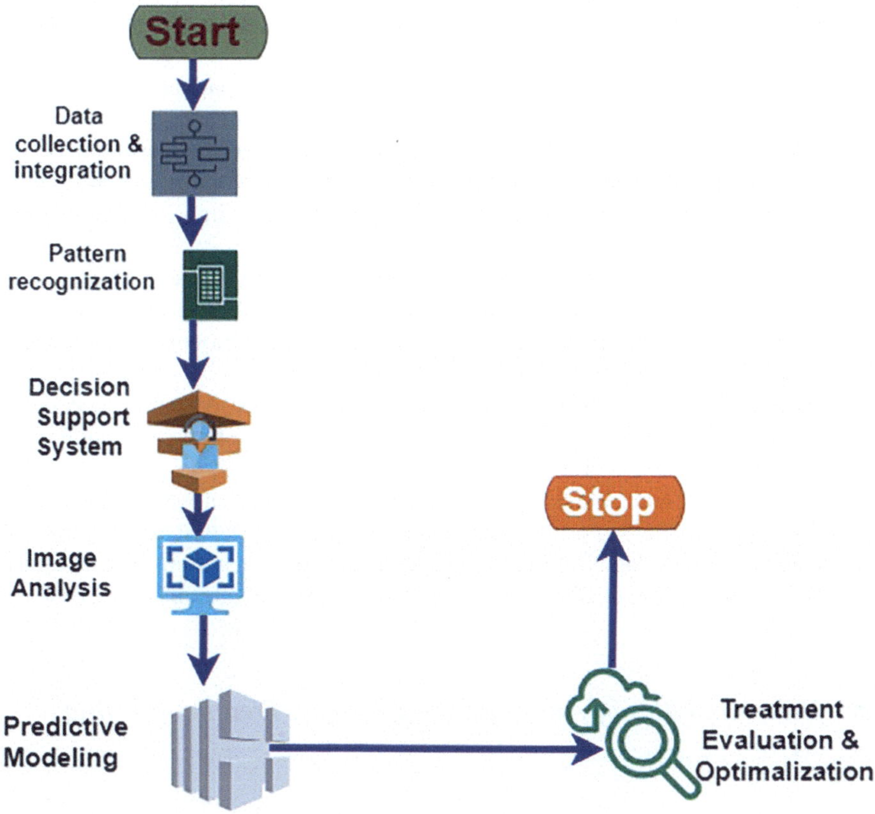

Fig. 5 Flow chart of data analytics of Autoimmune disease diagnosis using AI

8.5 Data Analytics Autoimmune Diseases Tracking Using AI

Data analytics and AI can also be leveraged for tracking autoimmune diseases, enabling better monitoring, management, and research. Here's how data analytics and AI can contribute to tracking autoimmune diseases:

#1. Data aggregation and standardization: AI algorithms can gather data from electronic health records, patient-generated data, wearable devices, and social media. AI analyzes autoimmune disease trends, demographics, and variables by standardizing and integrating this data.

#3. Real-time monitoring: AI-powered solutions can constantly monitor and analyze autoimmune disease data. Tracking symptoms, medication adherence, lifestyle, and physiological measures. Real-time monitoring may identify disease changes and exacerbations for early intervention and personalized care.

#4. Predictive analytics: AI models can forecast illness development, flare-ups, and consequences using historical and real-time data. These models may assist doctors and patients in choosing autoimmune disease treatments and lifestyle changes by spotting trends and risk factors.

#5. Adverse event detection: AI algorithms can analyze patient reports, social media, and healthcare databases to identify adverse events from autoimmune disease drugs and therapies. This helps detect adverse effects early, improving patient safety.

#6. Patient stratification: AI can stratify autoimmune disease patients by clinical features, genetics, and therapy response. AI algorithms may improve therapy and personalized medicine by detecting patient subgroups.

#7. Research and medication development: Data analytics and AI may help autoimmune disease researchers analyze vast datasets. AI algorithms can spot patterns, genetic markers, and therapy responses across varied patient groups, helping uncover novel therapeutic targets and improve treatment.

#8. Population-level autoimmune disease data analysis: AI-powered systems aid public health monitoring. This may detect illness clusters, follow epidemiological trends, and guide public health strategies.

Tracking autoimmune illnesses requires careful handling and compliance with privacy and security laws. For accuracy and efficacy, AI models should be verified and updated with fresh data. Data analytics and AI can monitor autoimmune illnesses, but healthcare practitioners, researchers, and data scientists must collaborate (Fig. 6).

8.6 Data Analytics of Autoimmune Diseases Treatment Using AI

Data analytics and AI can be valuable in optimizing the treatment of autoimmune diseases. By analyzing vast amounts of patient data and considering various factors, AI algorithms can contribute to personalized treatment strategies, medication management, and outcome prediction. Here's how data analytics and AI can be applied to autoimmune disease treatment:

#1. Treatment recommendations: AI models can analyze massive patient datasets, including demographics, medical history, test findings, genetic information, and treatment outcomes. AI algorithms may help doctors prescribe patient-specific treatments by finding patterns and relationships. Based on patient characteristics and evidence, this may involve prescribing drugs, dose modifications, or alternative treatments.

#2. AI can optimize autoimmune disease drug management: AI systems can detect genetic markers, biomarkers, and comorbidities that affect therapy response from patient data. This information may be used to choose the best treatments and doses for individual patients, eliminating trial-and-error and increasing results.

#3. Adverse event detection: AI systems may monitor patient data for autoimmune disease therapy side effects. AI models may detect issues early and adapt treatment plans to improve patient safety and well-being by analyzing symptoms, test results, and other data.

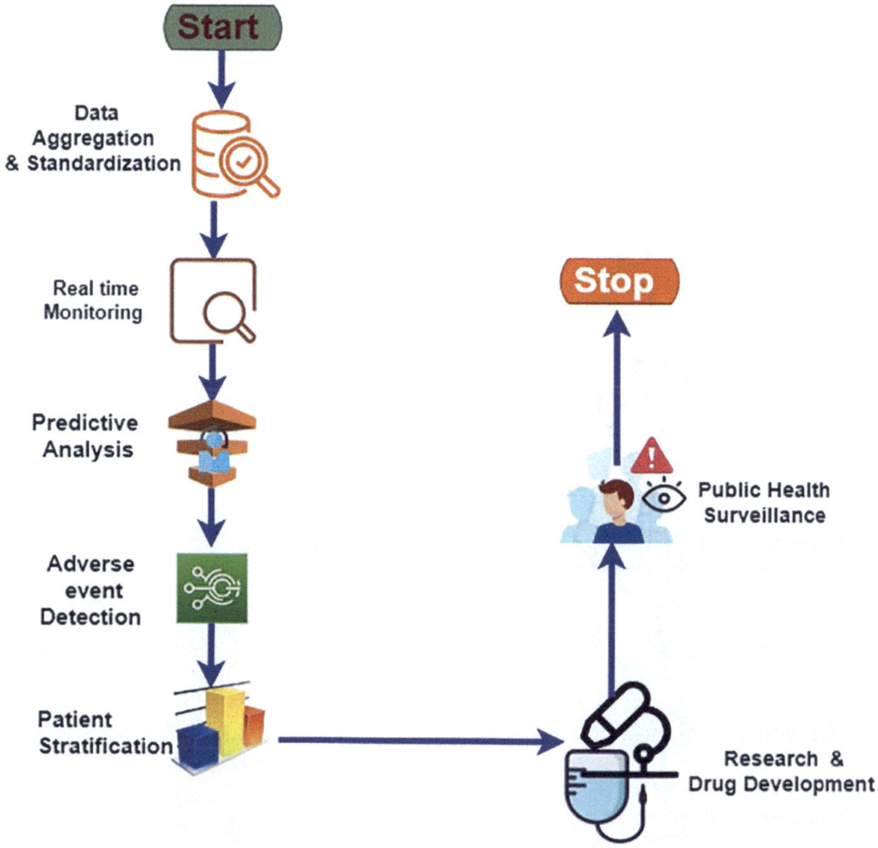

Fig. 6 Flow chart of data analytics of Autoimmune Disease tracking using AI

#4. AI predicts autoimmune disease therapy response: AI algorithms can predict therapy efficacy by analyzing previous data from comparable patients and treatment regimens. This may help doctors and patients choose the best therapy, saving time and money by eliminating useless treatments.

#5. Treatment adherence and patient engagement: AI-powered technologies may improve patient engagement and adherence. Virtual assistants and smartphone apps may remind, educate, and propose therapy to improve adherence. AI algorithms may analyze patient-generated data including symptom reports and lifestyle data to understand treatment adherence and participation.

#6. Clinical trial design: AI can optimize autoimmune disease clinical trials. AI systems may discover therapy-responsive patient subgroups by analyzing genetic data, patient characteristics, and treatment results. Researchers can design more focused and efficient clinical trials, speeding medication development and improving therapy alternatives.

It is crucial to note that while AI can provide valuable insights and recommendations, the final treatment decisions should be made by healthcare professionals in consultation with their patients. AI technologies should be considered as supportive tools to aid in treatment optimization, rather than replacing clinical expertise and judgment (Fig. 7).

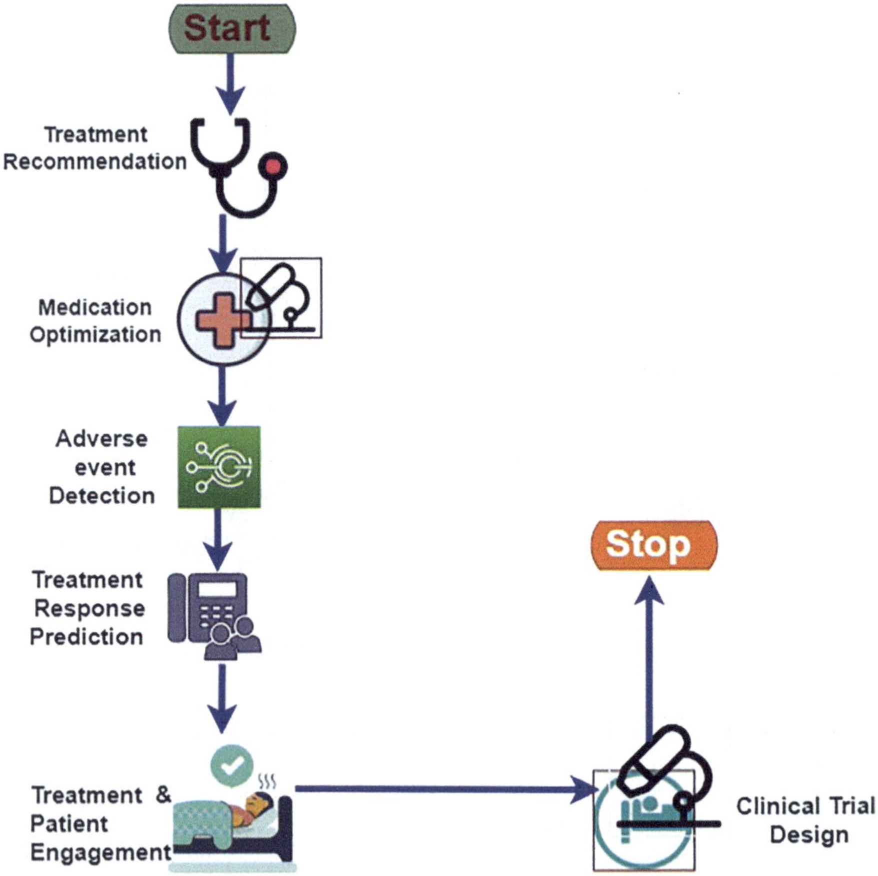

Fig. 7 Flow chart of data analytics of Autoimmune Disease treatment using AI

9 Deep Phenotyping and AI

In the field of precision oncology, artificial intelligence may be used to create a medicine combination based on a patient's personal biopsy and implement N-of-1 pharmaceutical recommendations. AI-based algorithms have already shown an increase in diagnostic accuracy and performance across a variety of subspecialties, most notably within the field of radiology. The Food and Drug Administration (FDA) in the United States has granted licenses to a number of AI systems in order to advance medical imaging assessment [26]. One of these systems may identify aberrant lesions that might develop into cancer. A recent piece of research demonstrates how AI and the evolution of technology combined are making it possible to move toward the goal of personalized and precision medicine. The use of machine learning is essential for the integration of data from many omics, and there are a number of facets in which different kinds of data may be merged and their associations investigated. The United Kingdom Biobank project is one of the biggest prospective cohort studies that has gathered extensive genetic and phenotypic data from a total of 500,000 people. This data includes biological measures, lifestyle indicators, blood and urine biomarkers, and brain imaging. This study has given researchers the chance to look for genetic connections with the likelihood of developing a disease and has led to the publishing of a number of papers according to [26]. In addition, a study on precision medicine screening that introduced a platform of deep quantitative multimodal phenotyping that included genomics, metagenomics, advanced imaging, metabolomics, clinical testing, and family history provided a comprehensive, predictive, and personalized assessment of an individual's health and the likelihood that they will develop a chronic disease. Recent research provided its participants with an extra behavioral coach in addition to providing them with large amounts of data acquired via deep phenotyping. An early effort to gather and analyze massive omics data sets in order to connect molecular networks in 108 healthy individuals was the purpose of the Pioneer 100 wellness project, often known as P100. During the course of this investigation, whole genome sequencing, proteome, microbiome, and metabolome sequencing were carried out. Additionally, clinical data, daily physical activity, and sleep patterns were collected every three months. The researchers carried out an integrated study of six different kinds of data using the personal data clouds that they created for each participant. These data clouds were dense and dynamic. In addition, the combination of these data-driven insights with behavioral coaching resulted in a significant improvement in the participants' overall health in terms of nutrition, inflammation, diabetes, and cardiovascular diseases.

10 Conclusions

In conclusion, gastrointestinal autoimmune diseases are life-threatening and have many causes. Despite being organ-specific, these autoimmune conditions affecting the gastrointestinal tract have increased in recent decades. These disorders require a multidisciplinary approach to diagnose and understand their cause. Antibodies are reliable indicators for specific disorders, but biotechnology investment is needed to develop more sensitive diagnostic tools. Beyond pharmacological and surgical treatments, a better understanding of the brain-digestive tract connection and other etiological factors could improve preventive medicine and patient quality of life. Nearly one in four people have chronic health issues, straining global healthcare systems and economies. Longitudinal cohort studies have improved human health by revealing disease progression, risk factors, and biomarkers. Biosensors and multi-omics have enabled more accurate disease classification, targeted therapeutics, and better prognoses for a variety of diseases. Digital medicine has helped find the causes of diseases in individual patients, advancing treatment. Lifestyle factors cause most chronic diseases, so adopting healthier lifestyles can reduce risk. Employment and education levels, geographic location, the built environment, social networks, and climatic conditions all affect lifestyle choices. To combat obesity and nutrition-related chronic diseases, food system socioeconomic determinants, environmental influences, and climate change must be examined. Targeted public health initiatives to reduce health disparities are also needed to address this global health issue. In conclusion, gastrointestinal autoimmune diseases and chronic illnesses require a multidisciplinary approach, advanced diagnostic technologies, and a thorough understanding of socioeconomic factors affecting lifestyle choices and health outcomes. These efforts could improve patient care and lower chronic disease rates.

References

1. Abeda BM, Kumar R (2022) Design a linear classification model with support vector machine algorithm on autoimmune disease data. https://doi.org/10.1109/iciem54221.2022.9853182
2. Bernstein CN (2016) Psychological Stress and Depression: Risk Factors for IBD? Dig Dis 34(1–2):58–63. https://doi.org/10.1159/000442929
3. Bragina VA, Guteneva NV, Znoyko SL, Gorshkov BG, Orlov AN (2018, Jun) Detection of autoimmune disease markers by optical label-free immunosensors. https://doi.org/10.1109/lo.2018.8435773
4. Caso F, Costa L, Nucera V, Barilaro G, Masala IF, Talotta R, Caso P, Scarpa R, Sarzi-Puttini P, Atzeni F (2018) From autoinflammation to autoimmunity: old and recent findings. Clin Rheumatol 37(9):2305–2321. https://doi.org/10.1007/s10067-018-4209-9
5. Corrado A, Monaco M (2017). Diagnostic approaches to autoimmune rheumatic diseases. J Immunol Res 1–3
6. De la C-M, U G-C, Gálvez-Romero M, L J (2017) Infections and autoimmunity. J Immunol Res 1–2
7. Dean J, Keshavan M (2017) The neurobiology of depression: an integrated view. Asian J Psychiatr 27(27):101–111. https://doi.org/10.1016/j.ajp.2017.01.025

8. Ehrenfeld M, Tincani A, Andreoli L, Cattalini M, Greenbaum A, Kanduc D (2020) Covid-19 and autoimmunity. Autoimmunity Rev. https://linkinghub.elsevier.com/retrieve/%20pii/S1568997220301610
9. Fitzgibbon G, Mills KHG (2020) The microbiota and immune-mediated diseases: opportunities for therapeutic intervention. Eur J Immunol 50(3):326–337. https://doi.org/10.1002/eji.201948322
10. Gaudino SJ, Kumar P (2019) Cross-Talk between antigen presenting cells and T cells impacts intestinal homeostasis, bacterial infections, and tumorigenesis. Front Immunol 10. https://doi.org/10.3389/fimmu.2019.00360
11. Hodson R (2016) Inflammatory bowel disease. Nature 540(7634):S97–S97. https://doi.org/10.1038/540s97a
12. Holdgate N, St Clair EW (2016) Recent advances in primary Sjogren's syndrome. F1000 Res 5:1412. https://doi.org/10.12688/f1000research.8352.1
13. Hujoel IA, Reilly NR, Rubio-Tapia A (2019) Celiac disease. Gastroenterol Clin North Am 48(1):19–37. https://doi.org/10.1016/j.gtc.2018.09.001
14. Kalantari M, Hollywood A, Lim R, Hashemi M (2020) Mapping the experiences of people with achalasia from initial symptoms to long-term management. Health Expect 24(1):131–139. https://doi.org/10.1111/hex.13160
15. Kany S, Vollrath JT, Relja B (2019) Cytokines in inflammatory disease. Int J Mol Sci 20(23):6008. https://doi.org/10.3390/ijms20236008
16. Lebwohl B, Haggård L, Emilsson L, Söderling J, Roelstraete B, Butwicka A, Green PHR, Ludvigsson JF (2021) Psychiatric disorders in patients with a diagnosis of celiac disease during childhood from 1973 to 2016. Clin Gastroenterol Hepatol 19(10):2093-2101.e13. https://doi.org/10.1016/j.cgh.2020.08.018
17. Lee SH (2015) Intestinal permeability regulation by tight junction: implication on inflammatory bowel diseases. Intestinal Res 13(1):11. https://doi.org/10.5217/ir.2015.13.1.11
18. Lenti MV, Miceli E, Cococcia S, Klersy C, Staiani M, Guglielmi F, Giuffrida P, Vanoli A, Luinetti O, De Grazia F, Di Stefano M, Corazza GR, Di Sabatino A (2019) Determinants of diagnostic delay in autoimmune atrophic gastritis. Aliment Pharmacol Ther 50(2):167–175. https://doi.org/10.1111/apt.15317
19. Loosen SH, Kandler J, Luedde T, Kostev K, Roderburg C (2021) Achalasia is associated with a higher incidence of depression in outpatients in Germany 16(4):e0250503–e0250503. https://doi.org/10.1371/journal.pone.0250503
20. Mankia K, Emery P (2016) Review: preclinical rheumatoid arthritis: progress toward prevention. Arthritis Rheumatol 68(4):779–788. https://doi.org/10.1002/art.39603
21. Maryam M, Taher M (2017) Automatic diagnosis of autoimmune diseases by classifying HEp-2 cells. https://doi.org/10.1109/icenco.2017.8289789
22. Massironi S, Zilli A, Elvevi A, Invernizzi P (2019) The changing face of chronic autoimmune atrophic gastritis: an updated comprehensive perspective. Autoimmun Rev 18(3):215–222. https://doi.org/10.1016/j.autrev.2018.08.011
23. Meroni MF, L P (2017)The impact of pregnancy on the autoimmune diseases. Best Practice Res Clin Rheumatol 31(3):397–412
24. Navegantes KC, de Souza Gomes R, Pereira PAT, Czaikoski PG, Azevedo CHM, Monteiro MC (2017) Immune modulation of some autoimmune diseases: the critical role of macrophages and neutrophils in the innate and adaptive immunity. J Trans Med 15(1). https://doi.org/10.1186/s12967-017-1141-8
25. Orme J., Scorza F. (2017) Diagnosis and management of multiple sclerosis: the present and the future. Ther Adv Neurol Disord 10(6):227–237
26. Raiteri A, Granito A, Giamperoli A, Catenaro T, Negrini G, Tovoli F (2022) Current guidelines for the management of celiac disease: a systematic review with comparative analysis. World J Gastroenterol 28(1):154–176. https://doi.org/10.3748/wjg.v28.i1.154
27. Rasha E, Rafea M, Elkafrawy P (2023) An approach for detecting missed tissue proteins in autoimmune diseases. https://doi.org/10.1109/lt58159.2023.10092296
28. Reddy V, Desai MC (2016) Lupus nephritis: an overview of recent findings. Autoim Dis 1–7

29. Reed CC, Dellon ES (2019) Eosinophilic esophagitis. Med Clin North Am 103(1):29–42. https://doi.org/10.1016/j.mcna.2018.08.009
30. Rieder E, Fernandez-Becker NQ, Sarosiek J, Guillaume A, Azagury DE, Clarke JO (2020) Achalasia: physiology and diagnosis. Ann N Y Acad Sci 1482(1):85–94. https://doi.org/10.1111/nyas.14510
31. Rooij WE, Bennebroek Evertsz' F, Lei A, Bredenoord AJ (2020) Mental distress among adult patients with eosinophilic esophagitis. Neurogastroenterology & Motility 33(7). https://doi.org/10.1111/nmo.14069
32. Rönnblom L, Eloranta M-L (2013) The interferon signature in autoimmune diseases. Curr Opin Rheumatol 25(2):248–253. https://doi.org/10.1097/bor.0b013e32835c7e32
33. Sairenji T, Collins KL, Evans DV (2017) An update on inflammatory bowel disease. Primary Care: Clin Office Pract 44(4):673–692. https://doi.org/10.1016/j.pop.2017.07.010
34. Singh K, Chang C, Gershwin ME (2014) IgA deficiency and autoimmunity. Autoimmun Rev 13(2):163–177. https://doi.org/10.1016/j.autrev.2013.10.005
35. Song H, Fang F, Tomasson G, Arnberg FK, Mataix-Cols D, Fernández de la Cruz L, Almqvist C, Fall K, Valdimarsdóttir UA (2018) Association of stress-related disorders with subsequent autoimmune disease. JAMA 319(23):2388. https://doi.org/10.1001/jama.2018.7028
36. Srikanth P (2016) Clustering algorithm of novel distribution function for dimensionality reduction using big data of OMICS: health, clinical and biology research information. https://doi.org/10.1109/iccic.2016.7919647
37. Tenca A, Massironi S, Pugliese D, Consonni D, Mauro A, Cavalcoli F, Franchina M, Spampatti M, Conte D, Penagini R (2015) Gastro-esophageal reflux and antisecretory drugs use among patients with chronic autoimmune atrophic gastritis: a study with pH-impedance monitoring. Neurogastroenterol Motil 28(2):274–280. https://doi.org/10.1111/nmo.12723
38. Tian Y, Wan-Jun Y, Zhang M, Zhang M, Tang J-Y (2020). The application of blockchain technology in the early warning and monitoring of infectious diseases. https://doi.org/10.1109/iciibms50712.2020.9336418
39. Torres J, Mehandru S, Colombel J-F, Peyrin-Biroulet L (2017) Crohn's disease. The Lancet 389(10080):1741–1755. https://doi.org/10.1016/s0140-6736(16)31711-1
40. Wakefield D, Wildner G (2020) Is glaucoma an autoimmune disease? Clin Trans Immunol 9(10). https://doi.org/10.1002/cti2.1180
41. Wei S-C, Sollano JD, Hui YT, Yu W, Santos PV, John L, Koram N (2021) Epidemiology, burden of disease, and unmet needs in the treatment of ulcerative colitis in Asia. 15(3):275–289. https://doi.org/10.1080/17474124.2021.1840976
42. Weitzmann MN (2014) T-cells and B-cells in osteoporosis. Current Opinion Endocrinol Diabetes Obesity 21(6):461–467. https://doi.org/10.1097/med.0000000000000103
43. Wiley Online Library (2019) Wiley Online Library | Scientific research articles, journals, books, and reference works. Wiley.com. https://onlinelibrary.wiley.com/
44. Zhang X, Zhang J, Sun K, Yang X, Dai C, Guo Y (2019). Integrated multi-omics analysis using variational autoencoders: application to pan-cancer classification. https://doi.org/10.1109/bibm47256.2019.8983228

Applications of Artificial Intelligence, Machine Learning, and Deep Learning in Diagnosis and Treatment of Rheumatoid Arthritis

K. R. Dasegowda, M. Y. Kavyasree, H. Prabhavathi, Majji Rambabu, Karthick Vasudevan, and Mohammed Abdul Kareem

Abstract Artificial intelligence (AI), machine learning, and deep learning are growing fields in healthcare and medicine. These techniques can be beneficial for treating chronic rheumatological disorders, such as rheumatoid arthritis (RA). RA is a systemic disease that can cause joint damage, disability, and polyarthritis. Machine learning a branch of AI, is used in the medical industry to assist patients and doctors. AI algorithms can help with phenotyping, diagnosis, treatment response evaluation, disease tracking, prognosis, medication discovery, and research. ML may also be able to suggest treatments and calculate the expected benefit. This book chapter summarizes machine learning techniques and applications in rheumatology, mainly supervised learning for e-diagnosis, illness detection, and medical image analysis. Supervised learning techniques such as support vector machine, random forest, natural language processing, and neural networks are discussed. Machine learning may help rheumatologists predict a patient's illness and identify risk factors in the future. Future collaborative decisions will consider the patient's perspective, the rheumatologist's experience and evidence, and machine-learned evidence.

Keywords Artificial intelligence · Machine learning · Deep · Rheumatoid arthritis

K. R. Dasegowda · M. Rambabu · K. Vasudevan
School of Applied Sciences, REVA University, Bangalore, Karnataka, India

M. Y. Kavyasree
Department of Biotechnology, Ramaiah Institute of Technology, Bangalore, KA, India

H. Prabhavathi
Department of Cytogenomics, Dr Lal Pathlabs, Bangalore, KA, India

M. A. Kareem (✉)
Department of Biochemistry, Indira Gandhi National Open University, New Delhi, India
e-mail: abdul.kareem@ignou.ac.in

K. Raza and S. Singh (eds.), *Artificial Intelligence and Autoimmune Diseases*, Studies in Computational Intelligence 1133, https://doi.org/10.1007/978-981-99-9029-0_12

1 Introduction

The second most common autoimmune condition is rheumatoid arthritis (RA), it is anticipated that by 2030, the number of individuals affected by arthritis will reach 67 million, as the population is projected to continue aging. An early diagnosis of disease activity allows healthcare professionals to provide appropriate care and treatment to patients [1]. If ignored, these destructive joint alterations may spread to larger joints. Reducing inflammation and joint damage is the goal of RA treatment. Nonsteroidal anti-inflammatory medicines (NSAIDs) and corticosteroids are used as initial treatments, followed by anti-rheumatic medications that are disease-modifying [2]. One of the most prevalent rheumatologic illnesses is RA, ultrasound, computed tomography (CT), and magnetic resonance imaging (MRI), are commonly used in the assessment of RA. The severity of the disorder is usually understood only in its advanced stages, leading to significant functional impairment. Early detection of disease provides appropriate care and treatment to patients [1].

The use of artificial intelligence (AI) in precision medicine is increasing. There are many machine learning (ML) and deep learning (DL) algorithms that could help doctors at every stage of RA treatment, including initial prevention, diagnosis, and treatment. However, there are other obstacles in the way of developing AI-guided precision medicine, particularly its application to RA, which might and should be overcome through multidisciplinary scientific work. The global market of AI in healthcare is estimated at 15.4 billion USD in 2022 and is projected to increase by 37.5% compound annual growth rate (CAGR) from 2023 to 2030. The study of AI is a subfield of computer science that includes a number of interdisciplinary strategies for improving the capabilities of machines. One of the subdisciplines of AI is ML, which involves techniques for solving complex problems by autonomously learning patterns of communication among variables, without the need for explicit computer programming. ML techniques learn directly from data and concentrate on making correct predictions rather than inference, in contrast to classic statistical models that are motivated by hypotheses and seek to uncover correlations between outcomes and data points. Deep learning, a subset of ML, is the process of finding patterns in data by employing layered artificial neural network structures. Due to improvements in computer power and the availability of large datasets over the last ten years, DL has become increasingly important in the fields of drug development, genetic research, and image analysis. DL models are capable of carrying out more sophisticated tasks in comparison to conventional ML approaches like logistic regression, support vector machines (SVM), and random forest, but they need more training data and take longer to train. Further DL models are excellent at processing high-dimensional data, such as that found in electronic health records (EHRs) and medical imaging [2].

2 Machine Learning in Rheumatoid Arthritis

With the use of data, systems can learn and develop through the application of ML, a subfield of AI. There are numerous applications for ML algorithms, such as image identification, natural language processing, and medical diagnosis. The two types of ML algorithms are supervised learning and unsupervised learning. The ML model looks for relationships between the input features or variables and the output features, which provide labels or classifications. Then it calculates a role that can forecast the value of an output given a series of unlabeled input values. In order to train models, supervised learning needs tagged data. Unsupervised learning is data-driven and does not require class labels to recognize the structure in the data. Unsupervised learning is the term for learning from unlabeled data.

Common supervised learning techniques include, the relationship between the input and output data is modeled by the linear regression technique as a linear function. Logistic regression classifies an algorithm that models the possibility of each output class as a function of the input structures. Using input features to predict the output class, decision trees construct models based on decision trees. Multiple decision trees are combined in the random forest algorithm, a sort of ensemble learning technique, to increase classification accuracy. Support vector machines (SVMs) organize algorithm and finds a hyperplane that separates the input data into different classes. Neural networks are a class of algorithms that use artificial neural networks to learn complex non-linear mappings between input and output data [3].

In recent years, ML has revealed promising results in the diagnosis and management of RA. ML models can analyze large amounts of data from electronic health records, imaging studies, and patient-reported outcomes to identify patterns and predict disease progression. ML algorithms can be trained to recognize patterns in medical imaging, such as X-rays and MRI scans, to aid in the diagnosis of RA. For instance, a recent study used a convolutional neural network (CNN) to identify RA-related changes in X-ray images of hands and wrists with high accuracy(2).

Disease activity prediction: ML models can be trained on patient data, including laboratory results, clinical assessments, and patient-reported outcomes, to predict disease activity and response to treatment. This can help clinicians make informed decisions about treatment options and adjust therapy as needed [4]. ML algorithms can be used to predict treatment response and adverse events based on patient characteristics and treatment history. This can help personalize treatment decisions and improve patient outcomes. ML is used to identify subgroups of patients with similar disease characteristics and outcomes, which can inform clinical trial design and personalized treatment strategies(5).ML models can analyze patient data to identify early signs of RA, which can help improve patient outcomes (6).ML algorithms can predict which treatment options are most effective for individual patients, based on their medical history and other factors. ML models can analyze patient data to track disease progression and identify patients who may be at risk of complications. The use of omics, imaging, clinical, and sensor data in ML applications for RA diagnosis is given in Table 1.

Table 1 ML algorithm for the assessment of RA and its applications [2]

Supervised machine learning algorithms	Types of data/ sample size	Application/outcome	References
LASSO regression	Omics Data/Total at risk = 127 ACPA-negative (not progressor) = 47 ACPA-positive (not progressor) = 63 Progressors = 17	RA susceptibility proteins were identified/Model 3 (validation, n = 34): Accuracy = 91.2%, AUC = 0.931	[7]
Random forest, XGBoost, Ridge regression, and SVM	16S rRNA sequencing or Shotgun metagenomics or both/ RA = 371	Prediction of RA, identifying microbial signature Random forest: AUC = 0.879, F1 = 0.664, XGBoost: AUC = 0.847, F1 = 0.650, SVM RFE: AUC = 0.845, F1 = 0.647, Ridge regression: AUC = 0.795, F1 = 0.628	[8]
Random forest	Mass spectrometry (plasma and synovial fluid samples)/ RA = 67, OA = 63 Non-RA inflammatory arthritis = 42 Controls = 53	Identification of RA patients with early-stage symptoms by profiling oxidized, nitrated and glycated proteins and amino acids in SVF and plasma / Early RA vs. other arthritis: Test set validation: AUC = 0.62 (0.5–0.75), sensitivity = 0.60 (0.42–0.76), specificity = 0.61 (0.46–0.72), NPV = 0.97, PPV = 0.23, PLR = 1.5, NLR = 0.67	[9]
CNN, SVM, ANN	Hand X-ray/ RA = 160 Controls = 130	RA diagnosis using hand X-ray/Using CNN: accuracy = 94.46%, sensitivity = 0.95, specificity = 0.82N	[10]
ANN	Laser imaging data/ RA = 22 (72 joints) Controls = 8 (64 joints)	Finger joint inflammation assess using laser-based imaging technique/Accuracy = 83%, sensitivity = 80%, specificity = 89%	[11]

A case study in cancer biology is shown to demonstrate the interchange between supervised and unsupervised learning and familiarize the concept of combination to advance the predictive models. Sage Bionetworks-DREAM developed a model for Breast cancer prognosis that predicts the models based on genomic, clinical, and survival outcome data from nearly 2000 patients. Predictive models for survival outcomes were created by participating organizations from over 35 different countries, and these models were subsequently validated on a new validation sample of 184 patients. The mode 127 was partially constructed from genomic traits discovered by using unsupervised learning on malignancies that had no genetic or biological connection to one another. The attractor metagenes technique, which was previously developed, found gene clusters that were comparable across numerous tumor samples. Numerous of these clusters coincided with biological events necessary for the development of cancer, such as chromosomal instability and mesenchymal transformation. The presence or absence of these characteristics, along with other clinical variables, were included by the authors in multiple predictive models for breast cancer outcomes as shown in Fig. 1. The authors employed a number of different supervised learning algorithms and blended the results of each algorithm to create a final prediction of survival outcomes since different learning algorithms may be more or less effective at predicting outcomes for particular categories of patients [12].

In machine learning, data imbalance is a challenge based on arthritis diagnosis. The datasets that are currently accessible are imbalanced, and the research publications do not discuss how they address this problem [3]. Some issues in implementing MLin medicine may potentially be a result of real statistical learning difficulties [12]. The application of ML to clinical practice faces a number of difficulties. The selection of reliable results is crucial but might be difficult. Algorithms that are frequently developed using retrospective studies yield superior performance measures than those that are frequently developed using applications to prospective, real-world data, making their implementation challenging and potentially unreliable [13].

ML has applications in various fields, including medical diagnosis and prognosis. Supervised learning requires labeled data, while unsupervised learning doesn't. In healthcare, ML has shown promise in diagnosing and managing RA. It can analyze patient data, imaging, and outcomes to aid diagnosis and predict disease progression. ML models can predict disease activity, treatment response, and personalized treatment options, ultimately improving patient care. A case study in cancer biology demonstrates how ML combines supervised and unsupervised learning to create predictive models for breast cancer prognosis. However, data imbalance and challenges in real-world implementation remain significant issues. ML faces challenges in selecting reliable results and applying algorithms to real-world, prospective data. Despite these challenges, ML holds great potential for advancing medical diagnosis and treatment.

2.1 *Early Diagnosis of Rheumatoid Arthritis*

In order to prevent inflammatory damage to the joints and improve results, it is important to diagnose RA as early as possible. Erythrocyte sedimentation rate (ESR) and C-reactive protein (CRP) are two biomarkers that can be used to diagnose RA. The ESR and CRP have limited specificity, and anti-citrullinated protein antibodies

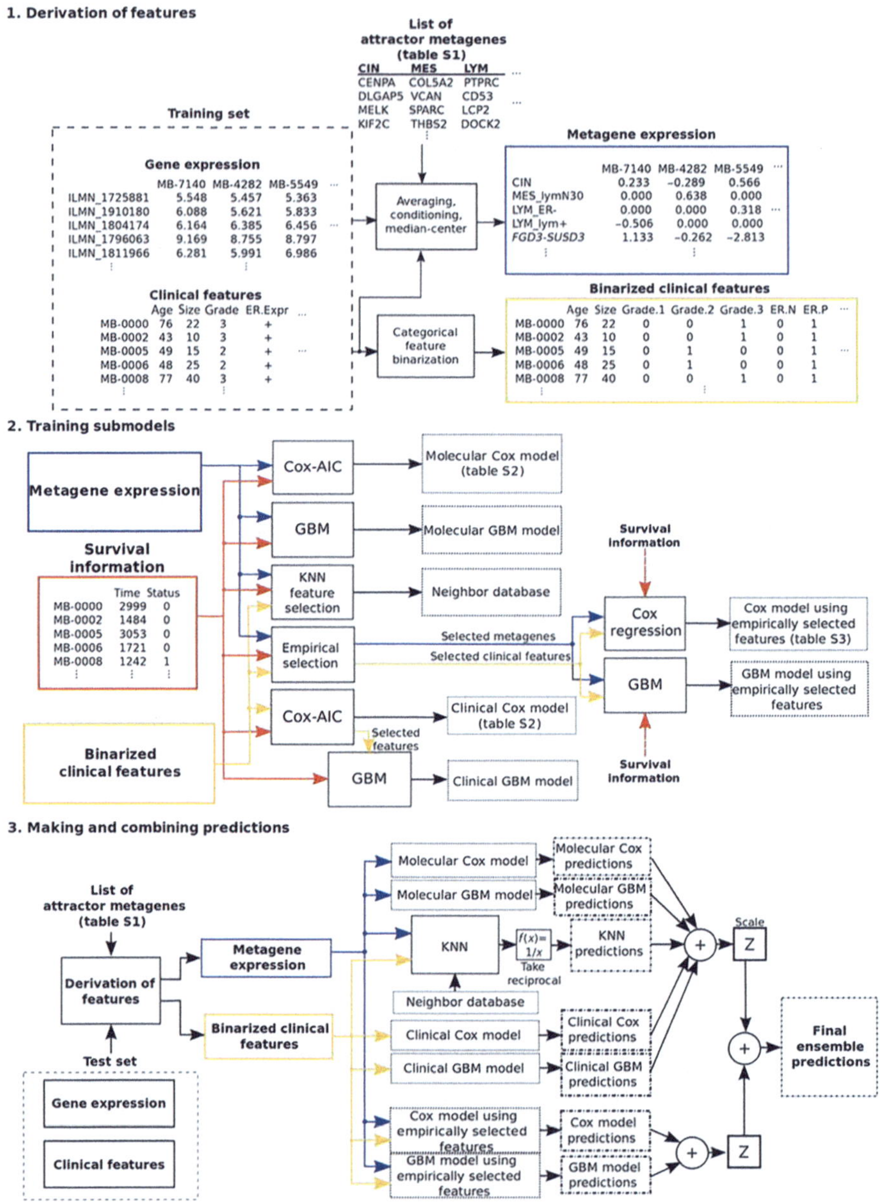

Fig. 1 Predictive ML model developed for breast cancer risk [12]

(ACPAs) or rheumatoid factor (RF) have subpar sensitivity. Due to the lack of a perfect biomarker with high sensitivity and specificity, the development of novel biomarker panels is necessary for the early identification of RA. It is possible to gain important insights into the molecular mechanisms underlying RA and support the diagnosis and treatment of the disease by using ML techniques to analyze omics data, which is a term used to describe large-scale data generated from different biological molecules, such as DNA, RNA, and proteins. Omics data such as genomes, transcriptomics, proteomics, metabolomics, lipidomics, glycomics, or metagenomic data, it is possible to examine the relationship between several different biomolecules and RA simultaneously [2].

Genome-wide association studies (GWAS) have found a large number of genetic variations linked to RA. An individual's risk of having RA can be predicted using these mutations to create polygenic risk scores (PRS). Additionally, genetic testing can help rule out other conditions that may have similar symptoms to RA [14]. RNA sequencing can be used to measure gene expression levels in blood, synovial tissue, and other tissues affected by RA. This can provide insights into the molecular pathways involved in RA and help identify potential biomarkers for diagnosis and monitoring disease progression [15]. Proteomics can be used to identify changes in protein expression and post-translational modifications in RA patients. This can help identify potential therapeutic targets and biomarkers for diagnosis and disease monitoring [16]. Metabolomics can be used to measure the small molecule metabolites present in blood and other tissues. Changes in metabolite levels can provide insights into the metabolic pathways involved in RA and help identify potential diagnostic and therapeutic targets [17]. Overall, omics data has the potential to provide valuable insights into the molecular mechanisms underlying RA and aid in the diagnosis and treatment of the disease. However, careful consideration of ethical and privacy issues is essential in the collection and analysis of omics data in healthcare. Additionally, omics data should be used in conjunction with other clinical and diagnostic tools to ensure accurate and effective diagnosis and treatment of RA.

A wide range of huge datasets, including personal information from genomics data, demographic data, and medication history are saved and used in diverse studies, raising possible ethical concerns regarding data privacy. This is especially true given the rise of ML applications in personalized medicine [5]. Four significant ethical concerns need to be resolved in order for AI in healthcare to completely realize its potential: Important things to think about include informed consent to utilize data, safety and openness, algorithmic fairness and biases, and data privacy [18].

3 Deep Learning in Rheumatoid Arthritis

Deep learning is a subclass of ML that seeks patterns in data by layering artificial neural networks as shown in Fig. 2 [2]. Artificial neural networks (ANNs) serve as the basis for deep learning, which aids in simulating human learning ability, using mathematical models of neurons and their connections [19]. DL has led the way in

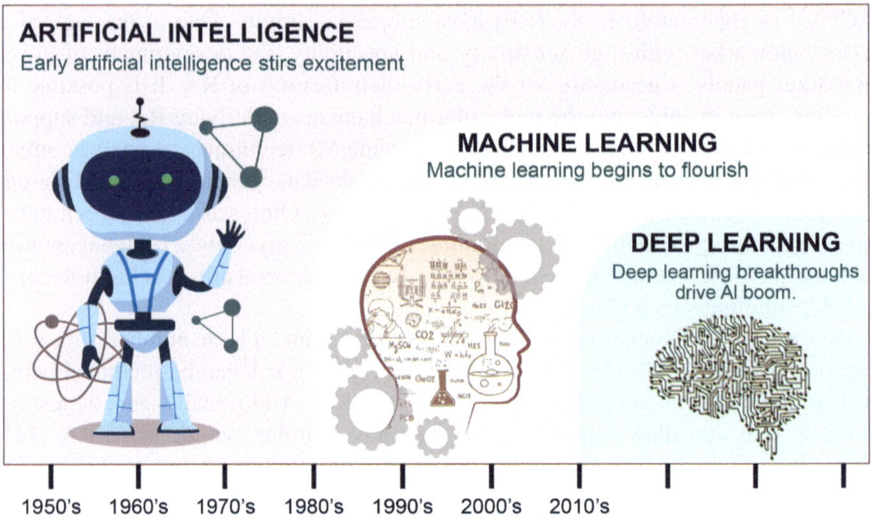

Fig. 2 Evolution of AI, Machine Learning and Deep Learning [2]

image analysis, genome research, and drug development during the past ten years as a consequence of enhancements in computer capacity and the accessibility of large datasets. Because they need more training data and more time, DL models are capable of handling more difficult jobs. Moreover, high-dimensional data, including EHRs and medical pictures, can be processed by DL models [2].

Deep learning models have more learning layers and a greater degree of abstraction than typical ML models. This benefit is further enhanced by the fact that all model components are directly learned from data. Traditional ML models experience limits as data size and the need for adequate insights from the data expand due to the algorithm they rely on. More advanced, quick, and precise learning algorithms have been developed as a result of the growth in data. DL can extract extremely precise representations of data from very big datasets, which makes it different from typical ML and data mining. Any DL technique must use data-driven modeling that is appropriate for the features of the raw data to be successful. A system must first be trained utilizing data and information related to the intended application using sophisticated learning algorithms before it can assist in intelligent decision-making [20].

Liu et al. have developed a DL approach for diagnosing knee osteoarthritis using X-ray images. Their model employs a region proposal network to identify joint regions, followed by object detection using Fast R-CNN. The model's architecture and integration of different components contribute to its ability to perform accurate and efficient osteoarthritis diagnosis. This approach represents a significant advancement in the field of medical image analysis and demonstrates the potential of DL techniques for improving medical diagnostics [3].

3.1 *Studies Related to Deep Learning Models on Rheumatoid Arthritis*

In the past few years, a number of DL researchers have presented their work on the subject of rheumatology, and more precisely in the context of RA. These researchers were working to create a method for automatically identifying medical images for RA diagnosis [21]. The application of AI in rheumatology for imaging has a long history, however, the majority of these approaches have still not been applied in real-world clinical situations. Recent experiments have shown that deep learning, a subset of AI methods, can analyze images more accurately than humans when done automatically. When it comes to image interpretation, rheumatologists and radiologists are unlikely to be replaced by AI; instead, a hybrid strategy that benefits both humans and AI is more likely to be developed [19].

Although DL models often require input images, radiographs (or X-rays) of the hands are typically utilized to calculate the SvH score for every image. In several investigations, the OMERACT-EULAR Synovitis Scoring (OESS) system and ultrasound imaging technology were both employed. Because they are inexpensive and simple to get, radiographs are the most often used medical modality for diagnosing RA and tracking its activity. Most models generally attempt to forecast if the condition is present and, if so, which of the two forms of joint injury such as erosion and narrowing will occur [21]. Fukae and colleagues used convolutional neural networks (CNNs) to make precise modifications to two-dimensional images created from a variety of clinical data from patients to determine whether or not they have RA. The groundwork for using DL to diagnose RA has been established by this work [22].

3.2 *Algorithms Based on Deep Learning*

3.2.1 Convolutional Neural Network (CNN)

It is employed in architectures with input layers, convolutional kernels, pooling layers, fully connected layers, and output layers utilized in the training, validation, and testing processes (Fig. 3). CNN's architecture is built in a way that enables it to study and distinguish between larger data sets. They analyze and identify arthritis using a total of 20 layered CNNs. In order to examine and grade the synovial region for the purpose of determining the presence of arthritis, CNN is utilized. DL is largely utilized to help doctors accurately diagnose and spot numerous clinical problems or diseases [1].

Sharp-van der Heijde scoring (SvH) approach was adopted in DL model to develop X-ray images in order to identify the radiographic finger joint to score in RA. The joint detection phase and the joint assessment step are the two tasks that this model follows. The very first step is Training a classifier to recognize the finger joints using Haar-like features. Later the second stage involves applying a joint space

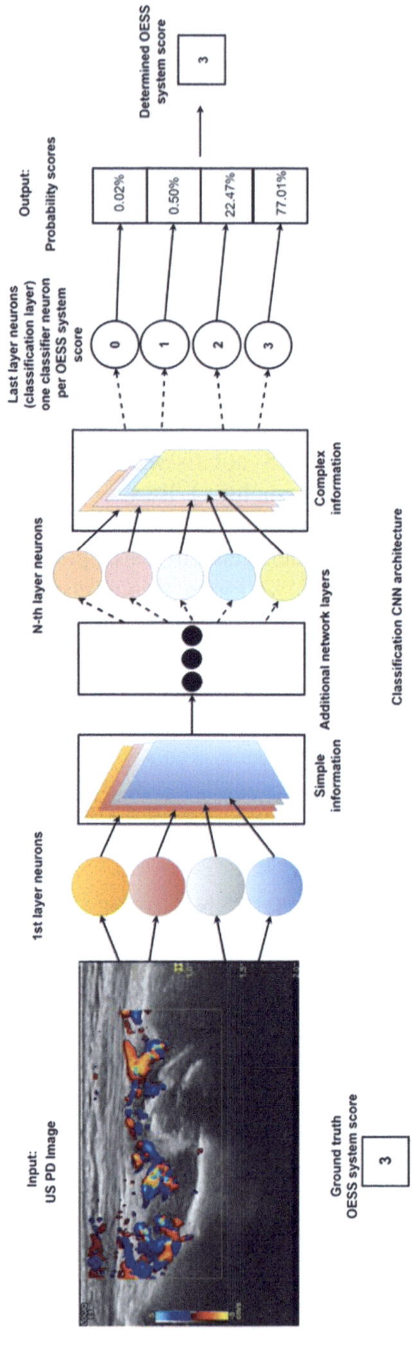

Fig. 3 Illustration of Convolutional neural network [23]

narrowing (JSN) score and an erosion score using a CNN model. This seven-layer model includes three fully connected layers, two pooling layers, two convolution layers, and two fully connected layers. To increase the size of the training data sets data augmentation i.e., horizontal flipping, and rotation was carried out. Both horizontal flipping and rotational data augmentation were carried out to enhance the size of the training datasets. Clinicians meticulously clipped and scored the images during training sets for JSN and bone erosion. Finally, the performance of the model was verified using a test dataset that was compared with the score provided by the model versus the score assigned by clinicians [21].

3.2.2 Artificial Neural Networks (ANNs)

Rheumatoid arthritis is diagnosed using ANN technology to support medical diagnostics. Backpropagation algorithms in artificial neural networks were looked at for the RA diagnosis in the Matlab R2015b environment. The algorithm correctly classifies the data that are obtained from persons who do not have RA as well as from RA sufferers. Performance comparisons were also made between the findings of the Perceptron method and the ANN backpropagation algorithm. In performance testing using the set of data, the accuracy is calculated using the Perceptron method, as opposed to the backpropagation approach, which yields an accuracy rate of 82% [24].

3.3 Applications

AI has made significant advances in a number of scientific fields in recent years. In therapeutic contexts, computer programs outperform humans at interpreting medical images. The use of deep learning, an AI subfield, for interpreting medical images has grown over time. The effectiveness of computer analysis over human research is well-known in various sectors; for example, AI is commonly used to analyze MRI data and predict an early RA (Fig. 4). Deep learning has various uses in computer vision, and it is crucial for the analysis of image data of melanoma, metastatic breast cancer, retinopathy, and other disorders. The most recent technique for longitudinal calculation and application in digital health record data is used in recurrent neural networks, a subset of deep learning. The integration of various patient data points to create AI-based models has demonstrated considerable promise for improving diagnosis accuracy and bringing about clinical advantages [22].

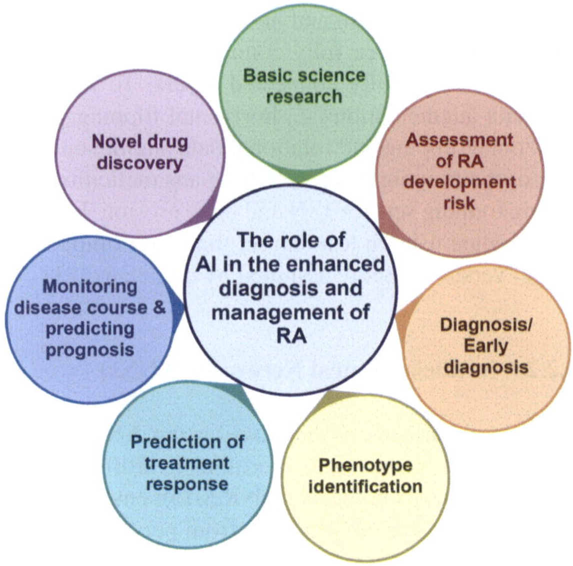

Fig. 4 AI's contribution to improved RA diagnosis and treatment [2]

4 Summary and Conclusion

Rheumatoid arthritis (RA) is the second most common autoimmune condition globally, affecting approximately 20 million individuals. The disease is identified by harmful joint variations that initially occur in the small joints of the extremities but can progress to larger joints if left untreated. The primary objective of RA treatment is to reduce inflammation and mitigate joint damage. AI is increasingly being employed in precision medicine for RA. These AI approaches have the ability to enhance precision and effectiveness in managing the disease. However, there are challenges that need to be addressed to further expand the use of AI-guided precision medicine, particularly in the field of RA. Overcoming these challenges will require collaborative efforts from multidisciplinary teams.

Image identification, natural language processing, and medical diagnosis are just a few of the many uses for ML. In the context of RA, ML has shown promising results in various areas. ML models can analyze extensive data from electronic health records, imaging studies, and patient-reported outcomes to identify patterns and predict disease progression. Moreover, ML techniques can be applied to omics data (genomics, transcriptomics, proteomics, metabolomics, etc.) to gain insights into the molecular mechanisms underlying RA. This can aid in early diagnosis by developing novel biomarker panels and predicting an individual's risk of developing RA using polygenic risk scores. DL has been widely used in many fields, including image analysis, genome research, and drug development. DL models excel at processing high-dimensional data, such as electronic health records (EHRs) and medical images. In rheumatology, DL has been explored for automatic identification of medical images for RA diagnosis, showing promising results compared to human interpretation.

The use of AI, particularly ML and DL algorithms, offers considerable promise for enhancing the accuracy and efficacy of RA treatment. These AI approaches can aid in primary prevention, accurate diagnosis, personalized treatment strategies, and efficient rehabilitation programs.ML has demonstrated its potential in improving the diagnosis and management of RA. By analyzing diverse datasets and identifying patterns, ML algorithms can support clinicians in making informed decisions, personalizing treatment approaches, and predicting disease outcomes. Incorporating ML techniques, especially in the analysis of omics data, can contribute to a better understanding of the molecular mechanisms underlying RA and facilitate early diagnosis. Deep learning techniques have shown promise in the field of rheumatology, particularly in RA diagnosis using medical images. These models have the potential to improve accuracy, aid in early detection, and provide valuable insights for clinicians. However, further research and validation are needed to ensure the reliability and clinical utility of DL models in real-world clinical settings. Applying ML to medical diagnostics, particularly in cases of arthritis diagnosis, faces several challenges. Data imbalance, real statistical difficulties, algorithmic performance disparities, and challenges in clinical implementation collectively present a complex landscape. As ML continues to be integrated into medical practice, it's important to address these challenges systematically and transparently to ensure that the promising potential of ML is realized in a meaningful and reliable manner.

References

1. Hemalatha RJ, Vijaybaskar V, Thamizhvani TR (2019) Automatic localization of anatomical regions in medical ultrasound images of rheumatoid arthritis using deep learning. J Eng Med 233(6):657–667
2. Momtazmanesh S, Nowroozi A, Rezaei N (2022) Artificial intelligence in rheumatoid arthritis: current status and future perspectives: a state-of-the-art review. Rheumatol Ther [Internet] 9(5):1249–1304
3. Imtiaz M, Shah SAA, ur Rehman Z (2022) A review of arthritis diagnosis techniques in artificial intelligence era: Current trends and research challenges. Neurosci Informatics [Internet] 2(4):100079
4. Norgeot B, Glicksberg BS, Trupin L, Lituiev D, Gianfrancesco M, Oskotsky B et al (2019) Assessment of a deep learning model based on electronic health record data to forecast clinical outcomes in patients with rheumatoid arthritis. JAMA Netw Open 2(3):e190606
5. Peng J, Jury EC, Dönnes P, Ciurtin C (2021) Machine learning techniques for personalised medicine approaches in immune-mediated chronic inflammatory diseases: applications and challenges. Front Pharmacol 12(September):1–18
6. Koo BS, Eun S, Shin K, Yoon H, Hong C, Kim DH et al (2021) Machine learning model for identifying important clinical features for predicting remission in patients with rheumatoid arthritis treated with biologics. Arthritis Res Ther 23(1):1–10
7. O'Neil LJ, Spicer V, Smolik I, Meng X, Goel RR, Anaparti V et al (2021) Association of a serum protein signature with rheumatoid arthritis development. Arthritis Rheumatol 73(1):78–88
8. Volkova A, Ruggles KV (2021) Predictive metagenomic analysis of autoimmune disease identifies robust autoimmunity and disease specific microbial signatures. Front Microbiol 12(March):621310

9. Ahmed U, Anwar A, Savage RS, Thornalley PJ, Rabbani N (2016) Protein oxidation, nitration and glycation biomarkers for early-stage diagnosis of osteoarthritis of the knee and typing and progression of arthritic disease. Arthritis Res Ther [Internet]. 18(1):1–11
10. Wang Z, Liu J, Gu Z, Li C (2021) An efficient CNN for hand x-ray overall scoring of rheumatoid arthritis. J Healthc Eng. 2021(1):10
11. Scheel AK, Krause A, Mesecke-Von I, Metzger G, Rost H, Tresp V et al (2002) Assessment of proximal finger joint inflammation in patients with rheumatoid arthritis, using a novel laser-based imaging technique. Arthritis Rheum 46(5):1177–1184
12. Deo RC (2015) Machine learning in medicine. Ahajournals 132(1):1920–1930
13. Nelson AE, Arbeeva L (2022) Narrative review of machine learning in rheumatic and musculoskeletal diseases for clinicians and researchers: biases, goals, and future directions. J Rheumatol 49(11):1191–1200
14. Martin AR, Kanai M, Kamatani Y, Okada Y (2019) Current clinical use of polygenic scores will risk exacerbating health disparities Alicia. Nat Genet 51(4):584–591
15. Lewis MJ, Barnes MR, Blighe K, Taylor PC, Townsend MJ, Pitzalis C et al (2019) Molecular portraits of early rheumatoid arthritis identify clinical and treatment response resource molecular portraits of early rheumatoid arthritis identify clinical and treatment. Cell Rep 8(1):2455–2470
16. Park Y-J, Chung MK, Hwang D, Kim W-U (2015) Proteomics in rheumatoid arthritis research. Immune Netw 15(4):177
17. Duarte-Delgado NP, Cala MP, Barreto A, Rodríguez CLS (2022) Metabolites and metabolic pathways associated with rheumatoid arthritis and systemic lupus erythematosus. J Transl Autoimmun 5(1):100150
18. Naik N, Hameed BMZ, Shetty DK, Swain D, Shah M, Paul R et al (2022) Legal and ethical consideration in artificial intelligence in healthcare: who takes responsibility? Front Surg 9(Mar):1–6
19. Stoel B (2020) Use of artificial intelligence in imaging in rheumatology-current status and future perspectives. RMD Open 6(1):1–10
20. Directions F (2023) Understanding of machine learning with deep learning: comput MDPI 12(91):1–26
21. Avramidis GP, Avramidou MP, Papakostas GA (2022) Rheumatoid arthritis diagnosis: deep learning versus humane. Appl Sci 12(1):1–21
22. Bai L, Zhang Y, Wang P, Zhu X, Xiong JW, Cui L (2022) Improved diagnosis of rheumatoid arthritis using an artificial neural network. Sci Rep [Internet] 12(1):1–7
23. Andersen JKH, Pedersen JS, Laursen MS, Holtz K, Grauslund J, Savarimuthu TR et al (2019) Neural networks for automatic scoring of arthritis disease activity on ultrasound images. RMD Open 5(1):1–5
24. Saritas I, Tok K (2016) The usage of artificial neural networks method in the diagnosis of rheumatoid arthritis. Int J Intell Syst Appl Eng 4(4):119–121

AI-Empowered Prediction of Prognosis and Treatment Response in Rheumatoid Arthritis

Isha Sharma, Ritu Karwasra, Usama Akram, Kapil Suchal, and Surender Singh

Abstract Rheumatoid arthritis (RA) is a debilitating autoimmune disease, necessitating precise prognosis and treatment response predictions for personalized care. Artificial intelligence (AI) has emerged as a transformative tool in RA management. This chapter discusses challenges in conventional assessment and the imperative integration of AI. Various AI techniques, like machine learning and deep learning, are examined for their capacity to analyze extensive patient data and uncover novel biomarkers. AI-powered prognostic models for RA are highlighted, considering patient characteristics, genetics, and disease activity markers to predict outcomes accurately. AI's role in tailoring treatment strategies based on genetics, biomarkers, and treatment histories is explored, enhancing therapeutic effectiveness. Moreover, AI's ability to forecast treatment responses aids healthcare providers in selecting optimal therapies. The integration of AI into clinical practice is discussed, addressing implementation challenges and ethical concerns, and emphasizing patient data security and responsible AI use. To summarize, AI holds immense potential for revolutionizing RA patient care and transforming diagnosis, management, and treatment. As AI gains acceptance, its incorporation into clinical practice will likely become commonplace, reshaping the landscape of RA healthcare.

Keywords Rheumatoid arthritis · Artificial intelligence · Disease progression · Patient outcomes · Clinical decision-making · Predictive modeling

---

I. Sharma
Department of Pharmaceutical Sciences, Gurugram University, Gurugram 122018, India

R. Karwasra (✉) · U. Akram
Central Council for Research in Unani Medicine, Ministry of Ayush, Government of India, New Delhi 110058, India
e-mail: rituccrum@gmail.com

K. Suchal
Department of Internal Medicine, School of Medicine, Texas Tech University Health Sciences Centre, Lubbock, TX 790430, USA
e-mail: fnu.Kapil@ttuhsc.edu

S. Singh
Department of Pharmacology, All India Institute of Medical Sciences, New Delhi 110029, India

K. Raza and S. Singh (eds.), *Artificial Intelligence and Autoimmune Diseases*, Studies in Computational Intelligence 1133, https://doi.org/10.1007/978-981-99-9029-0_13

1 Introduction

Rheumatoid arthritis (RA) is a chronic autoimmune disorder that affects approximately 1% of the global population, making it one of the most prevalent and debilitating joint diseases worldwide. Characterized by persistent joint inflammation, pain, and functional impairment, RA poses significant challenges to both patients and healthcare systems [1]. Recent statistics underscore the urgency of improving management strategies for this complex condition. As of the latest data available, it is estimated that over 23 million people are living with rheumatoid arthritis, with women being three times more likely to be affected than men [2]. The economic burden is substantial, with direct and indirect costs of RA exceeding billions annually, encompassing medical expenses, lost productivity, and reduced quality of life. The clinical course of RA is highly variable, with manifestations ranging from mild joint discomfort to severe joint destruction and systemic complications. Early diagnosis and aggressive treatment initiation are essential to prevent irreversible joint damage and improve long-term outcomes [3]. However, predicting the trajectory of RA and determining optimal treatment approaches remain formidable challenges due to the inherent heterogeneity of the disease and the varying responses to available therapies. In recent years, the rapid advancement of artificial intelligence (AI) and machine learning techniques has offered unprecedented opportunities to transform the landscape of medical research and clinical practice. By harnessing the power of AI, researchers and clinicians are exploring innovative ways to decipher the intricate patterns within the vast and complex datasets generated by RA patients. These efforts aim to uncover novel insights into disease progression, identify predictive biomarkers, and optimize treatment strategies, ultimately leading to more personalized and effective care [4].

This book chapter goes into the emerging subject of AI-powered prognosis and therapy response prediction in rheumatoid arthritis. We will examine the latest developments in AI techniques, ranging from machine learning to deep learning and integrative models, and their applications in RA research and clinical practice. Through the integration of clinical data, molecular profiles, and advanced analytical tools, AI has the potential to revolutionize the way we understand, predict, and manage RA. Furthermore, we will address the ethical considerations challenges, and future directions that arise with the integration of AI in RA management. As we navigate through the intricate interplay of AI and RA, we embark on a journey toward more accurate prognostic assessments and personalized treatment strategies. By merging cutting-edge technology with clinical expertise, we aspire to usher in an era where patients with RA experience improved quality of life, minimized disease burden, and enhanced therapeutic outcomes.

2 AI Techniques for Prognosis Prediction

2.1 Machine Learning Approaches

Machine learning (ML) has emerged as a powerful tool for prognostic prediction in RA. ML algorithms learn patterns from diverse datasets and make predictions based on these learned patterns. In RA, machine learning models leverage various clinical, demographic, and molecular features to predict disease progression and treatment outcomes. These models encompass a range of algorithms, such as decision trees, random forests, support vector machines, and gradient boosting, each offering a unique approach to identifying complex relationships within the data (Fig. 1). ML algorithms excel at identifying subtle patterns that may not be evident to clinicians, thereby aiding in the discovery of new prognostic factors. These models integrate both traditional clinical markers (e.g., disease duration, joint involvement) and novel biomarkers (e.g., gene expression profiles, and cytokine levels) to generate more accurate and personalized predictions. By harnessing the potential of machine learning, clinicians can potentially stratify patients into risk categories, enabling tailored interventions and optimizing long-term outcomes [5].

Machine Learning in Cancer Diagnosis, Prognosis, and Therapy

Machine learning has revolutionized cancer diagnosis, prognosis, and therapy by leveraging advanced algorithms to extract valuable insights from vast and complex medical data. In cancer diagnosis, machine learning models analyze diverse patient

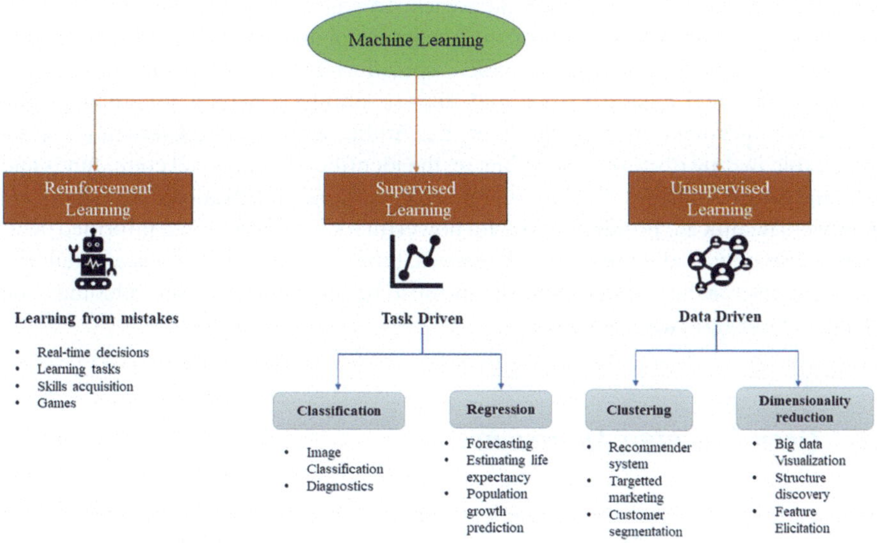

Fig. 1 Types of machine learning

data, including medical images, genomics, and clinical records, to assist in early detection and accurate classification of malignancies. These models can identify subtle patterns and anomalies, enabling oncologists to make more precise and timely diagnoses. Support vector machines (SVMs), artificial neural networks (ANNs), and deep learning approaches are well-known and commonly used AI methods for structured data. There are several AI techniques that have the ability to address difficult medical problems. For example, ANN has been used to diagnose breast, gastric, thyroid, and oral epithelial cancers, as well as radiographic and histopathological image analysis (computed tomography (CT) and magnetic resonance imaging (MRI) scans) and data interpretation in intensive care units (ICUs). Fuzzy logic (FL), another intelligent system, has been utilized to identify numerous malignancies, including lung cancer, utilizing tumor profile indicators. The genome-wide association study, an evolution-based algorithm, has been researched to predict outcomes for diseases such as lung cancer, and melanoma, and therapeutic responses (such as warfarin). The curators in the field of artificial intelligence in medicines (AIM) are the researchers, and it is their responsibility to provide credible and applicable proof that these strategies function on logical and sensible grounds. Nonetheless, there is still a gap between current and AI-based medical approaches. However, there is much proof demonstrating that AIM is more efficient and, as a result, is critical for making it a part of personalized healthcare [28].

In the realm of cancer prognosis, machine learning systems utilize patient-specific information to predict disease progression and survival rates. By integrating clinical variables, biomarkers, and treatment response data, these models empower clinicians to tailor treatment plans, enhancing patient outcomes. Furthermore, machine learning aids in identifying potential therapeutic targets, which is crucial for the development of personalized treatment strategies. In cancer therapy, machine learning contributes significantly by optimizing treatment plans and predicting therapeutic responses. It assists in designing patient-specific treatment regimens, taking into account individual characteristics and disease profiles, thereby minimizing side effects and improving overall quality of life. Additionally, machine learning plays a pivotal role in drug discovery, speeding up the identification of novel compounds and potential drug combinations. Overall, machine learning's integration into cancer care empowers healthcare professionals with powerful tools to make more informed decisions, ultimately leading to earlier diagnoses, more accurate prognoses, and tailored treatment approaches, which hold the promise of improving patient outcomes and advancing our fight against cancer.

2.2 *Deep Learning Approaches*

Deep learning, a subset of machine learning, has garnered significant attention for its ability to process and learn intricate patterns from complex and high-dimensional data. Convolutional neural networks (CNNs) and recurrent neural networks (RNNs)

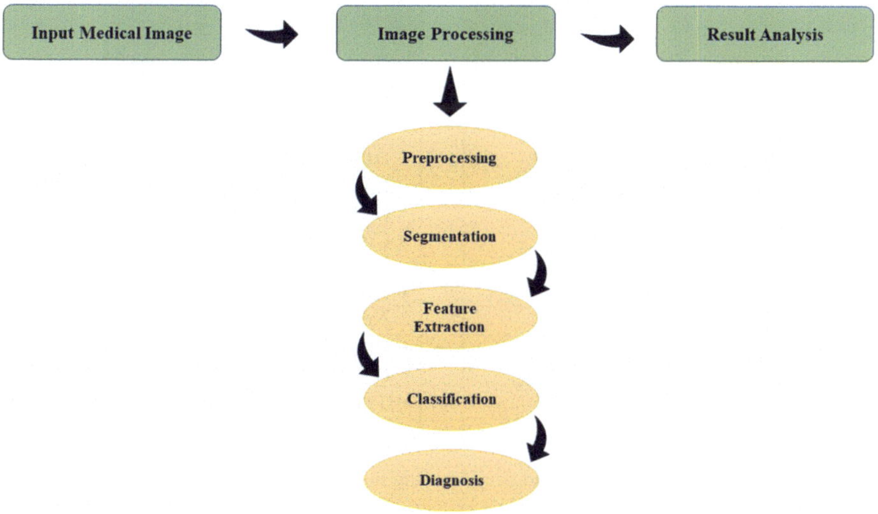

Fig. 2 Deep learning approaches in RA

are examples of deep learning architectures that have shown promise in RA prognosis prediction. These models can capture subtle temporal and spatial relationships within data, making them well-suited for analyzing longitudinal disease progression and treatment response [6]. Deep learning approaches excel at feature extraction, allowing them to automatically identify relevant features from raw data, such as medical images or time-series data. In RA, deep learning algorithms can be applied to medical imaging data, such as X-rays or MRI scans, to predict joint damage and monitor disease evolution (Fig. 2). Furthermore, deep learning models can uncover hidden patterns in multi-modal data sources, facilitating a more comprehensive understanding of RA pathogenesis and prognosis [7].

Applications of Machine and Deep Learning Models in RA

Machine learning and deep learning models have shown promising applications in the field of RA research and management. These models leverage the power of computational algorithms to analyze complex data and improve our understanding of RA. One common approach is the use of supervised machine learning techniques, such as support vector machines and random forests, to predict disease outcomes based on clinical and biological data. These models can help in early diagnosis and prognosis, aiding clinicians in making informed treatment decisions.

Deep learning models, particularly convolutional neural networks (CNNs) and recurrent neural networks (RNNs) have been employed to analyze medical imaging data like X-rays and MRIs (Fig. 3). These models can automatically detect and classify joint abnormalities associated with RA, facilitating quicker and more accurate diagnosis. Furthermore, natural language processing (NLP) techniques are utilized to extract valuable insights from electronic health records and medical literature. NLP

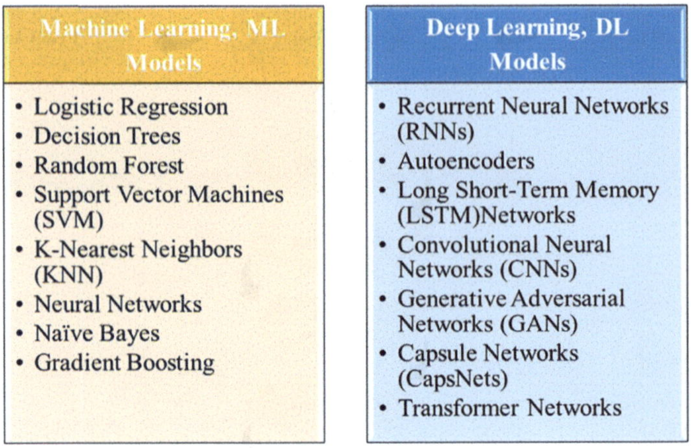

Fig. 3 Models of machine learning and deep learning in RA

models can assist in identifying trends, risk factors, and potential treatment options by mining vast amounts of textual data. Machine and deep learning models have become valuable tools in the study of rheumatoid arthritis. They enhance our ability to predict, diagnose, and understand this complex autoimmune disease, ultimately improving patient care and treatment outcomes.

2.3 Integrative Models: Combining Clinical and Omics Data

Integrative models represent a promising avenue for enhancing the accuracy of RA prognosis prediction by merging diverse datasets. These models combine clinical data, such as patient demographics and disease characteristics, with omics data, including genomics, transcriptomics, proteomics, and metabolomics. The integration of multiple data modalities allows for a holistic view of the disease, capturing both genetic predisposition and molecular responses [8]. By fusing clinical and omics data, integrative models can unravel intricate interactions between genetic variations and environmental factors, shedding light on personalized disease trajectories. These models can identify molecular signatures associated with disease progression, therapeutic response, and adverse outcomes. Integrative approaches hold the potential to uncover novel therapeutic targets and biomarkers, paving the way for more precise interventions and improved patient management [9]. Incorporating machine learning, deep learning, and integrative models into RA prognosis prediction empowers clinicians with advanced tools for informed decision-making. As AI techniques continue to evolve and mature, the ability to harness complex data and extract meaningful insights will drive a paradigm shift in the management of rheumatoid arthritis, offering patients a brighter prognosis and better quality of life.

Applications of AI in Diagnosing RA

Artificial Intelligence (AI) has emerged as a powerful tool in the field of healthcare, particularly in diagnosing Rheumatoid Arthritis (RA). AI applications have the potential to revolutionize the way RA is detected and managed. Machine learning algorithms can analyze vast datasets of patient information, including medical history, imaging scans, and blood test results, to assist in the early detection of RA. These algorithms can identify subtle patterns and correlations that might be missed by human practitioners, leading to quicker and more accurate diagnoses. Furthermore, AI can help monitor the progression of RA by analyzing real-time patient data, allowing for personalized treatment plans and early intervention when necessary. Additionally, AI-driven chatbots and virtual assistants can provide patients with information and support, enhancing their overall care experience. AI's applications in diagnosing RA offer the potential for earlier detection, improved management, and better outcomes for patients with this chronic autoimmune disease (Table 1).

Table 1 Applications of AI in Diagnosing RA [27]

Researches	AI approach	Imaging data used	Results
"Automated Detection of rheumatoid arthritis in hand radiographs"	Deep learning (CNNs)	Hand radiographs	Achieved high accuracy in RA detection based on radiographs
"Machine Learning for the diagnosis of early rheumatoid arthritis"	SVM	MRI and ultrasound Images	SVM-based model showed promising results in early RA diagnosis using imaging data
"Deep Learning for diagnosis of rheumatoid arthritis based on sonography"	Deep learning (CNNs)	Musculoskeletal ultrasound Images	Demonstrated the potential of deep learning to aid in RA diagnosis through sonography
"Automated Detection of synovitis in ultrasound images for early rheumatoid arthritis diagnosis"	Machine learning	Musculoskeletal ultrasound Images	Developed an automated system for detecting synovitis, a key RA indicator, in ultrasound images
"Improving the classification of rheumatoid arthritis using deep convolutional neural networks"	Deep learning (CNNs)	X-ray and ultrasound images	CNN-based model enhanced the accuracy of RA classification using both X-ray and ultrasound data

3 Biomarker Discovery and Validation in RA Management

3.1 Identification of Novel Biomarkers Through AI

The search for reliable and predictive biomarkers in RA has been a longstanding challenge. AI-driven approaches have revolutionized this quest by enabling the identification of novel biomarkers from vast and heterogeneous datasets. Machine learning and deep learning algorithms can uncover intricate patterns and associations within multidimensional omics data, facilitating the discovery of molecular signatures linked to disease progression and treatment response [10]. AI algorithms excel at processing high-dimensional data, such as gene expression profiles, single-cell sequencing data, and proteomic patterns. By integrating diverse data sources, AI-powered methods can unveil previously hidden relationships between genetic variations, molecular pathways, and RA phenotypes. These discoveries can lead to the identification of potential biomarkers that accurately reflect disease activity, severity, and the likelihood of treatment success [11].

3.2 Validation of Predictive Biomarkers in RA

Identifying candidate biomarkers is just the first step; robust validation is essential to ensure their clinical relevance and utility. AI technologies play a pivotal role in facilitating the validation process by enabling the analysis of large-scale patient cohorts and datasets. These technologies help researchers assess the reproducibility and generalizability of identified biomarkers across diverse populations. Validation of predictive biomarkers involves rigorous statistical analyses, cross-validation techniques, and external validation on independent cohorts. AI-driven validation can enhance the accuracy of assessing biomarker performance, minimizing the risk of false discoveries. Furthermore, machine learning models can develop predictive algorithms that combine multiple validated biomarkers, creating more robust and accurate prognostic tools for clinicians [12].

By accelerating the discovery and validation of biomarkers, AI contributes to the transformation of RA management from a one-size-fits-all approach to a personalized and targeted strategy. The integration of AI-powered biomarkers into clinical practice holds the promise of improving patient outcomes through early disease detection, tailored treatment selection, and continuous monitoring of disease progression and therapeutic response (Table 2).

Table 2 Different biomarkers of RA with AI applications [13]

Biomarker	Function	AI applications in RA research
Rheumatoid Factor (RF)	Antibody against the Fc region of IgG antibodies	AI has been used to analyze patient data to predict RA based on RF levels and other clinical parameters
Anti-Cyclic Citrullinated Peptide (Anti-CCP)	Antibodies against citrullinated proteins	AI algorithms have been employed to identify patterns and predict the presence of anti-CCP antibodies in RA
C-Reactive protein (CRP)	Marker of inflammation	AI has been used to analyze CRP levels in RA patients and assess their disease activity and response to treatment
Erythrocyte Sedimentation Rate (ESR)	Measure of inflammation	AI-based models have been developed to predict ESR values in RA patients and monitor disease activity
Matrix Metalloproteinases (MMPs)	Enzymes involved in tissue remodeling	AI has been applied to study MMP expression patterns in RA joints, aiding in understanding disease progression
Tumor Necrosis Factor-Alpha (TNF-α)	Proinflammatory cytokine	AI has been used to analyze genetic and molecular data to predict TNF-α levels and response to anti-TNF therapies
Interleukin-6 (IL-6)	Proinflammatory cytokine	AI models have been employed to assess the role of IL-6 in RA and predict its levels in patient samples
Vascular Endothelial Growth Factor (VEGF)	Promotes angiogenesis	AI has been used in the analysis of VEGF expression in RA synovium and its correlation with disease severity
MicroRNA Biomarkers	Regulatory molecules	AI has been used to identify microRNA signatures associated with RA and their impact on gene expression and pathways

4 Personalized Treatment Response Prediction of AI

4.1 Tailoring Treatment Strategies Using AI

The advent of AI has ushered in a new era of personalized medicine in rheumatoid arthritis (RA) treatment. Traditional treatment approaches often follow a trial-and-error paradigm, which can lead to delayed symptom relief, adverse effects, and suboptimal outcomes. AI-powered models offer a transformative solution by analyzing patient-specific data to predict treatment responses, allowing clinicians to tailor interventions for improved efficacy [14]. Machine learning algorithms can integrate diverse patient factors, including clinical history, genetics, biomarker profiles, and imaging data, to predict the most suitable treatment options for individual patients. These models can consider a multitude of variables that influence treatment response, such as disease activity, comorbidities, medication history, and lifestyle factors. By leveraging these insights, clinicians can make informed decisions about the most appropriate therapies for each patient, ultimately optimizing outcomes and minimizing potential side effects [15].

4.2 Real-Time Adaptive Treatment Algorithms

AI's capacity to process and analyze data in real-time opens the door to dynamic treatment adaptations. Real-time adaptive treatment algorithms continuously monitor patient's disease activity and treatment responses, allowing for timely adjustments based on evolving clinical conditions. This approach ensures that patients receive the most effective interventions at all stages of their disease journey [16]. By integrating patient-reported outcomes, wearable device data, and laboratory results, AI-driven adaptive algorithms can provide a comprehensive view of disease dynamics. These algorithms can alert clinicians to changes in disease activity, enabling swift modifications to treatment plans. Furthermore, continuous monitoring fosters a proactive approach to managing potential treatment failures or adverse events, enhancing patient safety and well-being.

The convergence of AI and personalized treatment response prediction is poised to revolutionize RA management. By tailoring treatments based on individual characteristics and disease progression, clinicians can achieve better disease control, higher patient satisfaction, and improved long-term outcomes [17]. The integration of real-time adaptive algorithms adds an additional layer of precision, enabling agile responses to changing clinical scenarios and further enhancing the quality of care provided to RA patients (Fig. 4).

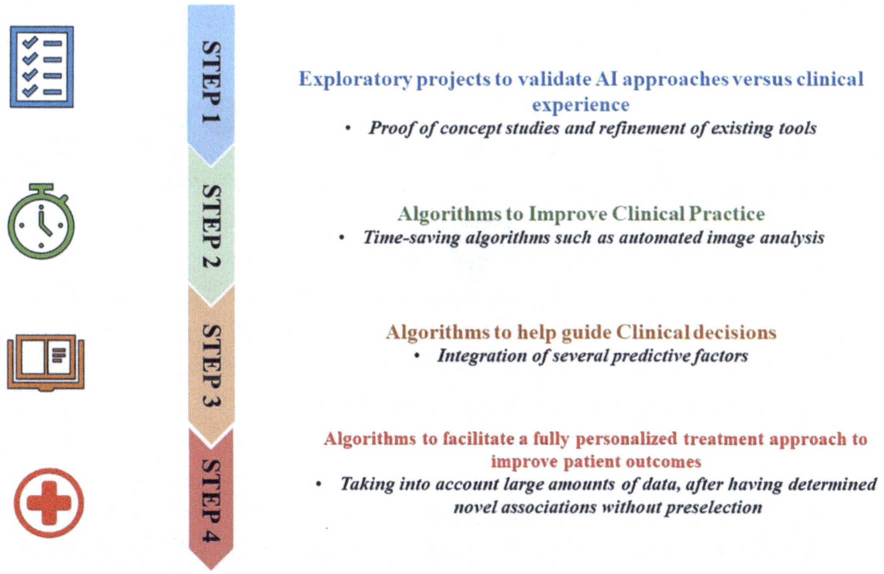

Fig. 4 Steps of AI in RA treatment

5 Clinical Decision Support Systems

5.1 AI-Powered Decision Support Tools for Healthcare Professionals

Clinical decision support systems (CDSS) are crucial in the complex landscape of RA management, where treatment decisions can be multifaceted and require careful consideration. AI-powered CDSS leverages patient-specific data, evidence-based guidelines, and advanced analytics to assist healthcare professionals in making informed choices. AI-driven CDSS can offer several benefits to clinicians [18]. They can provide real-time recommendations for treatment options, dosage adjustments, and monitoring intervals based on individual patient profiles. These systems integrate the latest research findings and clinical guidelines, ensuring that healthcare providers stay updated with the rapidly evolving field of RA management. Moreover, CDSS can help in identifying potential drug interactions, contraindications, and adverse events, enhancing patient safety (Fig. 5).

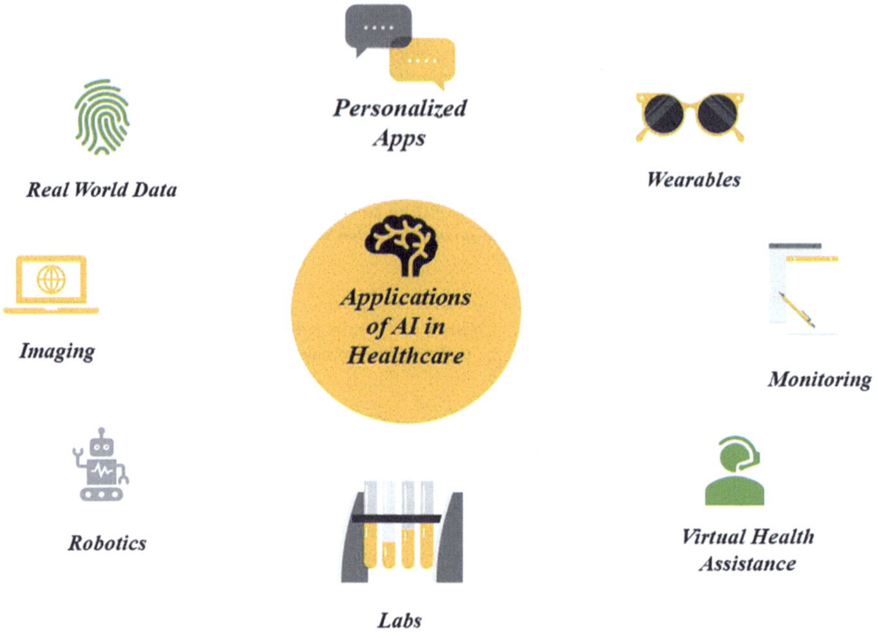

Fig. 5 Applications of AI in RA diagnosis, prognosis, and treatment

5.2 Enhancing Shared Decision-Making with Patients

CDSS plays a crucial role in enhancing shared decision-making between healthcare providers and patients in the context of AI-powered Rheumatoid Arthritis management. These systems leverage advanced algorithms and patient data to provide personalized treatment recommendations and prognostic insights. By presenting evidence-based information and treatment options in a comprehensible manner, CDSS empowers patients to actively participate in their care. This collaborative approach fosters informed discussions, aligns treatment plans with patient preferences and values, and ultimately leads to more effective management of Rheumatoid Arthritis, improving patient outcomes and quality of life [19].

6 Ethical Considerations and Challenges in AI

6.1 Data Privacy and Security

Ethical considerations and challenges in AI are increasingly prominent as artificial intelligence technologies become more integrated into our lives. One significant issue is data privacy and security. AI systems rely heavily on large datasets for training

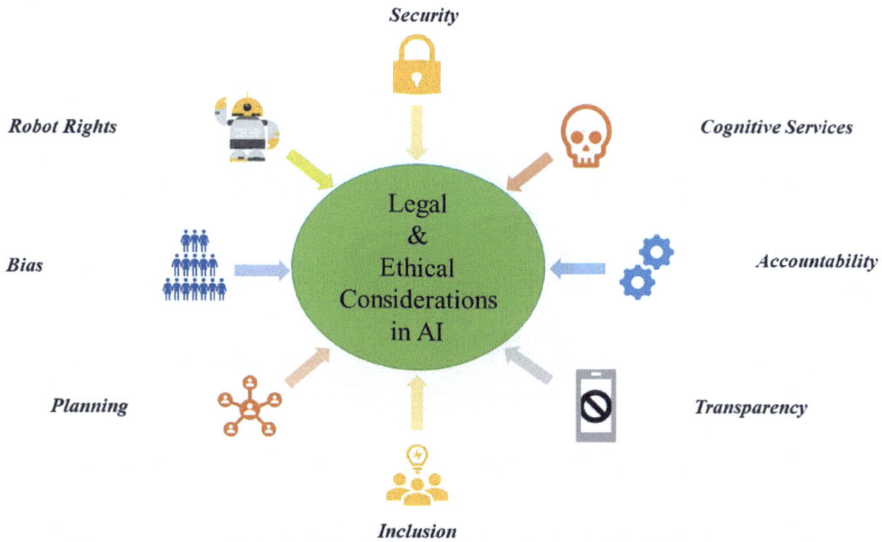

Fig. 6 Legal & ethical considerations in AI

and decision-making, raising concerns about how personal information is collected, used, and protected. Ensuring that data is anonymized and securely stored is essential to prevent unauthorized access or breaches. Additionally, the potential for bias in AI algorithms poses ethical dilemmas, as biased data can perpetuate discrimination and inequality [20]. Striking a balance between harnessing the power of AI and safeguarding individuals' privacy and security remains a critical challenge for the AI community and society as a whole. Robust regulations, transparency, and responsible data handling practices are essential to address these concerns (Fig. 6).

6.2 Future Directions in Bias and Fairness Research

Ethical considerations in AI models, particularly regarding bias and fairness, are paramount in ensuring responsible and equitable technology development. Bias can creep into AI models due to biased training data or algorithmic decisions, leading to unjust outcomes. Ensuring fairness requires proactive steps like data preprocessing, algorithmic transparency, and ongoing monitoring to detect and mitigate bias [21]. These efforts are vital to prevent reinforcing existing societal prejudices and to uphold principles of fairness and equity in AI applications, ultimately fostering trust and positive societal impact. However, addressing bias and fairness remains a complex challenge that requires collaboration among technologists, policymakers, and society to strike the right ethical balance [22].

Fig. 7 Challenges in AI

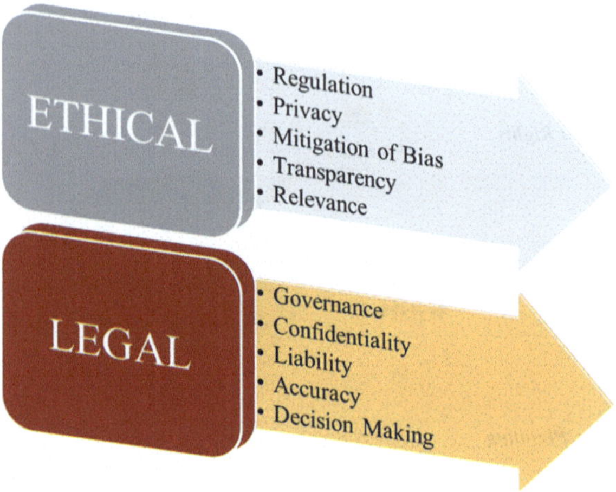

6.3 Regulatory and Clinical Adoption Challenges

Regulatory and clinical adoption challenges are significant ethical considerations in the field of healthcare AI. The integration of AI technologies into healthcare settings faces hurdles related to ensuring patient privacy, data security, and compliance with strict regulatory frameworks like HIPAA in the United States and GDPR in Europe [18]. Moreover, clinical adoption involves overcoming skepticism from healthcare professionals and patients, who may be concerned about the reliability, accountability, and potential biases of AI-driven diagnostic or treatment recommendations. Addressing these challenges requires clear and robust regulatory guidelines, comprehensive training for healthcare staff, and transparent communication to build trust in AI applications while upholding ethical standards in patient care (Fig. 7).

7 Future Directions and Conclusions

7.1 Prospects for AI in RA Management

The prospects for AI in Rheumatoid Arthritis (RA) management are promising and continue to evolve. AI-driven tools have the potential to revolutionize the field by enabling early and more accurate diagnosis, personalized treatment plans, and continuous monitoring of disease progression [23]. With advancements in machine learning algorithms and the integration of big data sources, AI can assist healthcare professionals in making data-driven decisions, improving patient outcomes, and ultimately enhancing the quality of life for individuals with RA. However, it is crucial to address challenges related to data privacy, model interpretability, and clinical validation to ensure the safe and effective implementation of AI in RA management. As research and development in this area progress, AI holds great potential as a valuable ally in the fight against RA [24].

7.2 Collaborative Efforts for Data Sharing and Model Validation

In the future, collaborative efforts for data sharing and model validation hold immense promise in advancing AI in Rheumatoid Arthritis (RA) management. By pooling resources, knowledge, and data, the healthcare community can accelerate the development of more accurate and reliable AI models for RA diagnosis, prognosis, and treatment. Furthermore, collaboration fosters transparency and trust in AI applications, ensuring that these technologies become integral tools in improving the lives of RA patients. Moving forward, it is essential to prioritize these collaborative initiatives, establishing standardized protocols for data sharing and rigorous model validation to unlock the full potential of AI in RA management [25].

7.3 Moving Toward Precision Medicine in RA

In conclusion, the integration of artificial intelligence in the pursuit of precision medicine for RA represents a significant step forward in healthcare. AI-driven tools and algorithms have the potential to revolutionize how we diagnose, treat, and manage RA by tailoring interventions to individual patients. As we continue to advance in this direction, the synergy between AI and precision medicine promises a brighter future for RA patients, offering them more effective and personalized treatments while minimizing potential side effects [26]. This paradigm shift is emblematic of the broader transformation underway in healthcare, where AI capacity to extract insights from vast datasets will drive innovations that benefit patients worldwide.

Acknowledgements The authors would like to thank the Central Council for Research in Unani Medicine (CCRUM), India for providing administrative and technical support.

References

1. Scott DL, Wolfe F, Huizinga TW (2010) Rheumatoid arthritis. The Lancet 376(9746):1094–1108
2. Aletaha D, Smolen JS (2018) Diagnosis and management of rheumatoid arthritis: a review. JAMA 320(13):1360–1372

3. Momtazmanesh S, Nowroozi A, Rezaei N (2022) Artificial intelligence in rheumatoid arthritis: current status and future perspectives: a state-of-the-art review. Rheumatology and Therapy. 9(5):1249–1304
4. Bird A, Oakden-Rayner L, McMaster C, Smith LA, Zeng M, Wechalekar MD, Ray S, Proudman S, Palmer LJ (2022) Artificial intelligence and the future of radiographic scoring in rheumatoid arthritis: a viewpoint. Arthritis Res Ther 24(1):1
5. Rajkomar A, Dean J, Kohane I (2019) Machine learning in medicine. N Engl J Med 380(14):1347–1358
6. Seneviratne MG, Shah NH, Chu L. Bridging the implementation gap of machine learning in healthcare. Bmj Innov 6(2) (2020)
7. McMaster C, Bird A, Liew DF, Buchanan RR, Owen CE, Chapman WW, Pires DE (2022) Artificial intelligence and deep learning for rheumatologists. Arthritis & Rheumatology. 74(12):1893–1905
8. Wang J, Tian Y, Zhou T, Tong D, Ma J, Li J (2023) A survey of artificial intelligence in rheumatoid arthritis. Rheumatol Immunol Res 4(2):69–77
9. Obayya M, Alamgeer MS, Alzahrani J, Alabdan RN, Al-Wesabi F, Mohamed A, Alsaid Hassan MI (2022) Artificial intelligence driven biomedical image classification for robust rheumatoid arthritis classification. Biomedicines 10(11):2714
10. McMaster C, Bird A, Liew DFL, Buchanan RR, Owen CE, Chapman WW, Pires DEV (2022) Artificial intelligence and deep learning for rheumatologists. Arthritis Rheumatol 74(12):1893–1905. https://doi.org/10.1002/art.42296. Epub 2022 Oct 26. PMID: 35857865; PMCID: PMC10092842
11. Hügle M, Omoumi P, van Laar JM, Boedecker J, Hügle T (2020) Applied machine learning and artificial intelligence in rheumatology. Rheumatol Adv Pract 4(1):rkaa005
12. Wang S, Hou Y, Li X, Meng X, Zhang Y, Wang X (2021) Practical implementation of artificial intelligence-based deep learning and cloud computing on the application of traditional medicine and western medicine in the diagnosis and treatment of rheumatoid arthritis. Front Pharmacol 23(12):765435
13. Yu R, Zhang J, Zhuo Y, Hong X, Ye J, Tang S, Zhang Y (2021) Identification of diagnostic signatures and immune cell infiltration characteristics in rheumatoid arthritis by integrating bioinformatic analysis and machine-learning strategies. Front Immunol 6(12):724934
14. Hu C, Dai Z, Xu J, Zhao L, Xu Y, Li M, Yu J, Zhang L, Deng H, Liu L, Zhang M (2022) Proteome profiling identifies serum biomarkers in rheumatoid arthritis. Front Immunol 6(13):865425
15. Chen Y, Liao R, Yao Y, Wang Q, Fu L (2021) Machine learning to identify immune-related biomarkers of rheumatoid arthritis based on WGCNA network. Clin Rheumatol 12:1–2
16. Stoel BC (2019) Artificial intelligence in detecting early RA. InSeminars in arthritis and rheumatism 2019 Dec 1, vol 49, No 3, pp S25–S28. WB Saunders.
17. Moingeon P (2023) Artificial intelligence-driven drug development against autoimmune diseases. Trends Pharmacol Sci
18. Bai L, Zhang Y, Wang P, Zhu X, Xiong JW, Cui L (2022) Improved diagnosis of rheumatoid arthritis using an artificial neural network. Sci Rep 12(1):9810
19. Duong SQ, Crowson CS, Athreya A, Atkinson EJ, Davis JM, Warrington KJ, Matteson EL, Weinshilboum R, Wang L, Myasoedova E (2022) Clinical predictors of response to methotrexate in patients with rheumatoid arthritis: a machine learning approach using clinical trial data. Arthritis Res Ther 24(1):1–1
20. Xiong Y, Mi BB, Liu MF, Xue H, Wu QP, Liu GH (2019) Bioinformatics analysis and identification of genes and molecular pathways involved in synovial inflammation in rheumatoid arthritis. Med Sci Monitor: Int Med J Exp Clin Res 25:2246
21. Xia J, Zhang L, Gu T, Liu Q, Wang Q (2023) Identification of ferroptosis related markers by integrated bioinformatics analysis and In vitro model experiments in rheumatoid arthritis. BMC Med Genomics 16(1):18
22. Üreten K, Erbay H, Maraş HH (2020) Detection of rheumatoid arthritis from hand radiographs using a convolutional neural network. Clin Rheumatol 39:969–974

23. Parashar A, Rishi R, Parashar A, Rida I (2023) Medical imaging in rheumatoid arthritis: a review on deep learning approach. Open Life Sci 18(1):20220611
24. Fukae J, Isobe M, Hattori T, Fujieda Y, Kono M, Abe N, Kitano A, Narita A, Henmi M, Sakamoto F, Aoki Y (2020) Convolutional neural network for classification of two-dimensional array images generated from clinical information may support diagnosis of rheumatoid arthritis. Sci Rep 10(1):5648
25. Cupek R, Ziębiński A (2016) Automated assessment of joint synovitis activity from medical ultrasound and power doppler examinations using image processing and machine learning methods. Reumatologia/Rheumatol 54(5):239–242
26. Witt M, Frielinghausen J, Mueller R, Mueller F, Proft F, Schulze-Koops H, Grunke M, Clevert DA (2016) Evaluation of a novel semi-automated ultrasound system for the detection of synovitis: a prospective study involving 45 patients with rheumatoid arthritis. Ultrasound Int Open 2(04):E117–E123
27. Hemalatha RJ, Vijaybaskar V, Thamizhvani TR (2019) Automatic localization of anatomical regions in medical ultrasound images of rheumatoid arthritis using deep learning. Proc Inst Mech Eng [H] 233(6):657–667
28. Qazi S, Iqbal N, Raza K (2021) Machine learning in cancer diagnosis, prognosis and therapy. Artif Intell Data-Driven Med Diag 8(3):103

Case Studies

Artificial Intelligence and Machine Learning Techniques in the Diagnosis of Type I Diabetes: Case Studies

Ahmad A. L. Ahmad and Ahmed A. Mohamed

Abstract The US Food and Drug Administration (FDA) approved the first AI-based medical device in 2012. Recently, there has been a notable surge in AI-based devices for diagnosing and managing diabetes. Although several AI-related devices are prevalent in diagnostic imaging and analysis, AI-driven devices for diabetes care are not yet widely available globally. AI technology is being explored in various aspects of diabetes management, encompassing self-management tools, automated retinal screening, clinical diagnosis aids, and risk assessment and categorization. Moreover, several studies have delved into utilizing AI for predicting diabetes, while there has been significant research into refining insulin dosage control. A noteworthy advancement includes AI systems alerting diabetic patients in advance about potential hypoglycemic attacks, marking a considerable stride in diabetes care innovations. This chapter discusses the application of AI and machine learning techniques in diagnosing Type I Diabetes, offering insights through case studies.

Keywords Diabetes · Diagnosis · Meal information · Complications

1 Introduction

Diabetes is a significant global public health challenge, resulting in substantial morbidity and mortality. The World Diabetes Federation reported 463 million individuals with diabetes in 2019, which is anticipated to reach 700 million by 2045 [1]. Type 2 (T2D) diabetes affects the majority, ranging from 85–95%, of individuals with diabetes, and a significant portion of the global diabetic population resides in socioeconomically disadvantaged regions, lacking adequate access to suitable diabetic care

A. A. L. Ahmad
Advanced Structures and Composites Center, University of Maine, 177 Aubert Hall, Orono, ME 04469, USA
e-mail: ahmad.ahmad@maine.edu

A. A. Mohamed (✉)
Department of Chemistry, University of Sharjah, Sharjah 27272, UAE
e-mail: amohamed61@gmail.com

K. Raza and S. Singh (eds.), *Artificial Intelligence and Autoimmune Diseases*, Studies in Computational Intelligence 1133, https://doi.org/10.1007/978-981-99-9029-0_14

[2–4]. Even within affluent communities, evidence-based therapies might be inaccessible or financially burdensome. Diabetes is categorized into two types, (T1D) and (T2D). T1D arises due to the demise of insulin-producing cells in the pancreas, while T2D diabetes results from insulin resistance or diminished insulin production. T1D and T2D are associated with various complications, including kidney and heart diseases, stroke, and blindness. Additionally, pregnant women with diabetes face a two- to fourfold increased risk of developing pre-eclampsia, heightening the chances of T2D, hypertension, and heart failure in both the mother and the child [2, 5, 6]. Timely detection of diabetes is imperative for effectively managing and preventing these complications.

Conventional methods of diabetes detection entail blood tests that measure glucose levels. Two main types of blood tests have been used for this purpose: the fasting plasma glucose test and the oral glucose tolerance test. The fasting plasma glucose test requires an individual to fast for at least eight hours. A blood sample is then taken, and the blood glucose level is measured, which signifies diabetes reported if the test results were 126 mg/dL or higher [7]. The second method is the oral glucose tolerance test, which involves the individual consuming a glucose solution, with blood samples drawn at intervals over the next two hours. Results showing 200 mg/dL or higher indicate diabetes. This test is beneficial for identifying diabetes in pregnant women at an elevated risk of developing gestational diabetes.

An alternative approach to diabetes detection is through the glycated hemoglobin (A1C) test. This assessment gauges the blood sugar level spanning the preceding three months, with a reading of 6.5% or higher indicating the presence of diabetes. The A1C test proves valuable in tracking diabetes progression and can pinpoint individuals who may be prone to complications. Beyond these conventional diabetes detection methods, more advanced alternatives exist. One such innovation is continuous glucose monitoring (CGM), which entails wearing a sensor for around-the-clock blood sugar level measurement. CGM proves advantageous for individuals actively managing diabetes who require close blood sugar level monitoring. Additionally, it can identify long-term trends in blood sugar levels, facilitating adjustments to treatment plans.

Genetic testing can play a role in identifying individuals with a heightened risk of developing diabetes, as specific genes such as TCF7L2 and PPARG have been linked to increased diabetes risk. While genetic testing is not typically employed as the primary method for diagnosing diabetes, it can be valuable in pinpointing individuals at elevated risk of developing the condition. In addition to these approaches, there are less commonly used methods for diabetes detection. For instance, random blood sugar or urine tests may be screening tools. A random blood sugar test assesses glucose levels in the blood at an unexpected time, regardless of the individual's last meal. A result exceeding 200 mg/dL indicates diabetes. The urine test aids in detecting elevated glucose levels, although it is notably unreliable for a definitive diabetes diagnosis.

2 AI and Machine Learning in Diabetes

Artificial intelligence (AI) and machine learning (ML) are transforming medicine, offering groundbreaking disease detection, diagnosis, treatment, and monitoring opportunities [8, 9]. These technologies have applications across various medical domains, including electronic health records (EHRs), drug discovery, imaging, and genomics. In medical imaging, AI and ML algorithms are being developed to analyze images from X-rays, MRIs, and CT scans, enabling the detection and diagnosis of diseases like heart disease, cancer, and neurological disorders [10, 11]. For instance, these algorithms have been employed to assess retinal images and diagnose conditions such as diabetic retinopathy [12]. Automating the analysis of medical images using AI and ML not only eases the burden on healthcare providers but also enhances diagnostic accuracy, leading to improved patient outcomes. Another significant area of progress for AI and ML is genomics. The vast amount of data within the human genome can be effectively analyzed by these algorithms, identifying intricate patterns and relationships that might be challenging for humans to discern [13]. Additionally, EHRs contain extensive patient data, which AI and ML algorithms can analyze to identify patterns indicative of specific diseases or conditions. By leveraging these technologies to analyze EHRs, healthcare providers can pinpoint patients at risk of developing specific conditions, allowing for early intervention and prevention. While AI and ML are still in their nascent stages of development, their potential to enhance patient outcomes, reduce costs, and expedite medical research is immense. Figure 1 provides an overview of the multifaceted applications of AI and ML techniques in assisting individuals with diabetes. This encompassing illustration explores various aspects, from personalized glucose monitoring and prediction to treatment optimization and early complication detection, contributing significantly to the improved care and management of diabetes patients.

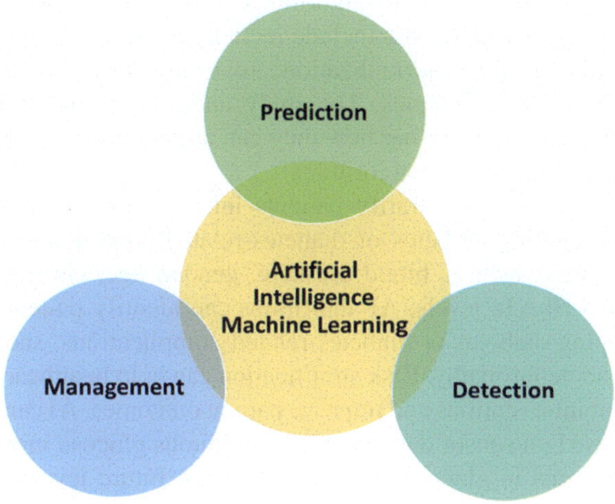

Fig. 1 AI and ML applications for Diabetes Care, covering personalized monitoring, treatment optimization, and early detection

3 Diabetes Prediction by AI and ML

AI and ML technologies offer new opportunities for the early detection and prediction of diabetes, allowing for personalized interventions and improved outcomes. One of the critical applications of AI and ML in diabetes prediction is the analysis of EHRs. EHRs contain vast patient data, including demographic information, laboratory results, and medical and medication history records. AI and ML algorithms can analyze this data and identify patterns indicative of diabetes or pre-diabetes. Diabetes risk assessment models and their respective algorithms have been extensively studied. Schwarz et al. conducted an exhaustive analysis of the specificity and sensitivity of these models [14]. As these risk-scoring models entail human intervention in determining criteria and risk score, albeit to a limited extent, the results may be susceptible to human error. In medical database systems, data mining is a prominent tool. This prospective method increases the sensitivity and specificity of disease diagnosis and detection by providing access to superior resources. It also significantly decreases associated expenses by avoiding unnecessary and costly medical examinations.

Accurate prediction of complications is essential for devising targeted interventions to prevent or delay their occurrence [15]. Utilizing AI with predictive analytics holds significant potential in enhancing the management of prevalent chronic conditions, which is crucial for individuals to maintain a healthy lifestyle, adhere to medication regimens, and monitor glycemic status effectively [16, 17]. Various AI algorithms, such as support vector machines, logistic regression, neural networks, and decision trees, can be employed for diabetes prediction [18]. These algorithms utilize diverse mathematical models to discern patterns in data and make predictions. For example, Rajendra and Latifi analyzed two datasets using the Logistic Regression algorithm: the PIMA Indians Diabetes dataset and the Vanderbilt dataset from a study involving rural African Americans in Virginia [19]. The accuracy reached 78% for Dataset 1 and 93% for Dataset 2. This research highlights that several factors, beyond the choice of algorithms, contribute to the accuracy and efficiency of the model. These factors include meticulous data preprocessing, eliminating redundant and null values, normalization, cross-validation, feature selection, and implementing ensemble techniques. The study underscores the significance of these additional elements, illustrating how they can augment the model's accuracy and runtime and select appropriate algorithms.

AI can also stratify patients into risk categories based on their likelihood of developing diabetes or diabetes-related complications. By analyzing various risk factors, such as blood pressure, gender, age, cholesterol level, body mass index, and HbA1c levels, AI algorithms can identify patients at substantial risk of developing diabetes or diabetes-related complications, such as retinopathy, neuropathy, and nephropathy. Risk stratification can help healthcare providers prioritize patients for interventions and improve patient outcomes. AI can forecast future glucose levels based on sensor data, such as continuous glucose monitoring. AI systems may find patterns in glucose levels and forecast future levels by examining CGM data. By changing their diet, increasing their physical activity, or tweaking their medication dosage, people may better control their diabetes. Also, depending on a patient's glucose trends, AI algorithms may provide tailored suggestions, such as alarms for hypoglycemia or hypertension or reminders to check blood sugar levels.

4 AI and ML for Diabetes Detection

Detecting glycemic episodes involves various methods for adequate blood glucose (BG) management, like BG prediction. These technologies enable the identification of glycemic events and prompt responses to their outcomes. Much of the existing research focuses on recognizing hyperglycemia or hypoglycemia in situations where monitoring blood sugar levels is challenging rather than predicting diabetes vulnerability [20–22]. Consequently, real-time techniques, rather than future event predictions, are predominant in this research. For insulin-dependent patients, daily tasks involve calculating accurate insulin doses, estimating planned carbohydrate intake, and considering patient-specific factors like insulin-to-carbohydrate ratio, insulin sensitivity, and carbohydrate quantity. Manual calculations of bolus dosages and carbohydrate counting require careful attention to maintain optimal glucose control, which can be complex. Inaccurate estimates might result in prolonged hyperglycemic episodes. New tools for bolus guidance and carbohydrate estimation were utilized to enhance patient carbohydrate estimation and insulin dosage selection. Advanced technologies, including AI, are employed to develop tools that improve the precision of carbohydrate calculations and determine the most appropriate insulin bolus amount for consumed meals.

4.1 Early Detection

People managing both types of diabetes require consistent support, and effective diabetes treatments are linked to solutions that offer high accuracy and minimal user interaction. Identifying critical glycemic control events like meals, exercise, or infusion set failures is essential for systematically automating closed-loop and open-loop systems. Individuals relying on insulin often use CGM devices to track glucose levels and calculate insulin infusion rates based on BG measurements. However, device malfunctions can lead to hyperglycemia or hypoglycemia episodes. Leal et al. proposed using Support Vector Machines (SVM) to differentiate between correct and incorrect measurements in real-time CGM, showing promising results in critically ill patients, especially in cases of sepsis [23]. Turksoy et al. pursued a similar goal using a k-nearest neighbor algorithm to identify faults, validating their approach with data from 51 patients [24]. Their algorithm automatically recognizes exercise type and intensity in an Artificial Pancreas (AP) system, demonstrating a sensitivity of 98.37%. Likewise, Jacobs et al. introduced a regression model to automatically identify physical exercise in patients equipped with an accelerometer and a heart rate sensor [25].

The identification of meals is essential within AP systems that lack manual meal notifications, acting as a safety measure for patients prone to forgetting manual meal inputs. Turksoy et al. work on developing a meal detection system using a fuzzy algorithm for estimating carbohydrate content by analyzing CGM signals [26]. This innovative approach underwent rigorous validation in simulated environments (in silico) and real-life (in vivo) scenarios. In silico validation involved 30 patients with T1D using the UVA/Padova simulator, showcasing a remarkable sensitivity of 91.3% in carbohydrate estimation. Subsequently, in vivo validation utilized data from 11 diabetes patients, indicating a sensitivity of 68.0% for snacks and 93.5% for meals.

Furthermore, recognizing the significance of timely detection of insulin pump failures is paramount, given their potential to cause prolonged hyperglycemia or diabetic ketoacidosis. Cescon et al. proposed an innovative solution employing a time-varying autoregressive model, crafting a patient alert system [27]. This system underwent meticulous validation using data from 9 patients over 18 weeks of wearing an infusion set. The results were promising, yielding a sensitivity of 50% and a specificity of 66%. This meticulous approach signifies a significant step toward early detection and prevention, ultimately reducing associated risks and enhancing the overall safety of diabetic patients.

4.2 *Lifestyle and Diabetes Management*

Effective lifestyle management is a pivotal component in diabetes therapy, crucial for averting complications and associated conditions. Upon diagnosis, patients are encouraged to optimize their lifestyles, and with the aid of current technologies and extensive data repositories, data-driven solutions are being developed. One such innovation is the Decision Support System (DSS), designed to empower patients and physicians to manage diabetes therapies. The DSS incorporates monitoring features encompassing diet, physical activity, medication, glucose measurements, and other pertinent factors. It provides tools to support patients and clinicians in improving therapeutic outcomes [25]. Figure 2 showcases the promising potential of wearable glucose sensors in tailoring diabetes management to individual needs. Integrating wearable multiplexed chemical sensing platforms with biophysical sensors feedback-driven automated insulin delivery systems, real-time cloud-based data storage and sharing mechanisms, and AI and ML-powered decision-making. The goal is to achieve precise, personalized insulin dosing and effectively regulate glucose levels.

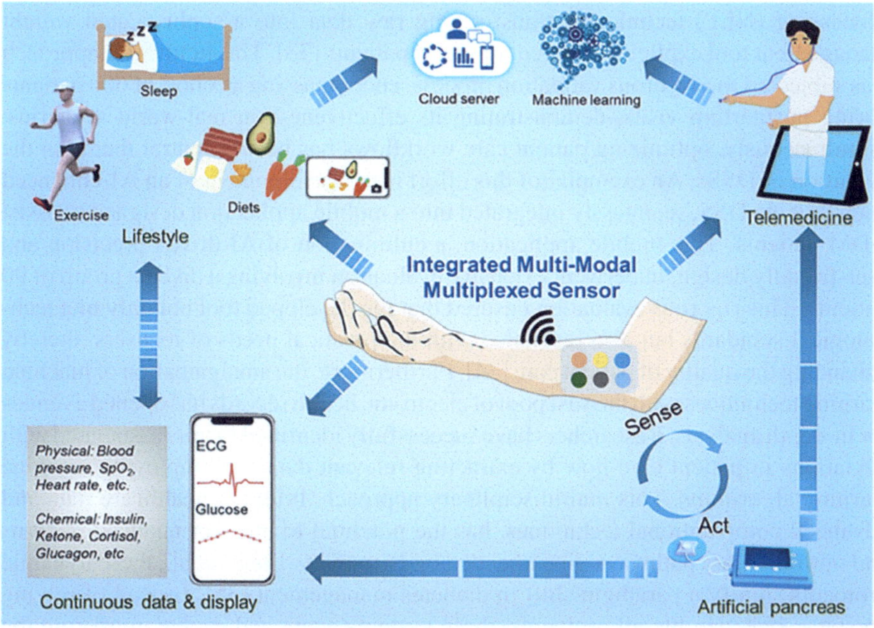

Fig. 2 Wearable glucose sensors for personalized diabetes management, integrating various technologies to achieve accurate insulin dosing and glucose regulation. Reprinted with permission from reference [36]. Copyright 2023 American Chemical Society

Since the beginning of this decade, DSSs have witnessed a surge in innovative studies, notably exemplified by the METABO project. This groundbreaking initiative has significantly shaped the landscape of diabetes management. This project stands out for its holistic approach, integrating real-time monitoring and cutting-edge tools designed to detect and prevent future glycemic fluctuations proactively. The METABO project boasts an impressive validation history, having undergone rigorous testing through a series of pilot trials. These trials included comprehensive usability assessments, engaging individuals managing T1D and T2D to ensure the practical applicability of the developed tools [28–31]. In parallel, everyday support systems have evolved substantially, incorporating intricate tools that utilize advanced technologies. Notable among these advancements is the introduction of a recommender system employing case-based reasoning. This cognitive technology refines its suggestions based on past cases, ensuring a personalized and practical approach to diabetes management. An integrated BG prediction tool, rooted in evolutionary computation principles, has been integrated into these support systems. Such tools represent a significant stride forward, leveraging artificial intelligence and evolutionary computation techniques to enhance the precision and reliability of diabetes management protocols [32]. Moreover, the application of ML and AI in gestational diabetes mellitus (GDM) has been a focus of recent research endeavors. For example, the MediClass system is a testament to the power of Natural Language

Processing (NLP) techniques, transforming raw data into a sophisticated weight management tool explicitly tailored for GDM patients [33]. This innovative approach was subjected to a rigorous validation process, encompassing a cohort of 600 patients during postpartum visits, demonstrating its effectiveness in real-world scenarios. Simultaneously, optimizing patient care workflows has been a central theme in the evolution of DSSs. An exemplar of this effort is the development of an AI-enhanced telemedicine DSS, seamlessly integrated into a mobile application designed to assist GDM patients. This mobile application, a culmination of AI-driven precision and user-friendly design, underwent extensive evaluation involving a diverse group of 90 patients. This rigorous evaluation ensured that the developed tool not only met technological standards but also resonated with the practical needs of its users, thereby enhancing the quality of patient care [34]. Furthermore, the amalgamation of machine learning techniques with the vast pool of electronic health records has opened avenues for in-depth analysis. Researchers have successfully identified factors associated with deviations in patient care flow by extracting relevant data and employing machine learning algorithms. This multidisciplinary approach, bridging healthcare data and advanced computational techniques, has the potential to uncover nuanced patterns and optimize care pathways. Spearheaded by Fernandez-Llatas et al., these dynamic protocols signify a paradigm shift in diabetes management [35]. Instead of relying on static, one-size-fits-all protocols, these systems adapt and evolve, mirroring the dynamic nature of diabetes and its management. This adaptability ensures that patient care remains responsive, providing tailored interventions responding to changing conditions and patient needs. In essence, the trajectory of DSS development in the diabetes management domain reflects a rich tapestry of technological innovation, interdisciplinary collaboration, and a steadfast commitment to enhancing patient outcomes vetitives not only pave the way for more effective diabetes management but also underscore the transformative potential of technology in shaping the future of healthcare.

Numerous innovations have been introduced to bolster the daily support for diabetes therapies, emphasizing the potential of machine learning techniques. These tools, designed to navigate the vast landscape of online discussion forums and social networks, utilize sophisticated algorithms to extract pertinent information. For instance, a study by Grieves et al. delved into a comprehensive comparison of machine learning techniques, encompassing decision trees, Support Vector Machines (SVM), bagging, and Bayes analysis. They aimed to assess patients' hospital performance by meticulously analyzing their online comments, thereby gaining valuable insights into their experiences and concerns [37]. Valdez et al. pioneered the application of k-means clustering analysis, a powerful data analysis method, to decipher intricate communication patterns within online platforms such as Facebook. Validated through an extensive cohort of 700 T2D diabetes patients, this approach provided invaluable insights into the nuances of patient interactions, shedding light on emotional and temporal aspects crucial for diabetes management [38]. A novel technique based on repeated bisecting k-means was proposed, offering a nuanced perspective on patient experiences and capturing the emotional and temporal dimensions of diabetes management journeys [39]. Beyond online interactions, these innovative tools have transcended into analyzing clinical appointments, medication adherence, and therapy compliance. Machine learning algorithms have been instrumental in scrutinizing medication adherence thresholds and assessing the risk of hospitalization. These systems employ automated feedback mechanisms, generating tailored messages to empower patients and reinforce therapy adherence. By leveraging the capabilities of machine learning, these tools not only provide valuable insights into patient behavior and encourage active patient engagement, ensuring a holistic approach to diabetes management [40]. Table 1 provides a range of diabetes risk prediction models, offering diverse examples that aid in foreseeing the likelihood of diabetes development symptoms. These models incorporate various factors and variables, providing valuable insights for assessing an individual's diabetes stages.

5 Conclusion

Utilizing AI and machine learning in diabetes management holds significant promise for enhancing patient outcomes and overall quality of life. Various tools have been created to analyze patient data, offering tailored recommendations for medication, therapy adherence, and lifestyle adjustments. These tools harness big data and advanced analytics, revealing insights that might be overlooked, leading to more informed decision-making and improved patient results. A key advantage of integrating AI and machine learning in diabetes management is real-time patient monitoring. Through wearable devices and connected health technologies, individuals can track their immediate blood glucose levels, physical activity, and other health metrics. AI algorithms process and analyze this data, enabling the provision of personalized medication dosages, dietary suggestions, and lifestyle changes. Furthermore, these tools assist healthcare providers in identifying patients at risk of diabetes-related complications. With this information, providers can adjust medication dosages and offer timely interventions, thus mitigating complications and enhancing patient outcomes.

Personalized treatment recommendations stand out as another significant benefit. By scrutinizing patient data and recognizing patterns, AI algorithms can propose individualized medication dosages, dietary modifications, and lifestyle adjustments tailored to each patient's needs. This high level of personalization empowers patients to manage their condition effectively, ultimately improving their overall health and well-being. However, challenges accompany the integration of AI and machine learning in diabetes management. Data quality is a significant hurdle, as AI algorithms demand error-free and unbiased data to offer precise recommendations. In diabetes management, where data is sourced from diverse channels and may be prone to inaccuracies, ensuring data quality becomes complex.

Additionally, interdisciplinary collaboration is crucial. Effective AI and machine learning tools for diabetes management require the cooperation of experts from various fields, including computer science, data science, healthcare, and patient advocacy. AI and machine learning deployment in diabetes management holds the

Table 1 Examples of diabetes risk prediction models

Study objective	Method used	Database (cases number)	Measuring progression	Output	References
Precise and readily understandable risk prediction models for advancing into Deep Convolutional	Random forest	Steno Diabetes Center Copenhagen, (648)	Baseline traits of participants categorized as progressors and non-progressors	Development of diabetic retinopathy	[41]
Automatically analyze retinal images to extract relevant features for assessing the level of diabetic retinopathy progression	Multi-input 2-dimensional deep belief network	Eye-PACS (88,702)	Modifications in the identified and relevant features from retinal images	Degree of progression	[42]
Forecasting the likelihood of late-stage AMD progression beyond the specified timeframe	Inception-v3 DCNN	Disease severity assessment over 12 years (31,262)	Identifying changes over time	AMD severity level and progression	[43]
Enhance the categorization of risk levels for diabetic retinopathy onset	Inception-v3 architectures	2-Year outcome (575,431)	Detecting indications of microvascular changes induced by diabetic retinopathy	Predict the development of mild-or-worse diabetic retinopathy	[44]

(continued)

Table 1 (continued)

Study objective	Method used	Database (cases number)	Measuring progression	Output	References
Develop algorithms capable of forecasting deterioration in untreated eyes compared to their baseline state over a 2-year timeframe	Inception-v3 architecture with transfer learning	Retrospective seven field fundus photographs obtained from RIDE and RISE studies	Identification of signals within the peripheral retinal fields, along with microvascular irregularities associated with the progression of diabetic retinopathy	Anticipate the severity level and future progression of diabetic retinopathy in a patient, considering a two-step or more worsening on the Early Treatment Diabetic Retinopathy Study scale at the 6, 12, and 24-month marks from the baseline	[45]
Integrate various geometric attributes from the retinal vasculature to enable early identification of the transition from diabetes without retinopathy to diabetic retinopathy progression	Statistical inferences were drawn using linear mixed models, while feature selection and classification stages involved the application of elastic-net logistic regression, Boruta algorithm, and regularized random forests	Diabetes that had not progressed to diabetic retinopathy was extracted, covering four years period (154)	Examining recorded bifurcations during consecutive stages of progression from diabetes without diabetic retinopathy to diabetic retinopathy, to pinpoint vascular modifications	Progression from diabetes without diabetic retinopathy to diabetic retinopathy	[46]

potential to revolutionize patient treatment and care. By harnessing the power of big data and advanced analytics, healthcare providers can gain valuable insights into individual patient needs, crafting personalized treatment plans that can potentially transform the lives of millions of people with diabetes worldwide.

References

1. Saeedi P, Petersohn I, Salpea P, Malanda B, Karuranga S, Unwin N, Colagiuri S, Guariguata L, Motala AA, Ogurtsova K, Shaw JE, Bright D, Williams R (2019) Global and regional diabetes prevalence estimates for 2019 and Projections for 2030 and 2045: results from the international diabetes federation diabetes atlas, 9th edn. Diabetes Research and Clinical Practice 2019, p 157. https://doi.org/10.1016/j.diabres.2019.107843
2. Hill-Briggs F, Adler NE, Berkowitz SA, Chin MH, Gary-Webb TL, Navas-Acien A, Thornton PL, Haire-Joshu D (2020) Social determinants of health and diabetes: a scientific review. Diabetes Care 44(1):258–279. https://doi.org/10.2337/dci20-0053
3. Whitmore C (2010) Type 2 diabetes and obesity in adults. Br J Nurs 19(14):880–886. https://doi.org/10.12968/bjon.2010.19.14.49041
4. Zhang P, Zhang X, Brown J, Vistisen D, Sicree R, Shaw J, Nichols G (2010) Global healthcare expenditure on diabetes for 2010 and 2030. Diabetes Res Clin Pract 87(3):293–301. https://doi.org/10.1016/j.diabres.2010.01.026
5. Kumar A, Bharti SK, Kumar A (2014) Type 2 diabetes mellitus: the concerned complications and target organs. Apollo Med 11(3):161–166. https://doi.org/10.1016/j.apme.2014.01.009
6. McCance DR (2015) Diabetes in pregnancy. Best Pract Res Clin Obstet Gynaecol 29(5):685–699. https://doi.org/10.1016/j.bpobgyn.2015.04.009
7. Association AD (2011) Diagnosis and classification of diabetes mellitus. Diabetes Care 34(Supplement_1), S62–S69. https://doi.org/10.2337/dc11-S062
8. Barragán-Montero A, Javaid U, Valdés G, Nguyen D, Desbordes P, Macq B, Willems S, Vandewinckele L, Holmström M, Löfman F, Michiels S, Souris K, Sterpin E, Lee JA (2021) Artificial intelligence and machine learning for medical imaging: a technology review. Physica Medica 83:242–256. https://doi.org/10.1016/j.ejmp.2021.04.016
9. Kumar K, Kumar P, Deb D, Unguresan ML, Muresan V (2023) Artificial intelligence and machine learning based intervention in medical infrastructure: a review and future trends. Healthcare 11(2):207
10. Castiglioni I, Rundo L, Codari M, Di Leo G, Salvatore C, Interlenghi M, Gallivanone F, Cozzi A, D'Amico NC, Sardanelli F (2021) AI applications to medical images: from machine learning to deep learning. Physica Medica, 83:9–24. https://doi.org/10.1016/j.ejmp.2021.02.006
11. Zheng D, He X, Jing J (2023) Overview of artificial intelligence in breast cancer medical imaging. J Clin Med 12(2):419
12. Grzybowski A, Brona P, Lim G, Ruamviboonsuk P, Tan GSW, Abramoff M, Ting DSW (2020) Artificial intelligence for diabetic retinopathy screening: a review. Eye 34(3):451–460. https://doi.org/10.1038/s41433-019-0566-0
13. Caudai C, Galizia A, Geraci F, Le Pera L, Morea V, Salerno E, Via A, Colombo T (2021) AI applications in functional genomics. Comput Struct Biotechnol J 19:5762–5790. https://doi.org/10.1016/j.csbj.2021.10.009
14. Schwarz PEH, Li J, Lindstrom J, Tuomilehto J (2009) Tools for predicting the risk of type 2 diabetes in daily practice. Hormone Metab Res 41(02):86–97. https://doi.org/10.1055/s-0028-1087203
15. Ljubic B, Hai AA, Stanojevic M, Diaz W, Polimac D, Pavlovski M, Obradovic Z (2020) Predicting complications of diabetes mellitus using advanced machine learning algorithms. J Am Med Inform Assoc 27(9):1343–1351. https://doi.org/10.1093/jamia/ocaa120

16. Behera A (2021) Use of artificial intelligence for management and identification of complications in diabetes. Clin Diabetol 10(2):221–225. https://doi.org/10.5603/DK.a2021.0007
17. Kosaki K, Tarumi T, Sugawara J, Tanahashi K, Kumagai H, Matsui M, Sugaya T, Osuka Y, Tanaka K, Kuro-o M, Saito C, Yamagata K, Maeda S (2021) Renal hemodynamics across the adult lifespan: relevance of flow pulsatility to chronic kidney disease. Exp Gerontol 152:111459. https://doi.org/10.1016/j.exger.2021.111459
18. Khanam JJ, Foo SY (2021) A comparison of machine learning algorithms for diabetes prediction. ICT Express 7(4):432–439. https://doi.org/10.1016/j.icte.2021.02.004
19. Rajendra P, Latifi S (2021) Prediction of diabetes using logistic regression and ensemble techniques. Comput Methods Programs Biomed Update 1:100032. https://doi.org/10.1016/j.cmpbup.2021.100032
20. Terao N (2023) A qualitative study of blood glucose and side effect self-management among patients with type 2 diabetes undergoing chemotherapy for cancer. Asia Pac J Oncol Nurs 10(2):100172. https://doi.org/10.1016/j.apjon.2022.100172
21. Peng Z, Xie X, Tan Q, Kang H, Cui J, Zhang X, Li W, Feng G (2022) Blood glucose sensors and recent advances: a review. J Innov Opt Health Sci 15(02):2230003. https://doi.org/10.1142/S1793545822300038
22. Tang L, Chang SJ, Chen C-J, Liu J-T (2020) Non-invasive blood glucose monitoring technology: a review. Sensors 20(23):6925
23. Taffese WZ, Espinosa-Leal L (2022) Prediction of chloride resistance level of concrete using machine learning for durability and service life assessment of building structures. J Build Eng 60:105146. https://doi.org/10.1016/j.jobe.2022.105146
24. Turksoy K, Roy A, Cinar A (2017) Real-time model-based fault detection of continuous glucose sensor measurements. IEEE Trans Biomed Eng 64(7):1437–1445. https://doi.org/10.1109/TBME.2016.2535412
25. Tyler NS, Mosquera-Lopez CM, Wilson LM, Dodier RH, Branigan DL, Gabo VB, Guillot FH, Hilts WW, El Youssef J, Castle JR, Jacobs PG (2020) An artificial intelligence decision support system for the management of type 1 diabetes. Nat Metab 2(7):612–619. https://doi.org/10.1038/s42255-020-0212-y
26. Samadi S, Turksoy K, Hajizadeh I, Feng J, Sevil M, Cinar A (2017) Meal detection and carbohydrate estimation using continuous glucose sensor data. J Biomed Health Inf 21(3):619–627
27. Cescon M, DeSalvo DJ, Ly TT, Maahs DM, Messer LH, Buckingham BA, Doyle FJ, Dassau E (2016) Early detection of infusion set failure during insulin pump therapy in type 1 diabetes. J Diabetes Sci Technol 10(6):1268–1276. https://doi.org/10.1177/1932296816663962
28. Fioravanti A, Fico G, Arredondo MT, Leuteritz J-P (2011) A mobile feedback system for integrated e-health platforms to improve self-care and compliance of diabetes mellitus patients. In: 2011 Annual international conference of the IEEE engineering in medicine and biology society, pp 3550–3553. https://doi.org/10.1109/IEMBS.2011.6090591
29. Fico G, Fioravanti A, Arredondo MT, Gorman J, Diazzi C, Arcuri G, Conti C, Pirini G (2016) Integration of personalized healthcare pathways in an ICT platform for diabetes managements: a small-scale exploratory study. IEEE J Biomed Health Inform 20(1):29–38. https://doi.org/10.1109/JBHI.2014.2367863
30. Fico G, Fioravanti A, Arredondo MT, Ardigó D, Guillén A (2010) A healthy lifestyle coaching-persuasive application for patients with type 2 diabetes. In: 2010 Annual international conference of the IEEE engineering in medicine and biology, pp 2221–2224. https://doi.org/10.1109/IEMBS.2010.5626185
31. Guillén A, Colás J, Fico G, Guillén S (2011) METABO: a new paradigm towards diabetes disease management. An innovative business model. In: 2011 Annual international conference of the IEEE engineering in medicine and biology society, pp 3554–3557. https://doi.org/10.1109/IEMBS.2011.6090592
32. Everett E, Kane B, Yoo A, Dobs A, Mathioudakis N (2018) A novel approach for fully automated, personalized health coaching for adults with prediabetes: pilot clinical trial. J Med Internet Res 20(2):e72. https://doi.org/10.2196/jmir.9723

33. Hazlehurst BL, Lawrence JM, Donahoo WT, Sherwood NE, Kurtz SE, Xu S, Steiner JF (2014) Automating assessment of lifestyle counseling in electronic health records. Am J Prev Med 46(5):457–464. https://doi.org/10.1016/j.amepre.2014.01.001
34. Rigla M, Martínez-Sarriegui I, García-Sáez G, Pons B, Hernando ME (2017) Gestational diabetes management using smart mobile telemedicine. J Diabetes Sci Technol 12(2):260–264. https://doi.org/10.1177/1932296817704442
35. Fernandez-Llatas C, Martinez-Millana A, Martinez-Romero A, Benedí JM, Traver V (2015) Diabetes care related process modelling using process mining techniques. Lessons learned in the application of interactive pattern recognition: coping with the spaghetti effect. In: 2015 37th Annual international conference of the IEEE engineering in medicine and biology society (EMBC), pp 2127–2130. https://doi.org/10.1109/EMBC.2015.7318809
36. Saha T, Del Caño R, Mahato K, De la Paz E, Chen C, Ding S, Yin L, Wang J (2023) Wearable electrochemical glucose sensors in diabetes management: a comprehensive review. Chem Rev 123(12):7854–7889. https://doi.org/10.1021/acs.chemrev.3c00078
37. Greaves F, Ramirez-Cano D, Millett C, Darzi A, Donaldson L (2013) Use of sentiment analysis for capturing patient experience from free-text comments posted online. J Med Internet Res 15(11):e239. https://doi.org/10.2196/jmir.2721
38. Valdez RS, Guterbock TM, Fitzgibbon K, Williams IC, Wellbeloved-Stone CA, Bears JE, Menefee HK (2017) From loquacious to reticent: understanding patient health information communication to guide consumer health IT design. J Am Med Inform Assoc 24(4):680–696. https://doi.org/10.1093/jamia/ocw155
39. Chen AT (2012) Exploring online support spaces: using cluster analysis to examine breast cancer, diabetes and fibromyalgia support groups. Patient Educ Couns 87(2):250–257. https://doi.org/10.1016/j.pec.2011.08.017
40. Fioravanti A, Fico G, Salvi D, García-Betances RI, Arredondo MT (2015) Automatic messaging for improving patients engagement in diabetes management: an exploratory study. Med Biol Eng Comput 53(12):1285–1294. https://doi.org/10.1007/s11517-014-1237-8
41. Al-Sari N, Kutuzova S, Suvitaival T, Henriksen P, Pociot F, Rossing P, McCloskey D, Legido-Quigley C (2022) Precision diagnostic approach to predict 5-Year Risk For Microvascular Complications In Type 1 diabetes. EBioMedicine 80:104032. https://doi.org/10.1016/j.ebiom.2022.104032
42. Tehrani AA, Nickfarjam AM, Ebrahimpour-komleh H, Aghadoost D (2021) Multi-input 2-dimensional deep belief network: diabetic retinopathy grading as case study. Multimed Tools Appl 80(4):6171–6186. https://doi.org/10.1007/s11042-020-10025-1
43. Yan Q, Weeks DE, Xin H, Swaroop A, Chew EY, Huang H, Ding Y, Chen W (2020) Deep-learning-based prediction of late age-related macular degeneration progression. Nat Mach Intell 2(2):141–150. https://doi.org/10.1038/s42256-020-0154-9
44. Bora A, Balasubramanian S, Babenko B, Virmani S, Venugopalan S, Mitani A, de Oliveira Marinho G, Cuadros J, Ruamviboonsuk P, Corrado GS, Peng L, Webster DR, Varadarajan AV, Hammel N, Liu Y, Bavishi P (2021) Predicting the risk of developing diabetic retinopathy using deep learning. Lancet Digit Health 3(1):e10–e19. https://doi.org/10.1016/S2589-7500(20)30250-8
45. Arcadu F, Benmansour F, Maunz A, Willis J, Haskova Z, Prunotto M (2019) Deep learning algorithm predicts diabetic retinopathy progression in individual patients. NPJ Digit Med 2(1):92. https://doi.org/10.1038/s41746-019-0172-3
46. Leontidis G, Al-Diri B, Hunter A (2017) A new unified framework for the early detection of the progression to diabetic retinopathy from fundus images. Comput Biol Med 90:98–115. https://doi.org/10.1016/j.compbiomed.2017.09.008

Computational Intelligence Methods for Biomarkers Discovery in Autoimmune Diseases: Case Studies

Nagmi Bano, Iqra Sajid, Syed Akramah Ahmad Faizi, Awelani Mutshembele, Debmalya Barh, and Khalid Raza

Abstract The discovery of biomarkers is a handy tool to improve diagnosis and therapeutic responses. It is used to determine disease onset, its progression, and treatment efficacy. Further, biomarker discovery has the potential to be used to find new potential drugs for personalized medicines. There is a plethora of methods for biomarker discovery, including data-driven bioinformatics approaches. Recent advancements in both high-throughput data generation techniques and computational intelligence methods witnessed the discovery of biomarkers in various diseases, including autoimmune diseases. This Chapter aims to systematically present computational intelligence-based approaches for biomarker discovery, along with case studies on the applications of computational intelligence methods for biomarkers discovery in Rheumatoid Arthritis, Systemic Lupus Erythematosus, and Multiple Sclerosis.

1 Introduction

Biomarkers, also called biological markers or molecular markers, are measurable indicators that can assess various biological processes, conditions, and diseases within an organism [35]. Usually, biomarkers are found in tissues and bodily fluids

N. Bano · I. Sajid · K. Raza (✉)
Department of Computer Science, Jamia Millia Islamia, New Delhi 110025, India
e-mail: kraza@jmi.ac.in

N. Bano
International Centre for Genetic Engineering and Biotechnology (ICGEB), New Delhi 110067, India

S. A. A. Faizi
Delhi Technological University, New Delhi 110042, India

A. Mutshembele
South African Medical Research Council (SAMRC), Pretoria, South Africa

D. Barh
Federal University of Minas Gerais, Belo Horizonte, Brazil

K. Raza and S. Singh (eds.), *Artificial Intelligence and Autoimmune Diseases*, Studies in Computational Intelligence 1133, https://doi.org/10.1007/978-981-99-9029-0_15

such as blood, urine, and saliva. Biomarkers provide valuable information about an individual's physiological state or disease's presence and progression [22]. The discovery of biomarkers in disease studies has pivotal importance, which helps us in (i) early detection and diagnosis, (ii) disease progression and prognosis studies, (iii) understanding disease mechanisms, treatment efficacy and personalization, (iv) drug development, predictive and preventive medicines, (v) monitoring response to therapy, and (vi) clinical trials [9, 38]. Hence, biomarkers are indispensable for disease studies, providing valuable information for healthcare professionals, researchers, and patients. These facilitate better understanding, more accurate diagnoses, and improved treatment strategies, ultimately leading to better patient outcomes and advancements in medical science.

Computational intelligence methods play a pivotal role in the discovery of disease biomarkers. These methods utilize advanced algorithms such as fuzzy logic, evolutionary algorithms such as genetic algorithms, and machine learning techniques such as artificial neural networks (ANNs), support vector machines (SVMs), and clustering methods to analyze complex biological data and identify potential biomarkers associated with specific diseases [35]. Computational intelligence methods can handle large-scale biological data from diverse sources, including genomics, proteomics, metabolomics, and clinical data. By integrating and analyzing these heterogeneous data types, it is possible to uncover the hidden patterns and relationships that may reveal potential biomarkers linked to disease development and progression [21]. Further, clustering and classification algorithms can identify distinct patterns or subgroups within the data that are associated with specific diseases or disease stages. These patterns may lead to discovering biomarkers characterizing different disease phenotypes or predicting disease outcomes. Once potential biomarkers are discovered, computational intelligence methods can also be used to validate their significance in independent datasets. Cross-validation techniques help assess the robustness and generalizability of candidate biomarkers, ensuring their reliability for clinical applications. Furthermore, machine learning algorithms can develop predictive models that estimate an individual's risk of developing a disease based on their biomarker profile and other relevant factors. Such models can aid personalized medicine and preventive strategies [25].

This chapter aims to provide a brief overview of biomarkers in autoimmune diseases, discuss computational intelligence methods for biomarker discovery including machine learning algorithms, data mining techniques, feature selection, and network analysis, and present case studies where computational intelligence methods were applied to discover biomarkers in specific autoimmune diseases. Further, challenges and limitations of computational intelligence methods for biomarker discovery in autoimmune diseases and future research directions in the field have been discussed.

2 Autoimmune Diseases: An Overview

An autoimmune disease is when the body's immune system mistakenly attacks and damages its healthy cells, tissues, and organs instead of protecting them from foreign invaders like bacteria and viruses, resulting in inflammation, tissue damage, and various clinical manifestations [15]. In autoimmune diseases, the immune system becomes dysregulated, and its ability to distinguish between "self" and "non-self" is compromised. As a result, immune cells and antibodies start attacking the body's cells and tissues, leading to symptoms specific to each autoimmune disorder [15].

As far as the classification of the disease is concerned, there are over 80 recognized autoimmune diseases that can affect virtually any part of the body, including the joints, skin, muscles, blood vessels, endocrine glands, and various organs such as the kidneys, heart, lungs, and brain [10, 41]. Autoimmune diseases can be chronic and lifelong, often involving periods of flare-ups and remission. The exact cause of autoimmune diseases is not fully understood, but a combination of genetic predisposition, environmental triggers, and immune system dysregulation is thought to contribute to their development [11]. Autoimmune diseases can be classified into two main categories: Organ-Specific Autoimmune Diseases and Systemic Autoimmune Diseases. In Organ-Specific Autoimmune Diseases, the immune response is primarily directed against specific organs or tissues. Examples of organ-specific autoimmune diseases include Type 1 Diabetes, Multiple Sclerosis [37], Hashimoto's Thyroiditis, and Rheumatoid Arthritis. Systemic Autoimmune Diseases affect multiple organs or organ systems throughout the body. They involve complex immune responses and may present with a variety of symptoms. Examples of systemic autoimmune diseases include Systemic Lupus Erythematosus (SLE), Systemic Sclerosis (Scleroderma), and antiphospholipid syndrome.

It is important to note that autoimmune diseases can have overlapping features, and individuals may have multiple autoimmune conditions simultaneously. Additionally, the exact cause of autoimmune diseases is often not fully understood, but genetic, environmental, and hormonal factors are thought to contribute to their development [11]. Proper diagnosis, management, and treatment of autoimmune diseases require a comprehensive and integrative approach.

2.1 Prevalence and Impact of Autoimmune Diseases

Globally, autoimmune diseases collectively represent a significant health burden, affecting millions of people of all ages and ethnicities. These impose a significant economic burden on healthcare systems and society. The cost of medical care, medications, and disability support can be substantial, especially in severe and poorly controlled cases. Additionally, indirect costs related to lost productivity and missed workdays can be considerable for patients and their families. The prevalence and impact of autoimmune diseases can vary depending on the specific condition, geographical location, and population demographics. It is estimated that around 5–10% of the global population is affected by one or more autoimmune conditions. Some autoimmune diseases are more prevalent in specific populations or ethnic groups, suggesting a genetic predisposition. Also, autoimmune diseases are more prevalent in females than males, with a female-to-male ratio often ranging from 2:1 to 9:1, depending on the specific disease [5]. Certain autoimmune diseases, such as rheumatoid arthritis and systemic lupus erythematosus, are more commonly diagnosed during women's childbearing years. Diagnosing autoimmune diseases can be challenging due to their diverse clinical manifestations and the lack of specific biomarkers for some conditions, resulting in delayed or missed diagnoses, potentially leading to more severe disease outcomes [5].

2.2 *Importance of Early Diagnosis and Effective Treatment:*

As discussed earlier, biomarkers play a crucial role in the early diagnosis and effective treatment of autoimmune diseases. They provide valuable information about disease presence, severity, and progression, helping healthcare professionals make informed decisions and improving patient outcomes. Autoimmune diseases often have nonspecific symptoms in their early stages, making diagnosis challenging. Biomarkers can serve as objective indicators of disease activity even before clinical symptoms become apparent. Early detection allows timely intervention and treatment, potentially preventing further damage and complications. Early diagnosis and targeted treatment based on biomarkers can save costs by reducing unnecessary tests, hospitalizations, and ineffective treatments [23]. Many autoimmune diseases have overlapping clinical features, making distinguishing between them based solely on symptoms difficult. Biomarkers can aid in differentiating between similar conditions, ensuring that patients receive the most appropriate diagnosis and treatment plan. Some autoimmune diseases have different subtypes or disease manifestations. Biomarkers can help identify specific subtypes, guiding personalized treatment strategies tailored to individual patient needs. Specific biomarkers can predict how an individual will respond to a particular treatment that allows for personalized medicine, where patients receive therapies that have a higher chance of being effective for their specific disease phenotype. In clinical research, biomarkers are crucial for selecting appropriate study participants and stratifying patient groups based on disease severity or treatment response, and they enhance the statistical power of clinical trials and improve the chances of identifying effective therapies [23]. Further, biomarkers are pivotal in understanding disease mechanisms and identifying potential therapeutic targets. They help researchers study disease biology, design preclinical experiments, and develop new therapies. Hence, biomarkers are indispensable tools in early diagnosis, effective treatment, and improved patient management, ultimately leading to better clinical outcomes and enhanced quality of life for individuals affected by autoimmune conditions.

3 Biomarkers in Autoimmune Diseases

In autoimmune illnesses, biomarkers are quantifiable signs that can reveal details about the presence, development, or response to therapy of these conditions, which may consist of cellular elements, chemicals, genes, proteins, or proteins discovered in body fluids, tissues, or imaging modalities. The potential of biomarkers to represent the underlying pathogenic mechanisms linked to autoimmune disorders distinguishes them from other diagnostic tools. They are essential in assisting with early diagnosis, forecasting illness outcomes, tracking disease activity, and determining the effectiveness of treatments. Biomarkers offer prospective targets for therapeutic interventions and significant insights into the complexity of autoimmune disorders. Various biomarkers have been used in autoimmune cases and have different roles as disease mechanisms.

3.1 Types of Biomarkers Used in Autoimmune Diseases

In autoimmune illnesses, various biomarkers help with diagnosis, prognosis, and treatment monitoring [42]. Autoantibodies, cytokines, and autoantigens are examples of serological biomarkers that can be found in blood. Single nucleotide polymorphisms (SNPs) and specific human leukocyte antigen (HLA) alleles are genetic biomarkers linked to higher risk or susceptibility to specific autoimmune disorders. Cellular biomarkers such as T, B, and regulatory cells are examined to measure immune system dysregulation. Imaging biomarkers, such as positron emission tomography (PET) and magnetic resonance imaging (MRI), offer visual representations of disease-related changes. Furthermore, non-coding RNA molecules known as microRNA biomarkers are being studied for their potential diagnostic and prognostic usefulness in autoimmune disorders [4]. In Fig. 1, we have provided a better insight into the autoimmune biomarkers.

3.2 Challenges and Limitations in Biomarker Discovery

The search for biomarkers in autoimmune illnesses is fraught with difficulties and restrictions. Finding common biomarkers is challenging due to the variability of autoimmune disorders, which differ in clinical presentations and disease processes. The absence of established validation criteria and methodologies hampers biomarker studies' reproducibility and comparability. Small sample volumes and laboratory heterogeneity may hamper the validation of prospective biomarkers. Furthermore, the patterns of autoimmune illnesses are dynamic and changeable, making longitudinal research necessary to understand the course of the disease entirely. The difficulties underscore the necessity for cooperative efforts, established protocols, and larger-scale studies to address the constraints in biomarker development [28].

Genetic Biomarkers

- Genetic variations, such as SNPs, are associated with susceptibility to autoimmune diseases where GWAS can help identify these genetic markers, which can shed light on the genetic factors contributing to disease development.

Serum Biomarkers

- Molecules in blood serum can reflect disease activity or severity. Examples include autoantibodies like anti-nuclear antibodies in systemic lupus erythematosus or specific cytokines and chemokines associated with inflammation.

Cellular Biomarkers

- Immune cells themselves can serve as biomarkers which can indicate disease progression. Flow cytometry and other techniques can quantify these cellular changes, providing insights into immune system dysregulation.

Epigenetic Biomarkers

- Epigenetic modifications, such as DNA methylation and histone modifications, can influence gene expression patterns in autoimmune diseases.

Microbiome Biomarkers

- Emerging research suggests that the gut microbiome plays a role in autoimmune diseases. Analysis of the microbiome composition and its metabolites can reveal biomarkers that contribute to disease development and progression

Imaging Biomarkers

- Techniques like MRI, PET scans, and ultrasound can provide visual insights into the affected tissues. In diseases like multiple sclerosis, these imaging biomarkers help assess disease activity and response to treatment.

Proteomic Biomarkers

- High-throughput proteomic analysis can identify overexpressed or under expressed proteins in autoimmune diseases. These proteins can serve as potential therapeutic targets or indicators of disease activity.

Fig. 1 Types of autoimmune biomarkers

3.3 Role of Computational Intelligence Methods in Biomarker Identification

Computational intelligence techniques significantly aid the identification of biomarkers in autoimmune illnesses. Large-scale omics data, including genomes, transcriptomics, proteomics, and metabolomics, can be analyzed using machine learning algorithms, data mining methods, and artificial intelligence techniques. These techniques make it easier to find the patterns, correlations, and forecasting models that can help with biomarker discovery. Creating customized medicine strategies can be aided by integrating numerous data sources to find complex biomarker signatures. These techniques improve the effectiveness and precision of biomarker identification, resulting in better autoimmune disease diagnosis, prognosis, and therapy approaches [8].

4 Computational Intelligence Methods

A branch of artificial intelligence known as computational intelligence (Monteiro et al.) aims to create algorithms and methods motivated by the inherent intelligence seen in people and other living things. It seeks to develop intelligent systems that can solve complicated issues without clearly stated rules. CI comprises a variety of techniques, including swarm intelligence, fuzzy logic, evolutionary algorithms, neural networks, and more [16]. The following are the four main foundations of computational intelligence:

Neural Networks: These are modeled by how the human brain is built and functions. Neurons, the interconnected nodes of neural networks, process and transfer information and are helpful for activities like picture recognition, language processing, and even playing games since they excel at spotting patterns and relationships in data [16].

Evolutionary Algorithms: Imitate the processes of mutation, selection, and reproduction to optimize solutions. They are modeled after the process of natural evolution. They resolve challenging optimization and search issues, from financial modeling to engineering design [17].

Fuzzy Logic: A framework for handling ambiguity and imprecision is fuzzy logic. Fuzzy logic provides subtle transitions between these values instead of conventional binary logic, which utilizes true or false values, allowing for more complex decision-making. It is frequently used in control systems and decision-making procedures when precise definitions are elusive [17].

Swarm Intelligence: Creating algorithms that simulate the cooperation and coordination seen in social species such as ants, bees, and birds. The group behavior of these creatures inspired swarm intelligence. Examples of optimization techniques used for routing and optimization problems are particle swarm optimization and ant colony optimization [16, 17].

4.1 Overview of Machine Learning Algorithms for Biomarker Discovery

Biomarker discovery has been transformed by machine learning algorithms, which have made it possible to identify key biological indications for various illnesses and ailments. Samples can be categorized based on recognized biomarker patterns using supervised algorithms like Random Forests, SVMs, and ANNs [27]. Without labels, unsupervised approaches like clustering and principal component analysis reveal hidden structures in data. Deep Learning models also perform exceptionally well at identifying complex patterns in enormous amounts of omics data. While Generative Adversarial Networks model complex biomarker distributions, Transfer Learning enables knowledge transfer between related tasks. These algorithms work together to provide a complete toolkit for biomarker identification, assisting early diagnosis, prognosis, and individualized therapy plans [12].

Machine learning algorithms have become crucial in biomarker development by making it possible to recognize important molecular, genetic, or imaging traits that have diagnostic, prognostic, or therapeutic relevance. These algorithms cover various methods that reveal underlying data patterns, including decision trees, k-means clustering, and Gaussian mixture models. Furthermore, sophisticated biomarker connections can be seen and understood using dimensionality reduction techniques like t-SNE and autoencoders. These methods not only expedite the finding of biomarkers but also help to understand disease mechanisms more thoroughly, ultimately advancing precision medicine and altering healthcare paradigms [24].

4.2 Methods for Feature Selection and Classification for Biomarker Discovery

The selection of features and the use of classification techniques are crucial in biomarker discovery. With models' increased effectiveness and interpretability, feature selection strategies seek to isolate the most informative qualities from high-dimensional data. These include mutual information-based techniques, which gauge the importance of features to desired results, LASSO, a regularization technique that promotes sparse feature sets, and recursive feature elimination (RFE), which iteratively prunes less relevant features. SVM, Random Forests, and Gradient Boosting are a few classification algorithms that use labeled data to classify samples according to recognized biomarkers. Convolutional neural networks (CNNs) and recurrent neural networks (RNNs) are examples of deep learning architectures that excel at extracting subtle patterns from complex biomolecular data, enabling highly accurate classifications. Combining these techniques enhances the basis for accurate disease diagnosis, prognosis, and therapy choice, in addition to assisting in developing biomarkers [19].

4.3 ANNs for Biomarker Prediction

A potent method for biomarker prediction using Artificial Neural Networks (ANNs) and Computational Intelligence (Monteiro et al.) methodologies has emerged. ANNs, modeled after the human brain's neural network, can capture complicated correlations in biomolecular data. CI approaches improve performance by optimizing network design, training settings, and feature selection. The prediction power of ANNs is improved by refining their hyperparameters and structures with the help of evolutionary techniques like genetic algorithms. Network parameters are adjusted by particle swarm optimization, improving biomarker predictions. Additionally, fuzzy logic-based methods help manage data ambiguity, improving the stability of predictions made [32] using ANNs. In addition to enabling precise biomarker prediction, the combination of ANNs and CI approaches also provides insights into disease causes, enabling well-informed medical decisions and promoting personalized medicine.

4.4 SVMs and Random Forests for Biomarker Identification

Support Vector Machines (SVMs) and Random Forests (RFs) are potent machine-learning methods frequently used to detect biomarkers. SVMs are skilled at determining the best decision boundaries to divide several classes of data points while increasing the margin between them. SVMs can discriminate between healthy and diseased samples in biomarker identification based on biomolecular characteristics [3]. They are excellent at handling high-dimensional datasets and situations where the data cannot be separated linearly. On the other hand, Random Forests build an ensemble of decision trees and combine their results to produce predictions. Random Forests can capture intricate correlations between biomarkers and their corresponding outcomes in biomarker identification, offering insights into the significance of features and potential interactions [36]. They can handle noisy data, are frequently present in biological datasets, and resist overfitting. SVMs and Random Forests provide valuable resources for identifying significant biomarkers and advancing our knowledge of numerous diseases at the molecular level. The decision between the two is based on the dataset's unique properties and the objectives of the biomarker identification study.

5 Case Studies

5.1 Case Study 1: Computational Intelligence Approach for Biomarker Discovery in Rheumatoid Arthritis

Rheumatoid arthritis (RA) is an autoimmune disease primarily affecting the synovium (lining of membranes surrounding joints), leading to joint damage and deformities over time. RA is a chronic condition that requires medication and self-management techniques. Current lab indicators of this disease have low efficiency and fail to differentiate between levels of disease potency. Computational intelligence uses algorithms to find potential biomarkers that aid in identifying the disease by analyzing clinical data. Computational intelligence, including machine learning, helps cure RA by detecting it early, allowing timely intervention, and providing precise treatment. Moreover, biomarkers assist in developing practical and innovative therapies by finding unique signs of RA in the patient's body [21].

Yu et al. [43] examine the diagnostic signatures of RA and their effect of immune cell infiltration using machine learning-driven approaches. They conducted a comprehensive analysis of gene expression data from the Gene Expression Omnibus (GEO) database (https://www.ncbi.nlm.nih.gov/geo/) to investigate RA. They retrieved datasets related to RA with specific criteria, such as genome-wide whole blood gene expression profiles, inclusion of both RA and healthy samples, and exclusion of samples treated with drugs. Three datasets, namely GSE100191, GSE17755, and GSE93272, were selected for further analysis, totaling 50 healthy controls and 119 RA patients. They identified differentially expressed genes (DEGs) using the limma package and robust DEGs using the Robust Rank Aggregation (RRA) method. Functional analysis of these genes was conducted through Gene Ontology (GO) and Kyoto Encyclopedia of Genes and Genomes (KEGG) pathway enrichment analysis, with a focus on pathways related to RA. To discover potential diagnostic markers, four machine learning algorithms were employed, including random forests, least absolute shrinkage and selection operator (LASSO) logistic regression, support vector machine-recursive feature elimination (SVM-RFE), and weighted gene co-expression network analysis (WGCNA). Further Quantitative PCR (qPRC) was carried out on blood samples from RA patients and healthy controls to validate the identified markers. Yu et al. [43] conclude that genes such as LSP1, GNLY, and MEOX2 may be used for diagnosing and treating RA.

In an another study, Chen et al. [13] explore to identify the potential diagnostic biomarkers of RA, and further study their pathological relevance pertaining to immune cell infiltration. They considered gene expression datasets from 35 RA patients and 29 controls from GEO database, applied a WGCNA method to shortlist differentially abundant genes, and applied machine learning techniques such as LASSO regression model and SVM-RFE to identify the candidate biomarkers in RA. Finally, Chen et al. [13] report 3 genes, namely FADD, CXCL2, and CXCL8, as potential RA diagnostic biomarkers.

In a recent study, Liu et al. [26] attempt to identify diagnostic gene markers for patients with aggravated atherosclerosis (AS) and RA. They obtained gene expression datasets from GEO and STRING interactome databases (https://string-db.org/), identified differentially expressed genes (DEGs) and module genes using limma and WGCNA packages. They applied machine learning algorithms such as LASSO regression and random forest to explore the immune-related hub genes. After further down-stream analysis, Liu et al. [26] report 6 immune-related hub genes (NFIL3, EED, GRK2, MAP3K11, RMI1, and TPST1) for AS with RA diagnosis.

Abdelati et al. [1] discover new diagnostic biomarkers for RA by analyzing serum peptidomic profiles using MALDI-TOF-MS. The research included 35 RA patients, 35 osteoarthritis (OA) patients as disease controls, and 35 healthy individuals. The analysis revealed 113 peaks distinguishing RA from OA and 101 peaks distinguishing RA from healthy controls. Additionally, 95 peaks identified OA from healthy controls, with 38 being significant. A genetic algorithm (GA) model exhibited the best sensitivity and specificity in all three comparisons. The findings indicate that peptidomic patterns can effectively differentiate RA from OA and healthy individuals, suggesting the potential for MALDI-TOF-MS combined with magnetic bead separation to identify novel serum protein biomarkers for RA.

5.2 Case Study 2: Computational Intelligence Approach for Biomarker Discovery in Systemic Lupus Erythematosus

A computational intelligence method was used to find biomarkers for Systemic Lupus Erythematosus (SLE) [11]. The initial phase was data gathering from a cohort of SLE patients, including clinical, genetic, and molecular data. Patient demographics, medical history, and laboratory test results were all included in the clinical data [5]. The genomic data contained details on genetic variants and markers linked to SLE. Gene expression levels discovered using high-throughput techniques like microarrays or RNA sequencing made up the molecular data. Preprocessing techniques were used to guarantee data uniformity and quality. Data has to be cleaned to perform such action of any inaccuracies or inconsistent entries, normalized to allow for differences in measurement scales and handled using imputation or exclusion techniques for missing values. Genetic data underwent quality control methods to find and eliminate potential outliers or technical artifacts, and clinical data had a comprehensive examination to verify accuracy. Molecular data were standardized to account for batch effects and other technical biases and ensure that the following analysis would produce relevant results.

Data preprocessing

After preprocessing the data, feature extraction and selection procedures were used to find the SLE biomarker variables that were most pertinent. The goal of feature selection was to isolate the subset of features that showed pronounced relationships with the illness. The statistical significance of each attribute was assessed using a variety of statistical tests, including t-tests and analysis of variance (ANOVA) [5]. Information gain and mutual information-based approaches were used to evaluate features' applicability and prediction ability. The minimized dimensionality of the data while keeping crucial information, feature extraction techniques like principal component analysis (PCA) or independent component analysis (ICA) were also used. These methods sought to identify the most insightful characteristics that might be used as SLE biomarkers.

Application of machine learning algorithms

After identifying the pertinent traits, several machine-learning techniques were used to look for potential SLE biomarkers. Predictive models were created using supervised learning methods like SVM, random forests, or logistic regression. Based on the chosen features, these models attempted to categorize patients into various disease subgroups or forecast illness outcomes. Unsupervised learning algorithms, such as k-means or hierarchical clustering, were used to find patterns and subgroups within the SLE cohort. These algorithms used the chosen variables to find groups of individuals who shared similar molecular profiles or clinical traits. Machine learning algorithms were used to find patterns and links in the data, leading to the identification of possible biomarkers and their connection to SLE.

Evaluation and validation of identified biomarkers

Several methods were used to assess and validate the found biomarkers. The effectiveness and generalizability of the machine learning models were evaluated using cross-validation techniques, such as k-fold cross-validation or leave-one-out cross-validation [5]. These strategies ensured the models were assessed on separate data sets by dividing the dataset into training and testing subsets. The effectiveness of the identified biomarkers was assessed using performance criteria like accuracy, sensitivity, specificity, and area under the receiver operating characteristic curve (AUC-ROC). Additionally, external datasets or independent validation cohorts were used to confirm the reliability and robustness of the discovered biomarkers. The opportunity to evaluate the generalizability of the found biomarkers in other populations or experimental conditions was made possible by these external datasets. Meticulous statistical analyses were carried out to ensure the importance and dependability of the findings.

A computational intelligence approach used in this case study showed the potential of machine learning algorithms in searching for biomarkers for SLE. Relevant variables were found and turned into valuable features using data collection, preprocessing, feature selection, and extraction procedures. Then, machine learning algorithms were used to categorize patients, forecast the course of the disease, or find subgroups within the SLE cohort. The reliability and reproducibility of the identified biomarkers were guaranteed by evaluation and validation. This case study demonstrates how AI may advance biomarker identification and potentially enhance SLE diagnosis, prognosis, and individualized therapy approaches.

5.3 Case Study 3: Computational Intelligence Approach for Biomarker Discovery in Multiple Sclerosis

Multiple sclerosis (MS) is a neurological disorder that mainly affects young people. A few common symptoms include vision problems, worsening the situation during high temperatures, and shock-like sensations in the spine or limbs. It impacts all major body systems, including motor, sensory, and visual nerves. The disease worsens at certain times in the CNS, where the protective myelin coating around nerve fibers is damaged. Diagnosing the disease involves T2 signal change detection by MRI. Here, the signal intensity of the tissue appears different from that of surrounding normal tissues. MRI uses strong magnets and radio waves to create images of the brain. Brighter signals correspond to longer relaxation times during imaging. Since the patient has demyelinated lesions, they take longer to respond, which aids in detecting the disease's progression [18, 25].

Computational intelligence offers significant advantages in MS diagnosis and prognosis. It enhances accuracy, reduces time and costs, and distinguishes between relapsing-remitting and progressive MS forms. It employs patient data, like age, sex, and clinical information, alongside MRI results to predict future disability. Machine learning, a subset of AI, is increasingly used for risk assessment, diagnosis, and prognosis. Models like SVMs, Random Forest, and convolutional neural networks (CNNs) analyze MRI images for MS lesions. Clinical data also aids in disease diagnosis and progression prediction. Linear classifiers and unsupervised learning refine subtype classifications, while machine learning extracts disability-related insights from clinical and radiological data [15]. A recent review on the application of AI and machine learning in the diagnosis of MS can be found in Nabizadeh et al. [29] and Vázquez-Marrufo et al. [39], respectively.

Saccà et al. [34] explored the application of various machine learning algorithms to support early diagnosis of MS. Using Independent Component Analysis on resting-state functional MRI data, 15 brain networks were identified. The sensorimotor I network proved most discriminative marker for early MS detection. Random Forest and SVM achieved the highest accuracy (85.7%) in distinguishing MS patients from controls using this network, offering promising prospects for clinical diagnosis and prognosis. Plati et al. [31] address MS severity estimation and disease progression prediction using machine learning. Data from 30 patients were collected that including demographic, clinical, test, treatment, and comorbidity information recorded at three time points. They applied various machine learning methods, however, Random Forest achieved impressive results, with 94.87% accuracy for MS classification and 83.33% for disease progression prediction.

In the twenty-first century, technological advancements have revolutionized the approach to managing RA, SLE, MS, and other autoimmune diseases. The abundance of biomedical data and rapid computational progress has ushered in a new era of informatics in healthcare. Utilizing statistical informatics, computational intelligence, machine learning, and biomedical software, healthcare providers can enhance all aspects of patient care, from diagnosis to treatment. Precision medicine is becoming the standard, particularly for complex diseases like MS, where individualized treatment plans are crucial. With a robust computational framework, the unique characteristics of each patient can be analyzed, allowing for tailored treatment and management strategies that align with their specific needs and disease profile.

5.4 Comparative Analysis of Computational Intelligence Methods in Biomarker Discovery

Application of computational intelligence methods in biomarker development for autoimmune disorders, particularly SLE, has produced encouraging results, according to a comparative review of the techniques used. Different computational methodologies' merits and weaknesses were highlighted through comparative study. SVM, random forests, and logistic regression are machine-learning techniques with great accuracy and predictive capacity in identifying SLE patients and forecasting illness outcomes based on specific criteria [10, 24, 38]. These algorithms successfully uncovered intricate connections and patterns in the data, assisting in the discovery of prospective biomarkers. The finding of distinctive molecular subtypes or illness clusters was made possible by unsupervised learning algorithms, such as clustering methods, highlighting the heterogeneity of SLE. Techniques for feature selection, such as statistical tests, information gain, and correlation analysis, were successful in locating pertinent SLE-related variables. Additionally, the dimensionality of the data was decreased by feature extraction techniques like principal component analysis (PCA) or independent component analysis (ICA), allowing the identification of the most informative features. The comparison analysis demonstrated the adaptability and complementary nature of several computational intelligence approaches in the search for autoimmune disease biomarkers [10, 24, 38].

Interpretation and significance of identified biomarkers in autoimmune diseases:

The discovery of biomarkers in autoimmune disorders like SLE using artificial intelligence methods has significant ramifications for diagnosis, prognosis, and individualized therapy. These biomarkers have the potential to provide an early and accurate diagnosis, allowing for prompt intervention and the start of the most suitable treatment plans. They can help increase diagnostic precision by helping to identify SLE from other autoimmune or inflammatory disorders. The discovered biomarkers also have predictive relevance by foretelling the development of the disease, organ involvement, and long-term results. They can support the stratification of patients into various risk groups, assisting in the direction of treatment choices and identifying individuals who might profit from more aggressive therapeutic measures. Additionally, by identifying molecular subtypes or clusters that react differently to particular medicines, the found biomarkers aid in creating tailored treatment approaches. It enables individualized treatment approaches, reducing unneeded side effects and enhancing therapeutic effectiveness by enabling precision medicine methods, enhancing patient outcomes, lowering healthcare costs, and identifying biomarkers that can revolutionize the management of autoimmune illnesses [2].

Potential implications for diagnosis, prognosis, and personalized treatment:

The outcomes of the computational intelligence approach to biomarker identification in autoimmune illnesses, mainly Systemic Lupus Erythematosus, show the efficacy and potential of this method for extending our knowledge of disease mechanisms and enhancing patient care. The comparison of computational approaches revealed their advantages and disadvantages, while the interpretation of discovered biomarkers gave crucial new information on the pathophysiology of autoimmune disorders. These biomarkers' importance for diagnosis, prognosis, and individualized treatment opens up significant opportunities for precision medicine in treating autoimmune illnesses, ultimately resulting in better outcomes [2].

6 Future Directions and Challenges

The landscape of biomarker discovery is changing due to new trends and future directions in computational intelligence, which has significant implications for healthcare and personalized medicine. There has been a noticeable shift toward integrating multi-omics data sources, which include genomes, proteomics, and metabolomics, as technology makes it possible to generate enormous and diverse biological information [7]. This integration improves the identification of significant biomarkers by enabling a more thorough understanding of intricate biological processes. Additionally, sophisticated patterns within these data are being uncovered by deep learning algorithms like neural networks, allowing the identification of subtle links that could have gone unnoticed by conventional approaches. Transfer learning and pre-trained models are being used to accelerate the identification of pertinent biomarkers by speeding the adaption of knowledge from related fields. Despite the enormous potential of these developments, issues with ethics, data privacy, and the efficient fusion of clinical and omics data must also be resolved. These new trends will alter how biomarkers are discovered, opening the door for more precise diagnoses, focused therapies, and better patient outcomes [7].

6.1 Integration of Multi-omics Data and Network Analysis in Autoimmune Diseases

Multi-omics data refers to the collective information from various biological systems. The term 'omics' specifically means the study of specific biological molecules or systems on a large scale. Some fields include—Genomics, Transcriptomics, Proteomics, Metabolomics and Epigenomics. Multi-omics data integration combines information from different layers to obtain a precise analysis. First, data is collected from multiple sources, such as DNA sequencing, RNA sequencing, or mass spectrometry. Then, it is processed to remove any disturbances and correct biases to be compatible across various platforms. Algorithms and Machine learning models integrate this data, making it biologically interpretable for researchers. A network depicts and analyses how a biological network interacts with other entities, such as genes, proteins, or metabolites. Highly connected proteins, frequently essential for disease diagnosis, can be analyzed through physical interactions between proteins. Gene expression and metabolic pathways give a deep understanding of disease phenotypes. Network analysis techniques involve identifying subnetworks called modules with specific functions representing pathways or detecting highly connected nodes of proteins and genes known as hubs [40].

The significance of multi-omics data integration and network analysis in autoimmune diseases is immense. They help identify potential biomarkers, provide effective treatments based on the patient's disease profile, and analyze network interactions to understand the disease mechanisms better. Multi-omics data understands how DNA is organized within the nucleus, revealing connections between regions that control gene expression and those that initiate gene transcription. This leads to detecting genes actively transcribed during the onset of diseases like Rheumatoid Arthritis. After analyzing these genes' expression levels and regulation, we can predict what drug targets to focus on. In autoimmune disorders, detecting highly related genes gives us a significant idea about the development and progression of the disease. These genes can function as potential molecules for drug-targeted therapies [40]. Functional enrichment of these genes highlights disturbances in pathways of the immune system. We can comprehend disease interactions better when considering the interactions between different cell types. The application of network analysis in treating autoimmune diseases allows us to understand the mechanisms and interactions of the disease, which eventually leads to potential discoveries in treatment. A few limitations of integrating data from various platforms include data preprocessing and standardization, as there are various formats and scales. Moreover, analyzing complex biological data requires advanced computational methods and extensive time. Finally, network analysis and multi-omics integration findings often need experimental validation in laboratories and clinical studies [10].

6.2 Ethical Considerations and Data Privacy Issues

AI has been used immensely in healthcare and medical diagnosis in the past few years. The application of AI and ML models has revolutionized patient care and allows researchers and healthcare providers to focus on more opportunities. However, strict ethical guidelines and data privacy laws are necessary to keep these innovations in check. A primary ethical concern is the lack of approval from patients before data collection and incomplete awareness regarding its purpose. Patients' data is used to train ML models by observing behavioral patterns. However, a significant population of patients is drastically unaware of what data is being retrieved from their records and if the ambiguity is maintained [14]. Most AI algorithms find solutions through unknown mechanisms,therefore, we cannot explain them to our patients. Hence, there is little to no clarity behind the research methods applied. Data sharing further weakens the security of the information being used; hence, ML models must be trained to be specific in data retrieval.

The data control should remain in the hands of patients, and they should have the power to provide access to it on a requirement basis. Ethical considerations regarding new technological discoveries such as at-home care services must be focused on. These are especially useful for patients suffering from long-term diseases where regular hospital visits can be costly and time-intensive. Moreover, after the pandemic, this has helped reduce the chances of human contact. Most importantly, due to immediate care being provided, there is a significant reduction in emergency visits to the hospital, and the patient's health is managed before any severe event. For this service, sensors are placed in the patient's home as devices or monitors that can track their activities and health data, and it is stored in a dataset that further learns from patterns and predicts future diagnoses. However, there are various limitations to this discovery. AI models make decisions solely based on the data it has been trained on but lack the reasoning ability humans have to consider the patient's present need and situation. Moreover, since the model is trained on a generally available dataset, there are several chances of wrong decision-making for groups with low data availability, leading to uneven results between patients. The chances of data being shared without proper privacy are very high; hence, patient consent is a must while explaining the various limits of this process. Data should be collected at home, modified to make it unrecognizable from actual patients' data, and then sent for model learning [30]. Improvements can be made by providing complete privacy and controlling the patients. However, there can be severe issues where the patient's health could drastically deteriorate.

In those cases, giving control to another known person can lead to data sharing and, hence, loss of privacy. Finally, the sensors for each patient could be specifically designed for their own body, allowing only genuine alerts and custom-made treatment action plans. Providing a real-world feel to our diagnosis is essential as it boosts the patient's moral support [20]. AI models analyze data to find patterns and then predict behaviors. However, it can also generate artificial data. This data is anonymous, reducing the risk of any data privacy issues. It is based on the behavior of actual patients, but the data produced is fake. This application is currently used in various fields, such as education and image analysis. In cases where we have a low population of data to train the model, this method is of great use and helps produce precise and impartial results. Future developments in this field include ensuring the replicated data is not confused with accurate data, leading to danger to patient medical records. Since the data produced is not original, it might be misused for immoral purposes as no rules will apply to it. A need to create a global ethical body to address and solve these issues is a must. Hence, the created data must differ from the original records [6].

6.3 Challenges in Implementing Computational Intelligence Methods

Computational intelligence is a branch of AI that is being widely utilized in almost all fields of research and innovation. Although this concept has multiple applications, we will discuss a few limitations and what solutions can be offered in the future [9]. As AI primarily involves data analysis, it should be provided with complete datasets, but in reality, all datasets have slight differences and impracticalities and lead to biased results and wrong predictions by the algorithm. Focus should be laid on the foundation of datasets that include all groups, be it population data of race/gender or cancer data with both primary and metastatic data. Different platforms have differently coded AI models, and this causes disturbances during data sharing or transfer. Publishing well-documented code files will aid others in reproducing the results and gaining a better understanding of the concept. Model training uses a large amount of data from multiple sources, such as graphics, big data, or EHR. However, although EHR data is most suitable for predictive analysis, it has a lot of noise/redundancy that might cause fluctuating outputs and can be solved using particular restructured databases that concisely arrange data [33].

Many researchers do not entirely trust the results of Computational Intelligence analysis due to the high uncertainty in the outcomes. It all depends on the type and fit of data being used and the correct analysis conducted. Most errors occur due to insufficient labeling of data. Researchers know that Deep Learning is an extension of ML and is used to predict patterns, but the mechanism of how this model predicts these outcomes is still not completely understood. Hence, the application of this method is not so prevalent that it affects its ability to evaluate medical assessment in the healthcare field. AI is being vastly applied in cancer studies, but finding high-quality datasets is difficult due to high cost and low sample availability/quality. For deep learning to be used in the lab, it should be explainable and avoid incomplete diagnosis, and instead, it should be redirected to ask for expert opinion in such cases [37].

7 Conclusion

This chapter explores the critical function of biomarkers in autoimmune illnesses and the importance of these markers in clinical practice. Using biomarkers, healthcare practitioners, researchers, and patients can make educated decisions about the existence, progression, and effectiveness of the disease. The chapter discusses the value of early detection, the efficacy of treatment, and the difficulty of locating biomarkers for complex and diverse autoimmune illnesses. Computational intelligence—a field encompassing methods like neural networks, evolutionary algorithms, fuzzy logic, and swarm intelligence—is introduced to evaluate complex biological data and find biomarkers. The chapter also discusses how machine learning algorithms categorize and extract pertinent aspects from data, highlighting them as practical tools in biomarker development. Additionally, it investigates the use of SVMs, random forests, and artificial neural networks in predicting and identifying biomarkers, demonstrating their effectiveness in identifying subtle correlations and intricate interactions in biomolecular datasets. These computational tools make identifying biomarkers easier, better-comprehending diseases, and developing precision medicine. This chapter emphasizes the potential to alter the diagnosis, treatment, and management of autoimmune disorders by fusing computational intelligence with clinical practice, ultimately resulting in better patient outcomes and advances in medical research.

In finding autoimmune disease biomarkers, computational intelligence techniques have become indispensable tools. Due to the complex nature of these disorders, which cause the immune system to target the body's cells and tissues mistakenly, they provide difficult hurdles. Extensive and varied data sets covering genomics, proteomics, metabolomics, and clinical records can be assimilated and decoded using computational approaches like network analysis, data mining, and machine learning. These methods enable the discovery of essential biomarkers by revealing hidden correlations, complex patterns, and interactions within these datasets. They significantly advance our understanding of these complicated conditions and enhance patient care by allowing researchers to identify disease subtypes, forecast disease progression, and optimize therapy approaches.

The potential for transforming clinical practice lies in integrating artificial intelligence approaches into the biomarker development process for autoimmune disorders. As these techniques evolve, they will probably help create exact and individualized diagnostic tools for early disease identification and intervention. Additionally, incorporating computational insights into clinical decision-making may result in individualized treatment plans that consider variances in each patient's disease presentation and response. Precision medicine's transition can improve therapeutic results while reducing side effects. However, for integration to be successful, it will be necessary for computational scientists, physicians, and researchers to work together across disciplines. It will also be necessary to address issues with data privacy, validation, and the dynamic nature of autoimmune illnesses. In the long run, combining clinical practice and computational intelligence can transform how autoimmune illnesses are identified, treated, and managed, resulting in better patient outcomes and a more efficient healthcare system.

References

1. Abdelati AA, Elnemr RA, Kandil NS, Dwedar FI, Ghazala RA (2020) Serum peptidomic profile as a novel biomarker for rheumatoid arthritis. Int J Rheumatol 2020:6069484. https://doi.org/10.1155/2020/6069484
2. Akhoon N (2021) Precision medicine: a new paradigm in therapeutics. Int J Prev Med 12
3. Anaissi A, Goyal M, Catchpoole DR, Braytee A, Kennedy PJ (2016) Ensemble feature learning of genomic data using support vector machine. PLoS ONE 11(6):e0157330

4. Anfossi S, Babayan A, Pantel K, Calin GA (2018) Clinical utility of circulating non-coding RNAs—an update. Nat Rev Clin Oncol 15(9):541–563
5. Angum F, Khan T, Kaler J, Siddiqui L, Hussain A (2020) The prevalence of autoimmune disorders in women: a narrative review. Cureus 12(5)
6. Arora A, Arora A (2022) Generative adversarial networks and synthetic patient data: current challenges and future perspectives. Futur Healthc J 9(2):190
7. Baum ZJ, Yu X, Ayala PY, Zhao Y, Watkins SP, Zhou Q (2021) Artificial intelligence in chemistry: current trends and future directions. J Chem Inf Model 61(7):3197–3212
8. Baxi V, Edwards R, Montalto M, Saha S (2022) Digital pathology and artificial intelligence in translational medicine and clinical practice. Mod Pathol 35(1):23–32
9. Bhinder B, Gilvary C, Madhukar NS, Elemento O (2021) Artificial intelligence in cancer research and precision medicine. Cancer Discov 11(4):900–915
10. Birga AM, Ren L, Luo H, Zhang Y, Huang J (2022) Prediction of new risk genes and potential drugs for rheumatoid arthritis from multiomics data. Comput Math Methods Med
11. Bosch X (2011) Systemic lupus erythematosus and the neutrophil. N Engl J Med 365(8):758–760
12. Cai C, Wang S, Xu Y, Zhang W, Tang K, Ouyang Q, Lai L, Pei J (2020) Transfer learning for drug discovery. J Med Chem 63(16):8683–8694
13. Chen Y, Liao R, Yao Y, Wang Q, Fu L (2022) Machine learning to identify immune-related biomarkers of rheumatoid arthritis based on WGCNA network. Clin Rheumatol 41(4):1057–1068. https://doi.org/10.1007/s10067-021-05960-9
14. Davis KD, Flor H, Greely HT, Iannetti GD, Mackey S, Ploner M, Pustilnik A, Tracey I, Treede R-D, Wager TD (2017) Brain imaging tests for chronic pain: medical, legal and ethical issues and recommendations. Nat Rev Neurol 13(10):624–638
15. Diakou I, Papakonstantinou E, Papageorgiou L, Pierouli K, Dragoumani K, Spandidos DA, Bacopoulou F, Chrousos GP, Goulielmos GN, Eliopoulos E (2022) Multiple sclerosis and computational biology. Biomed Rep 17(6):1–7
16. Engelbrecht AP (2007) Computational intelligence: an introduction. Wiley
17. Fulcher J, Jain LC (2008) Computational intelligence: a compendium, vol 21. Springer
18. Gelfand JM (2014) Multiple sclerosis: diagnosis, differential diagnosis, and clinical presentation. Handb Clin Neurol 122:269–290
19. He Z, Yu W (2010) Stable feature selection for biomarker discovery. Comput Biol Chem 34(4):215–225
20. Hine C, Nilforooshan R, Barnaghi P (2022) Ethical considerations in design and implementation of home-based smart care for dementia. Nurs Ethics 29(4):1035–1046
21. Hu C, Dai Z, Xu J, Zhao L, Xu Y, Li M, Yu J, Zhang L, Deng H, Liu L (2022) Proteome profiling identifies serum biomarkers in rheumatoid arthritis. Front Immunol 13:865425
22. Karwasra R, Khanna K, Singh S, Ahmad S, Verma S (2022) The incipient role of computational intelligence in oncology: drug designing, discovery, and development. In: Computational intelligence in oncology, vol. 1016. Springer, pp 369–384
23. Krzyszczyk P, Acevedo A, Davidoff EJ, Timmins LM, Marrero-Berrios I, Patel M, White C, Lowe C, Sherba JJ, Hartmanshenn C (2018) The growing role of precision and personalized medicine for cancer treatment. Technology 6(03n04):79–100
24. Ledesma D, Symes S, Richards S (2021) Advancements within modern machine learning methodology: impacts and prospects in biomarker discovery. Curr Med Chem 28(32):6512–6531
25. Li M, Chen H, Yin P, Song J, Jiang F, Tang Z, Fan X, Xu C, Wang Y, Xue Y (2021) Identification and clinical validation of key extracellular proteins as the potential biomarkers in relapsing-remitting multiple sclerosis. Front Immunol 12:753929
26. Liu F, Huang Y, Liu F, Wang H (2023) Identification of immune-related genes in diagnosing atherosclerosis with rheumatoid arthritis through bioinformatics analysis and machine learning. Front Immunol 14:1126647. https://doi.org/10.3389/fimmu.2023.1126647
27. Mann M, Kumar C, Zeng W-F, Strauss MT (2021) Artificial intelligence for proteomics and biomarker discovery. Cell Syst 12(8):759–770

28. Monteiro M, Carvalho M, Bastos M, Guedes de Pinho P (2013) Metabolomics analysis for biomarker discovery: advances and challenges. Curr Med Chem 20(2):257–271
29. Nabizadeh F, Masrouri S, Ramezannezhad E, Ghaderi A, Sharafi AM, Soraneh S, Naser Moghadasi A (2022) Artificial intelligence in the diagnosis of multiple sclerosis: a systematic review. Mult Scler Relat Disord 59:103673. https://doi.org/10.1016/j.msard.2022.103673
30. Ngiam KY, Khor W (2019) Big data and machine learning algorithms for health-care delivery. Lancet Oncol 20(5):e262–e273
31. Plati D, Tripoliti E, Zelilidou S, Vlachos K, Konitsiotis S, Fotiadis DI (2022) Multiple sclerosis severity estimation and progression prediction based on machine learning techniques. In: 2022 44th annual international conference of the IEEE engineering in medicine & biology society (EMBC). IEEE, pp 1109–1112
32. Putin E, Mamoshina P, Aliper A, Korzinkin M, Moskalev A, Kolosov A, Ostrovskiy A, Cantor C, Vijg J, Zhavoronkov A (2016) Deep biomarkers of human aging: application of deep neural networks to biomarker development. Aging (Albany NY) 8(5):1021
33. Rosman G, Rus D, Meireles OR Artificial intelligence in surgery
34. Saccà V, Sarica A, Novellino F, Barone S, Tallarico T, Filippelli E, Granata A, Chiriaco C, Bruno Bossio R, Valentino P, Quattrone A (2019) Evaluation of machine learning algorithms performance for the prediction of early multiple sclerosis from resting-state FMRI connectivity data. Brain Imaging Behav 13(4):1103–1114. https://doi.org/10.1007/s11682-018-9926-9
35. Sahu A, Qazi S, Raza K, Singh A, Verma S (2022) Machine learning-based approach for early diagnosis of breast cancer using biomarkers and gene expression profiles. In: Computational intelligence in oncology: applications in diagnosis, prognosis and therapeutics of cancers. Springer, Berlin, pp 285–306
36. Song M, Jung H, Lee S, Kim D, Ahn M (2021) Diagnostic classification and biomarker identification of Alzheimer's disease with random forest algorithm. Brain Sci 11(4):453
37. Tran KA, Kondrashova O, Bradley A, Williams ED, Pearson JV, Waddell N (2021) Deep learning in cancer diagnosis, prognosis and treatment selection. Genome Med 13(1):1–17
38. Tripathi MK, Ahmad S, Tyagi R, Dahiya V, Yadav MK (2022) Fundamentals of molecular modeling in drug design. In: Computer Aided Drug Design (CADD): from ligand-based methods to structure-based approaches. Elsevier, pp 125–155
39. Vázquez-Marrufo M, Sarrias-Arrabal E, García-Torres M, Martín-Clemente R, Izquierdo G (2022) A systematic review of the application of machine-learning algorithms in multiple sclerosis. Neurologia S2173–5808(22):00075-X. https://doi.org/10.1016/j.nrleng.2020.10.013
40. Wang X, Fan D, Yang Y, Gimple RC, Zhou S (2023) Integrative multi-omics approaches to explore immune cell functions: challenges and opportunities. iScience
41. Yadav MK, Ahmad S, Raza K, Kumar S, Eswaran M, Pasha KMM (2022) Predictive modeling and therapeutic repurposing of natural compounds against the receptor-binding domain of SARS-CoV-2. J Biomol Struct Dyn 1–13
42. Yaung KN, Yeo JG, Kumar P, Wasser M, Chew M, Ravelli A, Law AHN, Arkachaisri T, Martini A, Pisetsky DS (2023) Artificial intelligence and high-dimensional technologies in the theragnosis of systemic lupus erythematous. Lancet Rheumatol 5(3):e151–e165
43. Yu R, Zhang J, Zhuo Y, Hong X, Ye J, Tang S, Zhang Y (2021) Identification of diagnostic signatures and immune cell infiltration characteristics in rheumatoid arthritis by integrating bioinformatic analysis and machine-learning strategies. Front Immunol 12:724934. https://doi.org/10.3389/fimmu.2021.724934

SPRINGER NATURE

GPSR Compliance

The European Union's (EU) General Product Safety Regulation (GPSR) is a set of rules that requires consumer products to be safe and our obligations to ensure this.

If you have any concerns about our products, you can contact us on ProductSafety@springernature.com

In case Publisher is established outside the EU, the EU authorized representative is:

Springer Nature Customer Service Center GmbH
Europaplatz 3
69115 Heidelberg, Germany

The manufacturer's authorised representative in the EU is Springer Nature Customer Service Centre GmbH, Europaplatz 3, 69115 Heidelberg, Germany. If you have any concerns regarding our products, please contact ProductSafety@springernature.com

Printed and bound by CPI Group (UK) Ltd, Croydon, CR0 4YY
01/10/2026
02225896-0013